Cancer Chemotherapy

Rachel Airley

Cancer Research Scientist and Lecturer in Pharmacology

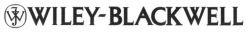

WILEY-BLACKWELL

A John Wiley & Sons, Ltd., Publication

This edition first published 2009
© 2009 by John Wiley & Sons Ltd

Wiley-Blackwell is an imprint of John Wiley & Sons, formed by the merger of Wiley's global Scientific, Technical and Medical business with Blackwell Publishing.

Registered office: John Wiley & Sons Ltd, The Atrium, Southern Gate, Chichester, West Sussex, PO19 8SQ, UK

Other Editorial Offices:
9600 Garsington Road, Oxford, OX4 2DQ, UK
111 River Street, Hoboken, NJ 07030-5774, USA

For details of our global editorial offices, for customer services and for information about how to apply for permission to reuse the copyright material in this book please see our website at www.wiley.com/wiley-blackwell

The right of the author to be identified as the author of this work has been asserted in accordance with the Copyright, Designs and Patents Act 1988.

Library of Congress Cataloguing-in-Publication Data

Airley, Rachel.
 Cancer chemotherapy / Rachel Airley.
  p. ; cm.
 Includes bibliographical references and index.
 ISBN 978-0-470-09254-5 (HB) – ISBN 978-0-470-09255-2 (PB) 1. Cancer–Chemotherapy. I. Title.
 [DNLM: 1. Neoplasms–drug therapy. 2. Antineoplastic Agents–therapeutic use. QZ 267 A298c 2009]
 RC271.C5A35 2009
 616.99'4061–dc22

                                                                                2008052079

ISBN: 978-0-470-09254-5 (H/B)
ISBN: 978-0-470-09255-2 (P/B)

A catalogue record for this book is available from the British Library.

Set in 10.5/12.5 pt Times by Thomson Digital, Noida, India.
Printed and bound in Great Britain by CPI Antony Rowe, Chippenham, Wiltshire.

First Impression 2009

Cancer Chemotherapy

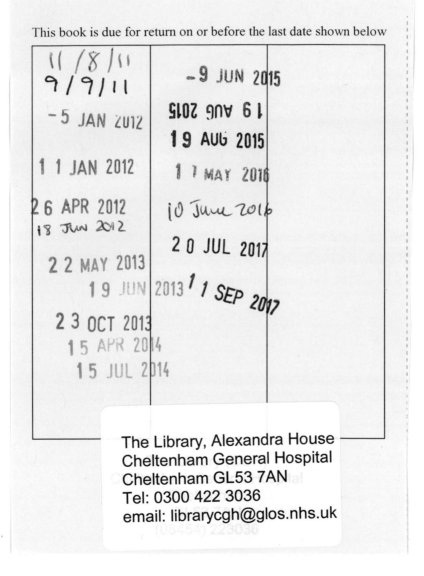

Contents

Preface

While researching this book, I came across a letter in the journal *Nature* asking for caution in the current trend for the use of humorous nomenclature for newly discovered genes[1], the author referring to the tumour suppressor gene *Pokemon*, which I have briefly described in Chapter 4. In this letter, the author reminded us that at a certain point, this name might have to be used by a health professional when discussing a clinical condition with a patient, a sobering thought that served as a reminder that every process started in the laboratory, however prolonged and seemingly removed from the clinic, potentially impacts on the lives of patients. I decided to compile this book after being asked on a number of occasions by pharmacy students at the School of Pharmacy and Chemistry, Liverpool John Moores University if there were a book available that offered a concise, relatively inexpensive and broad introductory text that covered the content of my lecture course in cancer chemotherapy. Specifically, their requests usually came following lectures describing the design, pharmacology and clinical development of novel anticancer agents for which there appeared to be only a limited range of reference sources suitable for undergraduates that didn't involve lengthy searches through the scientific journals. The research and treatment of cancer is a three-way collaboration between health professionals, clinical and experimental scientists, so I have tried to offer a text that unites the topics most pertinent to each group in order to foster a mutual understanding of the role of each at undergraduate level. To this end, the book is aimed at undergraduates of pharmacy, medicine, dentistry, nursing and the allied health professions; as well as providing a useful primer for those considering a career in cancer research, whether they are undertaking a final year dissertation or graduate research project in this area. I have attempted to summarize and consolidate the process behind the research and treatment of cancer, covering topics that range from the clinical aspects of cancer, such as its epidemiology and the role of the many of health professionals involved in its treatment, through to the currently accepted cancer chemotherapy regimens, in particular the classical cytotoxic anticancer agents

---

[1]Maclean, K. (2006) Humour of gene names lost in translation to patients. *Nature*, **439** (7074), 266.

and how they are applied according to cancer diagnosis and staging. I have devoted a large part of the book to the science of cancer research, encompassing basic research into the molecular pathways determining the course of the disease and the methodologies used in target validation, drug discovery and clinical trials. I have also included sections that represent the current state of the art of novel anticancer drug discovery and development. This covers what I would describe as targeted agents, such as the tyrosine kinase inhibitors, some of which have generated excitement and controversy in mainstream newsrooms in recent times. Cancer research is a rapidly evolving field, and although I have made every attempt to provide the most up to date information, it is inevitable that by the time this book comes to publication there will have been further important developments. In order to keep up to date with the progress of novel anticancer agents, I would recommend the web site www.clinicaltrial.gov, and to keep track of newly approved novel agents, the Food and Drug Administration web site provides a search facility www.fda.gov/search/databases.html. Finally, I have included some worked examples of structured essay questions, where I have tried to offer advice that goes beyond the regurgitation of complex chemical structures and offer some insight into exam technique.

It just remains for me to acknowledge the support I have had during this project; at Wylie, my commissioning editor Rachael Ballard and project editor Fiona Woods, who have both showed endless patience through many delays associated with transatlantic moves and working as a real life pharmacist; and the constant support through each new academic challenge of my parents Lorraine and Alan Airley MRPharmS. I would also like to thank the students at Liverpool John Moores University, now also real life pharmacists, who provided me with the original idea for this book.

R.A.
July, 2008

1

Cancer epidemiology

1.1 Cancer incidence, prevalence and mortality

Every year, more than 285 000 people are diagnosed with cancer in the United Kingdom, and the current estimate is that more than one in three people will develop a form of cancer at some point in their lifetime. There are more than 200 different types of cancer, but four particular tumour types: breast, lung, colorectal and prostate- constitute over half of all new cases diagnosed (Figure 1.1). Cancer incidence, defined as the number of new cases arising in a period of time, is gender and age specific. In males, prostate cancer is the most prolific, where almost 35 000 new cases were diagnosed in 2004, followed by lung cancer, with around 22 000, and bowel cancer, with around 20 000 new cases per year. However, in females, breast cancer continues to be the most common tumour type, the disease accounting for nearly one in three female cancers, with over 44 000 new cases diagnosed in the year 2004. Cancer incidence may be further defined by the lifetime risk of developing the disease. For instance, in females, the risk of developing breast cancer is 1 in 9, and in males, the risk of developing prostate cancer is 1 in 14. In some tumour types, there are considerable gender-related differences in cancer risk; for example, males are nearly twice as likely to develop lung cancer (1 in 13) than women (1 in 23). Cancer occurs mostly in older people, and the risk of developing cancer increases with age. For example, in the 25–34 age group, the rate of diagnosis in males is 1834 cases per 100 000 of the population, and in females, 2782 cases per 100 000. However, in the 75 + age group, the rate of diagnosis in males has risen sharply to 52 831 cases per 100 000 in males and 50 803 cases per 100 000 in females. Overall, in the 10 year period 1995–2004, cancer incidence rate has been relatively constant, with a slight increase of around 1% in males and a slight increase in females of 3%. Broken down by cancer type, the largest increases in incidence rate within this period have been seen in malignant melanoma (43%), uterine (21%), oral (23%) and kidney cancer (14%). Cancer is currently the cause of a quarter of United Kingdom deaths, and around two thirds of all deaths in adults under 65 years. In fact, cancer caused 27% of all deaths in the United Kingdom in 2006; that is 29% in males and 25% in females. Five particular tumour types: lung, colorectal, breast, prostate and oesophagus, are responsible for over half (52%) of all cancer mortality (Figure 1.2). Survival is usually defined as the

Cancer Chemotherapy   Rachel Airley
© 2009 John Wiley & Sons, Ltd.

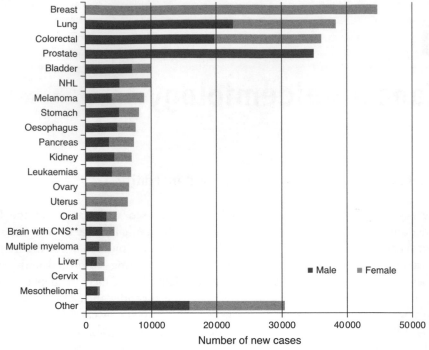

** central nervous system

Figure 1.1 The 20 most commonly diagnosed cancers diagnosed in the United Kingdom, 2004. NHL, non-Hodgkin lymphoma. Reproduced with permission from Cancer Research UK http://info. cancerresearchuk.org/cancerstats August 2008.

percentage of patients diagnosed with cancer still alive after a 5 year period. Survival rates vary according to cancer type (Figure 1.3), where cancers may be grouped into three survival bands: 50% or higher, which includes testicular (95%), female breast (77%) and cervix (61%) cancers; 10–50% survival, including colon (47% in males, 48% in females), renal (45% in males, 48% in females) and brain (12% in males, 15% in females); and cancers where less than 10% of all patients are alive after 5 years, notably oesophageal cancer (7% in men, 8% in women), lung (6% in men, 6% in women) and pancreatic (2% in men, 2% in women) cancers. In general, women have higher survival rates than men (43% in men compared to 56% in women), and among adults, survival decreases with increasing age (Table 1.1). This may be due, in part, to mortality that is non-specific to the disease. However, other factors may be contributory, such as the smaller proportion of elderly patients entered into phase I clinical trials. Exceptions to this trend usually occur where the age of the patient at diagnosis is a reflection of the molecular and pathological characteristics of the tumour, for example, breast tumours in premenopausal women tend to be more aggressive, therefore survival rates in these age groups are decreased relative to postmenopausal women.

Progress in the early diagnosis and treatment of cancer has positively affected cancer survival rates. In the United Kingdom, female breast cancer mortality rate has fallen

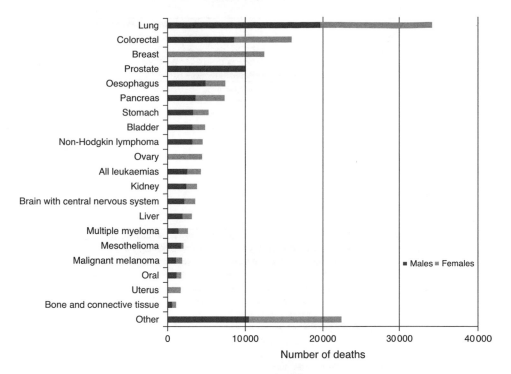

Figure 1.2 The 20 most common causes of death from cancer, persons, United Kingdom, 2006. Reproduced with permission from Cancer Research UK http://info.cancerresearchuk.org/cancerstats August 2008.

sharply, from 15 625 deaths from the disease in 1989 compared with 12 319 deaths in 2006. It is estimated that the National Health Service mammography breast screening programme saves around 1400 lives annually, detecting around 14 000 new cases of breast cancer per year. In prostate cancer, where tests for the biomarker prostate-specific antigen (PSA) have increased the proportion of PSA-detected asymptomatic prostate tumours diagnosed, and because these have an inherently good prognosis, the recorded survival rate has also increased dramatically. This is reflected by the change in 5-year survival rates over the period 1986–1999 (Figure 1.4), where the survival rate for breast cancer increased by an average of 5.4%, and for prostate cancer, by an average of 11.4% every 5 years.

1.2 Childhood cancers

By the age of 15 years, 1 in 500 children will be affected by childhood cancer, which in the United Kingdom means that around 1500 children are diagnosed with cancer every year. Childhood cancer is still relatively infrequent – the most common form being acute lymphoblastic leukaemia, though some rarer cancers are of embryological origin, such as retinoblastoma, rhabdomyosarcoma and neuroblastoma. Together, these were

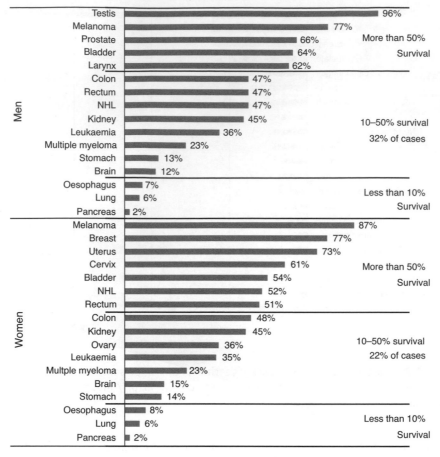

Five-year relative survival

Figure 1.3 Five-year age-standardized relative survival (%) adults diagnosed 1996–1999, England and Wales by sex and site. NHL, non-Hodgkin's lymphoma. Reproduced with permission from Cancer Research UK http://info.cancerresearchuk.org/cancerstats August 2008.

responsible for 1.8% of deaths in children under 15 in the United Kingdom in the time period 2000–2002 (Table 1.2), with an average total of 301 deaths per year (Table 1.3). Figure 1.5 shows mortality rate broken down by cancer type in Great Britain in the time period 1997–2001, where 32% of deaths were caused by leukaemias compared to 1% by retinoblastoma. In all cancer types, survival rates have risen dramatically, where between 1962 and 2001 death rates decreased by an average of 2.6% per year, amounting to a fall of more than half. There has been a steady increase in survival rates in all childhood cancer types, where almost 72% of the cases diagnosed in the time period 1992–1996 have survived for longer than 5 years. This is attributable to the continual refinement and validation of combination chemotherapy regimens made possible by the steady enrolment of children into phase III clinical trials, as well as improved diagnostic techniques. The best example of the sort of improvements in survival rates

Table 1.1 Five-year survival by site and age at diagnosis for patients diagnosed in England and Wales 1996–1999, follow up to 2001

Cancer type	Sex	Age at diagnosis (%)					
		15–39	40–49	50–59	60–69	70–79	80–99
Bladder	Men	90	84	77	70	62	48
	Women	78	70	75	65	53	40
Breast	Women	76	82	85	82	74	58
Cervix	Women	83	73	60	48	36	22
Colon	Men	61	54	50	50	47	40
	Women	58	54	54	52	48	39
Lung	Men	21	9	9	7	5	2
	Women	28	13	11	8	4	1
Ovary	Women	81	55	44	32	23	15
Prostate	Men	76	58	75	77	68	48
Rectum	Men	54	55	54	52	47	34
	Women	60	61	62	58	49	36
Stomach	Men	18	17	15	16	12	7
	Women	19	22	20	19	14	8
Testis	Men	97	96	95	86	67	55
Uterus	Women	77	81	85	78	67	45

Adapted from Cancer Research UK statistics available at http://info.cancerresearchuk.org/cancerstats/survival/age/?a=5441. Accessed 9 October 2008.

Table 1.2 Main causes of child mortality, ages 1–14, by sex and age group, in England and Wales 2000–2002

	Percentages			
	Males		Females	
	1–4 years	5–14 years	1–4 years	5–14 years
Infections	11	3	7	5
Cancers	14	23	13	24
Nervous system and sense organs	14	15	12	14
Circulatory system	4	5	7	6
Respiratory system	9	5	8	8
Congenital anomalies	14	7	15	9
Accident	17	30	16	19
Other	17	12	20	16
All deaths (= 100%) (numbers)	968	1444	752	1049

Taken from Cancer Research UK statistics available at http://info.cancerresearchuk.org/cancerstats/childhoodcancer/mortality/?a=5441. Accessed 9 October 2008.

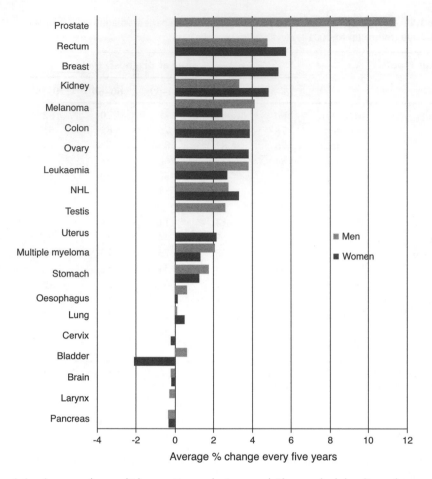

Figure 1.4 Average change (%) every 5 years in 5-year relative survival, by site and sex, adults diagnosed in England and Wales in time period 1986–1999. NHL, non-Hodgkin lymphomas. Reproduced with permission from Cancer Research UK http://info.cancerresearchuk.org/ cancerstats August 2008.

achieved is in acute lymphoblastic leukaemia (shown in Figure 1.6 alongside other cancer types), where 5 year survival rate has risen from 12% of cases diagnosed in the time period 1962–1971 to 80% of those diagnosed in the time period 1992–1996.

1.3 Global epidemiology

Global cancer incidence rate (per 100 000 population) for all cancers, as compared with the number of cancer deaths is shown in Figure 1.7, where crude rate is calculated by dividing the number of new cancers diagnosed during a given time period by the number of people in the population at risk. The number of cancer deaths is highest in the United States, which is partially due to large population. However, from the crude incidence rates, it is easily apparent that the population of China, which is significantly

Table 1.3 Annual average number of deaths from cancer before age 15, United Kingdom, 2000–2002 (average rounded to nearest whole number)

Country	Males	Females	Total
England and Wales	148	119	267
Scotland	16	9	25
N Ireland	8	2	9
UK	172	129	301

Taken from Cancer Research UK statistics available at http://info.cancerresearchuk.org/cancerstats/childhoodcancer/mortality/?a=5441. Accessed 9 October 2008.

larger than that of the United States, is considerably less affected by cancer, particularly in women. Incidence rates are broken down by gender, cancer type (lung, bladder, leukaemia, melanoma) and country (United Kingdom, United States, Australia, China, France, Germany and the Netherlands) in Figures 1.8–1.11. These may be explained by differences in lifestyle factors. These include diet, where the chemopreventive properties of soy beans in the Chinese diet, particularly with reference to bladder cancer, have been documented and are reflected in Figure 1.9; and the environment, where there is a notably higher rate of melanoma incidence in Australia due to the risks of sun exposure (Figure 1.11).

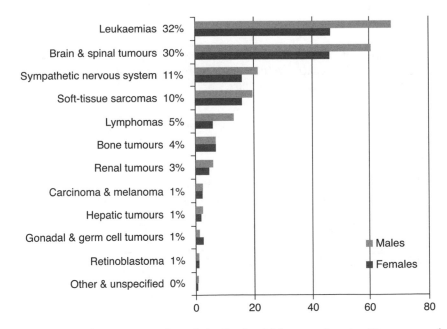

Figure 1.5 Annual average number of deaths in children aged under 15 years previously diagnosed with cancer, by diagnostic group and sex, Great Britain 1997–2001. Reproduced with permission from Cancer Research UK http://info.cancerresearchuk.org/cancerstats August 2008.

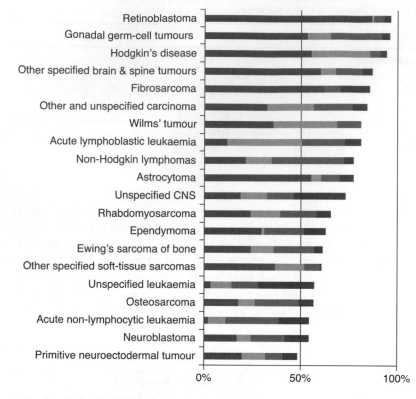

Figure 1.6 Survival of childhood cancer patients diagnosed in successive periods, Great Britain, 1962–1996. Reproduced with permission from Cancer Research UK http://info. cancerresearchuk.org/cancerstats August 2008.

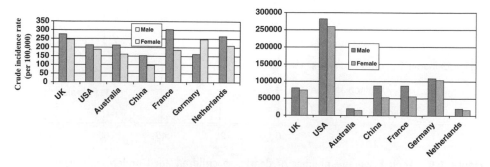

Figure 1.7 World cancer incidence, showing crude incidence rate (left) and number of deaths for all cancers (right) in 1998. Compiled using data from CANCERMondial http://www-dep.iarc.fr. Accessed October 2002.

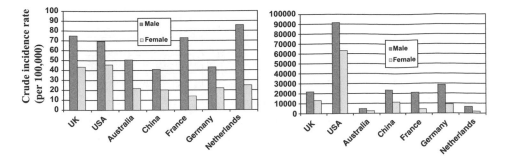

Figure 1.8 World cancer incidence, showing crude incidence rate (left) and number of deaths (right) for lung cancer in 1998. Compiled using data from CANCERMondial http://www-dep.iarc.fr. Accessed October 2002.

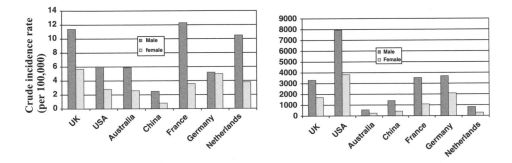

Figure 1.9 World cancer incidence, showing crude incidence rate (left) and number of deaths (right) for bladder cancer in 1998. Compiled using data from CANCERMondial http://www-dep.iarc.fr. Accessed October 2002.

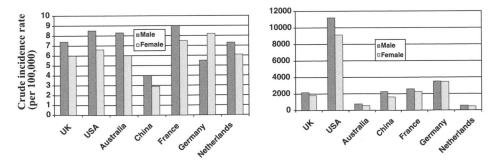

Figure 1.10 World cancer incidence, showing crude incidence rate (left) and number of deaths (right) for leukaemia in 1998. Compiled using data from CANCERMondial http://www-dep.iarc.fr. Accessed October 2002.

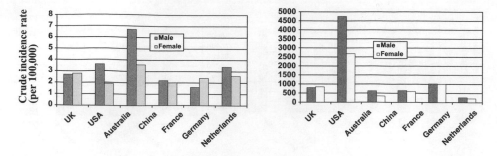

Figure 1.11 World cancer incidence, showing crude incidence rate (left) and number of deaths (right) for melanoma in 1998. Compiled using data from CANCERMondial http://www-dep.iarc.fr. Accessed October 2002.

2

Histopathology of cancer

2.1 Introduction

Tumours are characterized by a set of histological changes displayed by the tumour cells themselves, as well as the microenvironment in which they develop and function. The general term used to describe a tumour is *neoplasm*, the literal meaning being 'new growth'. A neoplasm refers to an abnormal mass of cells with uncoordinated or deregulated growth or cellular proliferation. Deregulation of cellular proliferation stems from a set of heritable changes in the expression of genes which control either cell division or cell survival, where the population of cells within the tumour has arisen from one cell. Tumours are made up of two components- the proliferating cells, or parenchyma; and the stroma, which includes the connective tissue and blood vessels. Malignant progression depends upon the ability of cells to invade into surrounding tissue, a process influenced by the expression of enzymes such as matrix metallo-proteinases that degrade surrounding host tissue. Advanced cancers will show progression to metastasis, which involves breakdown of tumour cells and intravasation or leaking of these cells from blood capillaries to sites distant from the primary tumour. Malignant progression also involves angiogenesis, or the growth of a tumour-derived blood supply to provide oxygen and nutrients to the growing tumour.

2.2 Malignant, benign and normal (non-malignant) tissue

Transformation to malignancy brings with it certain alterations in morphology, growth characteristics and tissue architecture (Figure 2.1). Malignant cells become immortalized, and depend less upon cell density, that is, contact and communication with other cells, to maintain growth rate. *In vitro*, there is a decreased requirement for serum in the growth medium, which is usually needed to provide growth factors. In contrast to normal cells, which require a basement membrane or solid surface *in vitro*, tumour cells are capable of anchorage-independent growth. Tumour cells are usually de-differentiated and de-specialized, that is, they lose the morphology and functionality of the host tissue. Tumour tissue is often laid out in tumour 'nests', surrounded by stroma which contains the vasculature necessary to supply oxygen and nutrients to the proliferating cells.

Cancer Chemotherapy Rachel Airley
© 2009 John Wiley & Sons, Ltd.

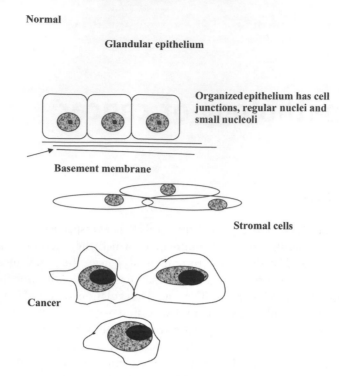

Figure 2.1 Histology of normal and malignant tissue. Adapted from King (2000).

The extent and functional integrity of this vasculature may be determined by the rate of angiogenesis, or new blood vessel growth (discussed in Section 5.6.1 and Chapter 13), which is either host or tumour tissue-derived. Tumour nomenclature depends upon the tissue of origin, and whether it is benign or malignant (Table 2.1). Benign tumours usually have the suffix *oma*, whereas malignant tumours may be a *carcinoma*, if derived from epithelial tissue, or an *adenocarcinoma*, if derived from glandular tissue. If the tumour is of mesenchymal origin, for example, muscle, the correct term is *sarcoma*. It is also normal practice to state the tissue of origin. For example, a tumour arising from the buccal cavity that produces cells of identifiable squamous type may be described as an oral squamous cell carcinoma, or a tumour with a glandular pattern in the cervix is classified as an adenocarcinoma of the uterine cervix.

2.3 Cell death

The rate of cell death is an important factor in determining the rate of growth and biological behaviour of a tumour, this applying not just to tumour cells but also the supporting tumour matrix, which includes fibroblasts, vascular endothelial cells and tumour associated monocytes such as macrophages. Programmed cell death is tightly controlled by dedicated signalling pathways. The most well-characterized type of programmed cell death is apoptosis, which takes place during tissue remodelling,

Table 2.1 Tumour nomenclature

Cell/tissue type	Benign	Malignant
Epithelial		
Epidermis (surface)	Papilloma	Carcinoma
Epithelial lining of glands	Adenoma	Adenocarcinoma
Renal	Renal tubular adenoma	Renal cell carcinoma
Hepatic	Liver cell adenoma	Hepatocellular carcinoma
Urinary tract epithelium (transitional)		Transitional cell carcinoma
Placenta	Hydatidiform mole	Choriocarcinoma
Non-epithelial		
Mesenchymal		
Connective tissue	Fibroma	Fibrosarcoma
Cartilage	Chondroma	Chondrosarcoma
Bone	Osteoma	Osteogenic sarcoma /osteosarcoma
Smooth muscle	Leiomyoma	Leiomyosarcoma
Striated muscle	Rhabdomyoma	Rhabdomyosarcoma
Neuroectodermal		
Nerve cells	Ganglioneuroma	Neuroblastoma
Melanocytes	Nevus	Malignant melanoma
Retina		Retinoblastoma
Endothelial		
Blood vessels	Hemangioma	Angiosarcoma
Lymph vessels	Lymphangioma	Lymphangiosarcoma
Synovium		Synovial sarcoma
Mesothelium		Mesothelioma
Brain coverings	Meningioma	Invasive meningioma
Blood cells		
Haematopoietic		Leukaemias
Lymphoid tissue		Lymphomas

Reproduced from Van Cruchten, S., Van Den Broeck, W. *Anat. Histol. Embryol.* 2002;31:214–23, copyright Blackwell Publishing Ltd 2002.

for example, during embryological development and metamorphosis in animals such as tadpoles. Apoptosis may also take place in response to physiological stimuli such as DNA damage by anticancer agents or the withdrawal of growth factors. Necrotic cell death, however, is a 'passive' process leading to cell lysis, this taking place in response to hypoxia, nutrient shortage, temperature change and heat stress. Apoptosis tends to target single, damaged cells and allows the recycling of cellular components, for example specific cleavage of DNA leads to the 'DNA ladder' effect seen when agarose gel

Table 2.2 Morphological, physiological and microscopic changes observed in apoptosis and necrosis

	Apoptosis	Necrosis
Morphology		
Affected cells	Single	Groups
Cell volume	Shrinkage	Swelling
Chromatin	Condensed	Fragmented
Lysosomes	Intact	Degraded
Mitochondria	Functional	Not functional
Inflammation	No	Yes
Physiological changes		
Gene activity	Required	Not required
DNA cleavage	Specific	Random
Intracellular Ca^{2+}	Increased	No change
Ion pumps	Retained	Lost
Microscopic changes		
	Budding and formation of apoptotic bodies, which are organelles and nuclear material packaged in membrane-bound vesicles	Swelling and leakage of lysosomal contents

electrophoresis is carried out using DNA extracts from apoptotic cells. Necrosis, on the other hand, takes place in groups of cells, observable microscopically as areas of non-viable or damaged tissue where the release of inflammatory mediators upon cell lysis often causes localized inflammation. The distinct differences in the morphological, physiological and molecular changes taking place in cells undergoing apoptosis or necrosis are described in Table 2.2.

Until recently, the terms apoptosis and programmed cell death were used interchangeably. However, it is now thought that programmed cell death take place via a range of possibly cell-type dependent mechanisms such as autophagy, necroptosis and paroptosis. These show cell morphology characteristics of both apoptosis and necrosis (Figure 2.2). Further, necrosis is sometimes referred to as oncosis, used to define cell death accompanied by marked cellular swelling and increased membrane permeability, restricting the term necrosis to those tissue effects taking place after cell death. Because cell death occurs in response to exposure to anticancer agents, exploring how each mode of cell death may be modulated or exploited may be useful therapeutically as a means of overcoming chemoresistance.

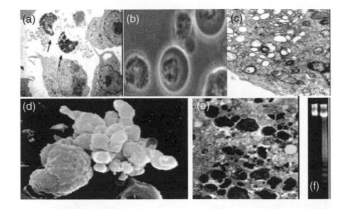

Figure 2.2 Programmed cell death is a tightly controlled physiological process that allows recycling of cellular components and regeneration of tissue, whereas necrosis involves cell lysis. The most well-characterized type of programmed cell death is apoptosis, where until recently apoptotic pathways were used exclusively to describe how it took place. However, there are now a range of known mechanisms, each displaying characteristic morphological changes and involving discrete signalling pathways. Shown here are (a) necroptosis in Jurkat cells, arrows indicating dead cells (reprinted with permission from Degterev *et al.* (2005)); (b) necrosis in *Dictyostelium* cells; (c) autophagy in HeLa cells (reprinted with permission from Golstein and Kroemer (2007)); (d) membrane blebbing, and (e) chromatin condensation in T-cells undergoing apoptosis; and (f) agarose gel electrophoresis of T-cell DNA extracts showing the DNA ladder, the hallmark of nucleotide fragmentation taking place during apoptosis. Reproduced from Zimmermann, K.C., Bonzon, C. and Green, D.R. *Pharmacol Ther.* 2001;92:57–70, © Elsevier 2001.

2.3.1 Apoptosis

Apoptosis takes place via two major pathways: the extrinsic or death receptor pathway, triggered in response to death promoting signals; or the intrinsic or mitochondrial pathway, in response to cellular stress or exposure to radiation or anticancer agents (Figure 2.3). Activation of both pathways occurs in three stages: the induction phase, where damage signals are detected; the commitment phase, where damage signals are integrated and modulated by pro- or anti-apoptotic factors and initiator caspases, for example, through activation of caspase 8 and 9; and the degradation phase, involving the activation of effector or executioner caspases (for example, caspase 3), which degrade the laminin matrix and the actin cytoskeleton; and endonucleases, which cleave DNA. The extrinsic pathway is initiated by ligand binding to several types of death receptor that possess a characteristic intracellular death domain, such as the tumour necrosis factor receptor (TNFR) family, CD95 (APO-1/Fas), TRAIL and DR3 receptors. Binding of the corresponding death ligand, such as TNF, TNF-related apoptosis inducing ligand (TRAIL) or Fas ligand, activates the initiator caspase 8, or FLICE (FADD-like interleukin-1B-converting enzyme). In the case of CD95-mediated apoptosis, activation of caspase 8 occurs when ligand binding to the receptor causes a conformational change allowing the formation of the death-inducing signal complex

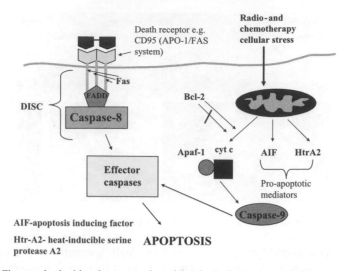

Figure 2.3 The extrinsic (death receptor) and intrinsic (mitochondrial) apoptosis pathways.

(DISC), composed of the CD95 receptor death domains, the adapter molecule FADD (Fas-associated death domain) and the enzyme precursor procaspase 8. The intrinsic pathway depends upon changes in mitochondrial membrane permeability, possibly as a result of signalling by reactive oxygen species (ROS), which releases the pro-apoptotic mediators apoptosis-inducing factor (AIF), heat-inducible serine protease HTR-A2 and cytochrome C. This in turn may be modulated by the bcl2 (B-cell/lymphoma-2) family of proteins, which function as pro- or anti-apoptotic proteins according to the sequence homology of four BH (Bcl-2 homology) domains, where the oncogenes Bcl-2 and bcl-xl are anti-apoptotic and others such as Bax and Bak are pro-apoptotic, the latter showing a loss of sequence homology in BH4 and conservation of the critical death domain BH3. It is believed that the pro-apoptotic proteins are able to insert into the mitochondrial membrane and increase permeability by forming pores, whereas the anti-apoptotic proteins are able to counter this by blocking them. Some pro-apoptotic proteins, such as Bid, Bad, NOXA and PUMA (p53-up-regulated modulator of apoptosis) share only the BH3 domain (BH3-only proteins) and these are thought to assist the assembly of Bax and Bak into mitochondrial pores. Upon release, cytochrome c and Apaf-1 form a complex with dATP, called the apoptosome, which converts the precursor procaspase-9 to caspase-9, this in turn activating effector caspase 3. Bcl2 proteins may function as homodimers, where the Bax homodimer promotes apoptosis but the Bcl-2 homodimer promotes cell survival. However, the sequence homology existing between members of the BCl-2 family means they are capable of interacting and forming heterodimers, for example, the Bax/Bcl-2 heterodimer, which disrupts the functionality of the individual proteins (Figure 2.4). Therefore, the relative levels of Bcl2 and Bax protein expression influence the rate of apoptosis versus the rate of cell survival. There is also evidence that the two apoptotic pathways do not take place independently, where caspase-8 activated via the death-receptor-mediated pathway is capable of activating Bid, altering mitochondrial permeability and ultimately leading to activation of caspase-9.

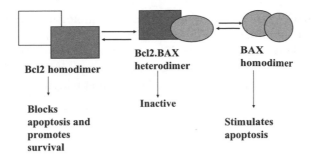

Figure 2.4 The relative levels of Bcl2 and Bax protein expression influence the rate of apoptosis versus the rate of cell survival. Formation of a homodimer of the pro-apoptotic Bax stimulates apoptosis, whereas formation of a Bcl2 homodimer promotes cell survival. The bcl2/Bax heterodimer is inactive.

2.3.2 Autophagy and paroptosis

Cell death by autophagy is characterized by the appearance of vacuoles, inside which degradation of cellular components takes place (Figure 2.2). Autophagy is initiated by the formation of autophagosomes, or double membrane-bound vesicles, which are able to capture and enclose cytoplasmic material. This process is regulated by enzymes such as the GTPases and phosphoinositol kinases and involves conjugation with ubiquitin. The autophagosomes fuse with lysosomes, leading to the degradation of cellular components. Lysosomal degradation is restricted to an intracellular compartment and takes place before the eventual loss of plasma membrane integrity, therefore autophagy is not accompanied by inflammation. Paroptosis is another non-apoptotic form of programmed cell death which is caspase-9, but not APAF-1-dependent. Instead, it has been proposed that caspase 9 is activated via the insulin-like growth factor 1 receptor (IGF1R). Although paroptotic cells resemble necrotic cells morphologically (that is, show characteristic cell swelling), the process also shares features of programmed cell death, such as the requirement for gene expression and protein synthesis, cell vacuolization and mitochondrial swelling.

2.3.3 Necroptosis

Necroptosis, or programmed necrosis, is a form of non-apoptotic programmed cell death morphologically similar to necrosis, in that it is characterized by cellular swelling, loss of plasma membrane integrity, lack of specific DNA cleavage and abnormal mitochondrial function; however, there are some characteristics of autophagy. Unlike apoptosis, the process is not dependent upon the activation of caspases; however it is induced via death receptors such as APO-1/Fas and TNFR. Necroptosis was discovered in studies that attempted to unravel the mode of action of necrostatin-1, an inhibitor of death-receptor-mediated non-apoptotic cell death. Subsequently, it was revealed that the target of this compound and other necrostatins was RIP 1 kinase, a death domain receptor-associated adaptor protein that plays a part in NFκB signalling and the formation of DISC. Whereas RIP kinase interacts homologously with death domain receptors via its C-terminal death domain, necroptosis is induced via its N-terminal serine/threonine kinase domain. RIP kinase may effect downstream execution of necroptosis in a number of ways, for example, via the formation of a complex with the rho family GTPase Rac1 (Ras-related C3 botulinum toxin substrate 1) and NADPH oxidase.

3

Carcinogenesis, malignant transformation and progression

3.1 Introduction

The cause of cancer may be chemical, physical or biological. Chemical carcinogenesis may take place following exposure to carcinogens, which may be occupational (for example, bladder cancer caused by exposure to nitrosamines); environmental (for example, exposure to cigarette smoke); or dietary. Major physical causes include exposure to ultraviolet or ionizing radiation, whereas biological causes include infection with oncogenic viruses, which can trigger mechanisms that lead to the deregulation of genes critical for the growth and survival of malignant tissue.

3.2 Chemical carcinogenesis

Carcinogenesis is a collection of independent but co-operative, unrepaired or mis-repaired, heritable changes that lead to the formation of the neoplastic phenotype in somatic cells. Three stages of chemical carcinogenesis are described (Figure 3.1), the first being *initiation*, or the formation of a mutation following exposure to a carcinogen (Table 3.1). This often results from the alkylation of just one guanine base, leading to methylation at the O6 or N7 position. However, for this to happen an activation step may be necessary, where the *procarcinogen* is activated by metabolizing enzymes such as those in the cytochrome P450 family of mixed function oxidases, to form the *ultimate carcinogen*. This may also involve a *cocarcinogen*, which is analogous to the co-enzyme sometimes appearing in an enzymic reaction involved in electron transfer. Initiation leads to a DNA mutation, of which there are several types. If one base is substituted for another, it is described as a *transition* if it is a purine/purine or pyrimidine/pyrimidine substitution, or a *transversion* if a purine/pyrimidine substitution takes place.

Other possible mutations arise when a base is added (*insertions*) or missed out (*deletions*). These mutations may occur when methylation of a base causes misreading of the DNA sequence during replication. Base mispairings are a common feature of

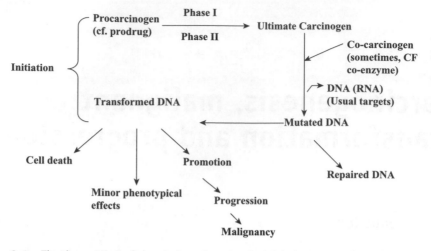

Figure 3.1   The three stages of chemical carcinogenesis: initiation, promotion and progression.

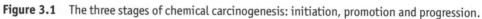

Table 3.1   Examples of carcinogenic compounds and promoting agents

Initiating agents – carcinogens	Exposure
Aflatoxins	Fungus *Aspergillus flavus*
Antitumour alkylating agents	Medical use
Asbestos	Fire retardant (occupational exposure)
Benzopyrene	Tobacco smoking
Benzidine	Dyes
β-naphthylamine	Production of aniline dyes
Chloroform (trichloromethane)	Medical use, occupational carcinogen
Dimethylnitrosamine	Preserved foods, e.g. cured meat
Ethidium bromide	Experimental DNA intercalating agent (research)
Formaldehyde	Occupational exposure
Lead	Paint
Metronidazole	Medical use (antibiotic)
Phenol phthalein	Chemical indicator
2-amino-1-methyl-6-phenylimidazo [4,5-b]pyridine (PhIP)	Food carcinogen
Thiourea (thiocarbamide)	Flame retardants, toners and photochemicals
Vinyl chloride (chloroethene)	Plastic products
Promoting agents	
Tetradecanoyl phorbol acetate (TPA)	Croton oil, from seeds of Asian croton tree (*Croton tiglium*).
Phenobarbital	Barbiturate used as sedative and treatment for epilepsy

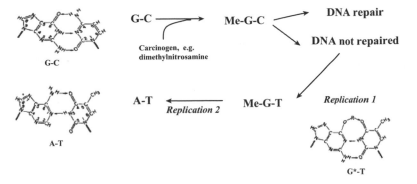

Figure 3.2 G–C to A–T transition occurring when methylation of guanine allows mispairing with thymine. Chemical structures from Drake and Baltz (1976); reprinted, with permission, from the *Annual Review of Biochemistry*, Volume 45 ©1976 by Annual Reviews www.annualreviews.org.

chemical carcinogenesis, where methylated bases may mispair with alternative bases. For instance, methylation of DNA bases by alkylating agents may lead to a GC–AT transition (Figure 3.2), when at replication, subsequent mispairing with thymine occurs. At the second replication, normal pairing will take place, where the mispaired thymine base will pair with adenine. Therefore the mutation will be apparent two replications downstream of the carcinogen-induced DNA damage. Cells that have undergone the initiation stage of carcinogenesis are described as *transformed* cells.

The second stage is *promotion*. Promotion is defined as the clonal expansion of transformed cells, a process induced by promoting agents (Table 3.1). A mutational event may give rise to a cell with altered functionality, for example, the expression of a receptor, enzyme or carrier protein. Promoting agents are not themselves tumorigenic, but provide the selection conditions to allow transformed cells to gain a survival advantage by virtue of this functional change, promoting proliferation and formation of a tumour mass.

The third stage of carcinogenesis is *progression*, which follows an accumulation of tumorigenic changes occurring in transformed cells that give the cell mass or tumour the characteristic loss of differentiation and tissue morphology, together with the ability to invade surrounding tissue and form metastases.

4

Molecular biology of cancer: oncogenes and tumour suppressor genes

4.1 Introduction

Tissue mass is tightly regulated to ensure that the balance between cell proliferation and cell death is maintained. A deregulation of this balance may lead to a net increase in cell numbers, or hyperplasia, and the beginnings of neoplastic formation. Uncontrolled cell division may result from genetic changes that effect progress through the cell cycle, or the rate of differentiation. Cell death, however, may occur by at least two mechanisms: necrosis, involving cell lysis; or apoptosis, a tightly controlled, genetically programmed cell death are the most well characterised. Apoptotic death involves shrinkage of cells, with retention of cellular components such as lysosomes and ionic pump mechanisms, and is more analogous to cell recycling. In general, a gene that promotes cell proliferation, either directly or by removing an inhibitory signal is described as an *oncogene*. A *tumour suppressor gene*, sometimes referred to as an 'anti-oncogene', inhibits cell division. This may be achieved through antagonism of oncogenic pathways, for example, by encoding phosphatases that run counter to kinase pathways involved in oncogenesis. Tumour suppressor genes may also be involved in DNA repair, where they are activated by DNA damage caused by exposure to carcinogens or radiation. Defective DNA repair machinery may give rise to mutation, and depending upon the function and location of the mutated gene within the genome, may ultimately lead to cancer. DNA repair is one of a number of safety nets to minimize the risk of malignancy upon exposure to carcinogens – the other key mechanism is the ability of a cell to undergo apoptosis, where this process is controlled via cell cycle checkpoints, a collection of signalling pathways that are triggered in response to DNA damage and subsequent failure of DNA repair. There are four checkpoints and one restriction point (Table 4.1), each serving as a biological hurdle to prevent any DNA damage incurred at a specific phase of the cell cycle from being replicated and passed onto future generations of cells. These are controlled by a series of highly specific cyclins and cyclin-dependent kinases (CDKs), which control

Table 4.1 The cell cycle and its regulation

Checkpoint	Transition	Action	Regulation
G1 restriction point	G0–G1	Allows re-entry of quiescent or G0 cells into cell cycle	Mitogens: Ras/Raf/MAPK pathway stimulates cyclin D production
G1	G1–S	Cell cycle arrest in response to DNA damage to prevent replication in S phase	G1 progression – cyclin D1–D3/CDKs 2,4,6

G1–S transition-cyclin E/CDK2. These CDKs phosphorylate the transcriptional inhibitor pRb, leading to subsequent release and activation of its binding partner, transcription factor E2F1, regulator of genes controlling DNA synthesis. |
S replication checkpoint	S	Monitors and slows progression through S-phase	S-phase progression limited by cyclin A/CDK2, which signals for E2F1 inactivation and degradation. Activation of ATM and ATR kinases– prevents mitosis in response to DNA damage via phosphorylation of chk1 and -2 and cdc25c. This causes inactivation of cyclin B/CDK1 complex and prevents further progression through G2 and S-phases.
G2	S–G2	Cell cycle arrest in response to DMA damage to ensure satisfactory completion of S-phase	Activation of cyclin A/CDK1 (cdc2), cyclin B/CDK1 complexes
M	G2–M	Arrest of chromosomal segregation in response to misalignment on mitotic spindle	Anaphase-promoting complex (APC), degradation of cyclin B, polo and aurora kinases monitor mitotic spindle and centrosome formation

Adapted from Schwartz and Shah (2005).

progression through first the cell cycle phase and then on through the next checkpoint. CDKs have become a focus for the development of novel anti-cancer drugs, with the rationale that CDK inhibition can induce cell cycle arrest in tumour cells.

4.2 Oncogenesis

Oncogenic transformation takes place when the expression of a *proto-oncogene* becomes deregulated. A proto-oncogene is defined as a normal gene carrying out an essential cellular function, that when mutated, may trigger tumorigenic pathways. Mutation is often of biological origin, taking place when certain tumorigenic viruses integrate into the host genome. Human tumour viruses may be RNA viruses, such as the retroviruses and flaviviruses; or DNA viruses, examples of these being the herpes, papilloma and polyoma viruses. These are often associated with certain cancer types (Table 4.2). Conventionally, the proto-oncogene is represented by the nomenclature *c-onc*, whereas *v-onc* represents a viral oncogene, where *onc* is the name of the gene. Such a gene may code for a receptor or enzyme intermediate involved in signalling pathways controlling

Table 4.2 Oncogenic viruses and cancer

Virus	Virus family	Associated cancer
Animal models		
MMTV (mouse mammary tumour virus)	RNA virus	Breast tumour models expressing Mtv-1, Mtv-2, notch gene family, Wnt and Fgf.
RSV (Rous sarcoma virus)	Avian RNA tumour virus	Solid tumours expressing *c-src* produced in chickens
MSV (murine sarcoma virus)	RNA virus	Has been used to model oncogenesis by *v-Ras*, *v-fos*
Human		
RNA virus		
HTLV-1 (human T-cell leukemia virus)	Retrovirus	Adult T-cell leukaemia
HCV (hepatitis C virus)	Flavivirus	Hepatocellular carcinoma
HMTV (human mammary tumor virus)	Retrovirus	Breast
DNA virus		
SV40 (simian virus 40)	Polyoma	Brain, bone, mesothelioma
HPV (Human papilloma virus)	Papilloma	Cervix, anogenital
KSHV (Kaposi's sarcoma-associated herpesvirus)	Herpes	Kaposi's sarcoma
EBV (Epstein-Barr virus)	Herpes	Nasopharyngeal, Burkitt's lymphoma, B and T cell lymphomas, Hodgkin's lymphoma

proliferation or cell death, for example, a growth factor receptor or phosphokinase enzyme; or direct the response to cellular damage inflicted by carcinogens (for example, DNA repair enzymes or apoptosis). A proto-oncogene becomes an oncogene when one of two mutational events occurs. This may be a qualitative change, where the mutation affects the coding region of the gene, culminating in the production of a protein with abnormal structure or function; or a quantitative change, where the mutation alters the regulation of the gene, leading to an abnormal level of the gene product. An increased level of normal product is described as *amplification*, common in the advanced stages of carcinogenesis, that is, tumour progression, but only occasionally associated with the events of early carcinogenesis.

4.2.1 Viral oncogenesis

Viral oncogenesis may follow infection with RNA or DNA viruses. RNA viruses infect cells and use cellular machinery to undergo reverse transcription to DNA, forming the DNA provirus, which becomes incorporated into the host genome. The DNA provirus may act in two ways, either forming an oncogene such as *v-ras* or *v-fos*, or by carrying out insertional mutagenesis where viral regulatory sequences interfere with the activity of host genes. DNA viruses code for protein products which may bind to and inactivate host proteins. For instance, human papilloma virus (HPV), the transforming virus linked with cancer of the cervix, produces a double-stranded circular DNA that integrates into the host genome and codes for the oncoproteins E6 and E7 (Figure 4.1). In non-malignant cells, the tumour suppressor gene *p53* protects against DNA damage by inducing transcription of the protein p21, which induces cell cycle arrest in the G1 phase and gives DNA repair enzymes sufficient opportunity to carry out their DNA repair function. If this is not successful, the pro-apoptotic protein Bax offers an alternative safeguard. E6, however, inhibits the p53-mediated transcription of both these proteins. Progression from G1 to S-phase of the cell cycle is regulated by the tumour suppressor protein pRb (retinoblastoma protein), which is phosphorylated by the checkpoint CDKs. In its hypophosphorylated state, pRb binds and inactivates E2F, a transcription factor that allows progression through to S-phase. However, when pRb is phosphorylated, it is unable to maintain the complex with E2F, leaving the transcription factor free to carry out its function. The E7 oncoprotein is able to bind and inactivate pRB, inhibiting the formation of the E2F/pRb complex and therefore affording E2F the ability to induce cell cycle progression by a mechanism that is independent of the activity of the G1–S checkpoint CDKs. Removal of these protective safeguards allows cellular proliferation to become deregulated and to take place unchecked. Cigarette smoking, the use of oral contraceptives for longer than 5 years and infection with other sexually transmitted diseases are all cofactors for oncogenesis by HPV.

HPV is known to be the causal agent of cervical cancer, with one study showing that over 99% of cases are due to HPV infection. This provided the rationale to develop a HPV vaccine for the prophylaxis of cervical cancer, for which two formulations were recently approved by the FDA: Gardasil (summer 2007) and Cervarix (early 2008). Whilst there are over 100 strains of HPV, 15 strains are designated as high risk. Of these, four strains have been targeted: HPV-16 and HPV-18, which together cause around

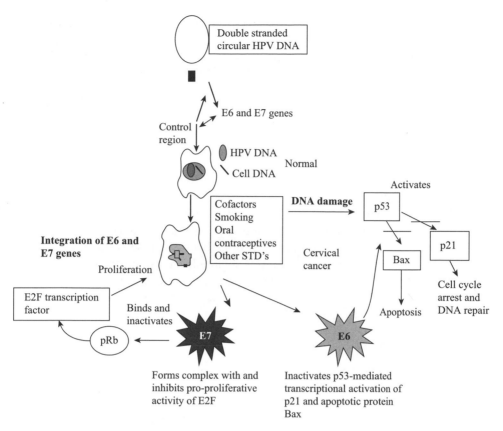

Figure 4.1 Effects of oncogenic transformation by human papilloma virus.

70% of cases of cervical cancer; along with HPV-6 and HPV-11, which have been linked with 90% of cases of genital warts. Gardasil, a quadrivalent vaccine, targets all four high risk HPV strains and so provides protection from genital warts, HPC-associated cervical cancer and the pre-cancers cervical intraepithelial neoplasia (CIN), squamous intraepithelial lesion (SIL), and dysplasia. Cervarix, however, is a bivalent vaccine that targets HPV-16 and HPV-18 only and is therefore not expected to provide immunity to genital warts. Both vaccines are prepared from non-infectious recombinant L1 capsid virus-like particles (VLPs), which are identical to native virions but modified to provide an 'inactivated' formulation. The quadrivalent vaccine has been evaluated in the FUTURE (Females United To Unilaterally Reduce Endo/Ectocervical Disease) studies, where the results of FUTURE I and II, which involved young women between the ages of 15 and 26 years, have been published. FUTURE III, which extends the study to women aged up to 45 years, is currently in progress. These are large-scale phase III clinical trials involving thousands of women, where those involved in FUTURE II will also be reassessed during long term follow up of a minimum of 14 years post vaccination. Whether the bivalent or quadrivalent vaccine is eventually adopted into general clinical practice is a matter of debate. Although it is established that HPV-16 and HPV-18 are the causal agents for cervical cancer, the non-oncogenic strains HPV-6 and HPV-11, aside from being the cause of genital warts, are also believed to be associated with recurrent respiratory papillomatosis and Buschke–Lowenstein tumours of the vulva, penis and anus, which have a low risk of malignancy but are potentially fatal. Further vaccines in the pipeline include those targeting E6 and E7 oncoproteins.

4.2.2 Amplification of a normal gene product

Amplification occurs when the promotor sequence regulating the expression of the gene is perturbed, one mechanism being via a chromosomal rearrangement. A good example is the deregulation of the protein product of the proto-oncogene *c-myc* (Figure 4.2), expressed in Burkitt's lymphoma and many other cancer types. The locus of c-myc is found on the q chromatid of chromosome 8, controlled by its promotor region. In some circumstances, infection with the Epstein–Barr virus (EBV) induces a chromosomal translocation between chromosomes 8 and 14, so that *c-myc* is subsequently under the control of the promotor region of an immunoglobulin found on the q chromatid of chromosome 14. Amplification of *c-myc* is believed to increase its pro-proliferative effects whilst suppressing c-myc-induced apoptosis, via the inactivation of the tumour suppressor proteins ARF, p53 and Bim.

4.2.3 Altered product

An altered product may be achieved through a mutation or the production of a fusion product, which is derived from portions of two separate functional genes. A good example of oncogenic transformation achieved through mutation occurs with the ras oncogene, named for the causative agent rat sarcoma virus. Ras codes for the protein p21, a GTPase with a role in signal transduction. There are three classic forms: *H* (Harvey)-*ras*, *K* (Kirsten)-*ras* and *N* (neuroblastoma)-*ras*, which are mutated at codons 12, 13 or 61. The region between codons 12 and 69 are important for normal activity, where the proto-oncogene or nascent form of ras cycles between its active and inactive

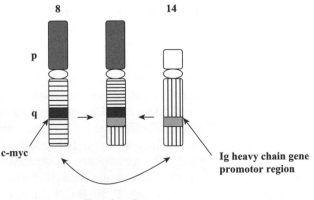

Figure 4.2 Translocation of portions of chromosomes 8 and 14 leads to amplification of the proto-oncogene *c-myc* by promotor swapping.

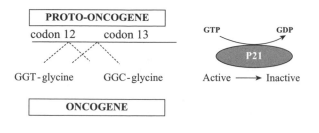

Tumour type

	Colon $n = 60$	Lunh $n = 14$	Pancreas	
			$n = 28$	$n = 50$
K12 GGT				
-AGT	12′	43	36	0
-TGT	12	0	0	0
-CGT	0	0	4	31
-GAT	16	21	28	31
-GTT	37	29	32	36
-GCT	7	7	0	2
K13 GGC-GAC	21	0	0	0

GGT-glycine
AGT- serine
TGT-cysteine
GAT-aspartic acid
GTT-valine
GCT-alanine
GGC-glycine
GAC-aspartic acid

Figure 4.3 Mutation of the *ras* proto-oncogene may exert a change in the sequence of codon 12, 13 or 61, leading to the production of a protein that has lost the capacity for inactivation. The nature of the mutation is characteristic of tumour type. Reproduced from Bos, J.L. (1989) ras oncogenes in human cancer: a review. *Cancer Res.* 49: 4682–4689, published by the American Association for Cancer Research.

form (see Chapter 15). The mutated form, however, cannot be inactivated, leading to uncontrolled signal transduction and therefore stimulation of cellular proliferation. A high incidence of *ras* mutations has been detected in samples from colon, lung and pancreatic tumours, and although each tumour type varies in the frequency of each type of mutation, they all involve a sequence change of just one base (Figure 4.3). For instance, a mutation specific to colon tumours where the sequence of codon 13 changes from GGC to GAC, leads to the substitution of a glycine for an aspartic acid residue. However, a change in codon 12 from GGT to AGT substitutes a glycine residue for serine, a mutation more often detected in lung tumours.

Fusion proteins, like c-myc, are produced through chromosomal rearrangement (Figure 4.4). These occur where functional units of the gene sequence are flanked by breakpoints, or fragile sites of genomic DNA which have a tendency to break as a result of errors in DNA synthesis. Whereas c-myc is subject to promotor swapping, fusion genes are formed when the chromosomal translocation juxtaposes the coding regions of two functional genes, forming a chimeric transcript that produces a fusion protein with tumorigenic activity. For this to occur, the necessary double strand breaks at the two coding regions must be coordinated spatially and temporally, with the fusion gene pair orientated in the correct fashion to produce the functional fusion protein following transcription and translation. The *bcr-abl* (breakpoint cluster region-Abelson) fusion oncogene is expressed in chronic myeloid leukaemia and is generated by the translocation of chromosome 9 to chromosome 22, forming the Philadelphia chromosome. The

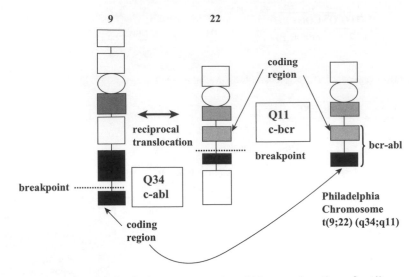

Figure 4.4 Formation of the fusion oncogene *bcr-abl* by translocation of coding sequences between chromosomes 9 and 22. This gives rise to the Philadelphia chromosome, a biomarker of chronic myeloid leukaemia.

bcr-abl oncogene codes for a fusion protein with potent tyrosine kinase activity, which is the target for newly developed tyrosine kinase inhibiting anticancer agents such as imatinib (Gleevec) (see Chapter 14).

4.3 Tumour suppressor genes

In normal tissue, cellular proliferation is restricted by suppressor proteins encoded by tumour suppressor genes. Whereas oncogenes are positive growth regulators, that is, promote cellular proliferation, tumour suppressor genes are negative growth regulators, where malignant transformation may occur due to the inactivation of such proteins. This is generally a result of a mutation in the tumour suppressor gene, which may take place when the gene is bound by viral oncoproteins.

4.3.1 p53

The tumour suppressor gene *p53* is described as 'the guardian of the genome', where a TP53 mutation or a defect in p53-dependent pathways is found in virtually all cancers. The decision to undergo cell cycle arrest or apoptosis in response to cell damage is influenced by the level of p53 and is dependent on separate pathways. The mechanism of p53-induced cell cycle arrest is linked to its transcriptional activation of p21, a protein that binds and inhibits the cyclin–CDK complex at the G1–S checkpoint, leaving the protein pRb in its hypophosphorylated state and consequently disabling the E2F transcription factor, which is necessary for cell cycle progression. High levels of p53, however, are believed to promote apoptosis via effector proteins such as Bax, a member of the bcl-2 family, and the release of the apoptogenic factor cytochrome C, key events in the mitochondrial (intrinsic) apoptotic pathway that is triggered in response to cellular stress and results in the activation of caspase 9. There may also be involvement of p53 in the extrinsic apoptotic pathway, activated by ligand binding to death receptors. These are a family of receptors that include the CD95/APO-1/Fas, tumour necrosis factor and the TRAIL (tumour necrosis factor-related apoptosis-inducing ligand) receptor, their activation signalling for downstream apoptosis via the death inducing signalling complex (DISC) (see Section 2.3.1). There is evidence that p53 promotes increases the expression and cycling of the death receptors, and promotes FADD-independent activation of caspase 8.

The activity of p53 is regulated by a set of feedback mechanisms that help to maintain a strict balance between the rate of cellular proliferation and the rate of cell death (Figure 4.5). The *MDM2* oncogene encodes a E3 ubiquitin ligase which packages p53 for proteasomal degradation, and has itself become a target for anticancer strategies (see Section 18.2). The activity of MDM2 is limited, however, by the tumour suppressor ARF (alternate reading frame tumour-suppressor protein), which re-establishes p53 function by sequestering MDM2. Recently, another control mechanism has been identified, where the newly discovered oncogene *Pokemon* (an abbreviation of the POZ and Kruppel family erythroid myeloid ontogenic factor, or alternatively referred to as *LRF*, *OCZF*, or *FBI-1*), a transcription factor that negatively regulates ARF expression, ultimately feeding back to suppress p53 and promote tumorigenesis.

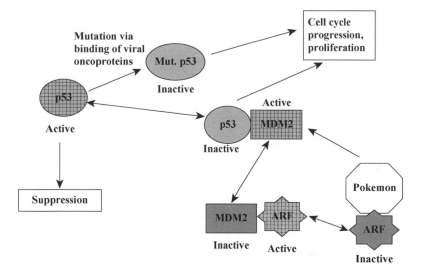

Figure 4.5 Regulation of the tumour suppressor protein p53: activity is fine-tuned by a set of feedback mechanisms. The *MDM2* oncogene binds and promotes degradation of p53, allowing normal cell division to resume but increasing the likelihood of malignancy if overexpressed. MDM2 protein is itself inactivated by the tumour suppressor protein ARF, the activity of which is in turn attenuated via overexpression of the newly discovered oncogene *Pokemon* (*LRF10*, *OCZF11* or *FBI-1*).

4.3.2 The Knudson two-hit hypothesis

A genetic mutation may be described as a *germ-line* mutation, where it is transferred via egg or sperm DNA, and is therefore present in all cells of the resulting offspring; or a *somatic* mutation, which affects only specific cells within a tissue or an organ. Predisposition to cancer may be caused by a range of hereditary syndromes involving inheritance of a germ-line mutation. For a mutation to cause cancer, the mutation has to affect the function of a gene critical to the proliferation and maintenance of cells. A simple analogy may be that a mutation within groups of genes that changes eye colour or the ability to role one's tongue is probably not critical for the development of cancer. However, mutation of a gene that encodes a growth factor such as transforming growth factor-β, or DNA repair, such as the breast cancer oncogene *BRCA1*, are strongly associated with malignancy. For a mutation to show phenotypically, it is necessary for both alleles to be affected. The proposed mechanism, proposed by the Knudson two-hit hypothesis, is that a predisposition to cancer encoded by a germline mutation that affects one allele of a critical gene will be 'converted' to an inducer of malignant transformation only after a subsequent somatic mutation (or hit) of the other allele.

4.3.3 Cancer susceptibility syndromes

Germ-line mutations of a crucial gene may lead to familial clustering of certain types of cancer, or inheritance of a *cancer susceptibility syndrome*. These may be caused by the loss of function of a tumour suppressor gene, affecting the ability to regulate cell proliferation and survival; or a defect in genes coding for proteins involved in DNA repair pathways or crucial for the maintenance of genomic stability. Whereas the former are usually dominantly expressed, the latter are mostly recessive. Table 4.3 shows examples of cancer susceptibility syndromes, notably Li–Fraumeni, caused by an inherited loss of p53 function and characterized by predisposition to a range of cancers that includes breast and brain cancers, sarcoma and rhabdomyosarcoma. Most Li–Fraumeni cases are caused by a mis-sense mutation, resulting in an altered p53 protein subunit. Because p53 forms a tetramer, the defective subunit acts as a dominant negative (see Section 10.2.2). Therefore, the second somatic mutation is not necessary for malignant progression and individuals with the heterozygous genotype are still affected, that is, the mis-sense mutation has high penetrance. The von Hippel–Lindau tumour suppressor gene is associated with the proteasomal degradation of oncogenic proteins such as the hypoxia-inducible factor HIF-1α (see Section 18.3). Von Hippel–Lindau disease is caused by a germline mutation of this gene and gives rise to a predisposition towards renal cancers and haemangioma, where the resulting tumours show a highly angiogenic phenotype due to the hypoxia-independent transcription of the gene encoding vascular endothelial growth factor (VEGF). The recessive disorders, caused by germ-line mutations in DNA repair genes or those involved in the maintenance of the genome, include Fanconi anaemia (FA), xeroderma pigmentosum (XP) and ataxia telangiectasia (AT). These disorders are characterized by a range of clinical characteristics as well as susceptibility to cancer. FA is caused by a mutation disrupting the functionality of DNA repair enzymes, leading to hypersensitivity to cross-linking agents, a factor that would have to be accounted for when treating tumours associated

Table 4.3 Genes and their associated cancer predisposition syndromes

Tumour suppressor gene	Locus	Function	Predisposition syndrome	Type of cancer
TP53	17q11	Transcriptional regulator, apoptotic signalling, growth arrest, DNA repair	Li–Fraumeni	Breast, brain, sarcoma, rhabdomyosarcoma
BRCA1	17q21	Transcription factor, DNA repair	Familial breast, ovarian cancer	Breast, ovarian
BRCA2	13q12	Transcription factor, DNA repair	Familial breast, ovarian cancer	Breast, ovarian
PTEN	10q23	Dual specificity phosphatase (antagonizes PI3 kinase-dependent pathways)	Cowden syndrome, Bannayan–Zonana syndrome, Lhermitte–Duclos syndrome	Breast, prostate,
NF1	17q11	Ras-GAP activity	Von Recklinghausen	Neurofibroma, neurofibromatosis
NF2	22q12	Cytoskeletal regulator	Neurofibromatosis type 2	Schwannoma, meningioma
Wt1	11p13	Transcriptional regulator	Wilms tumour	Nephroblastoma
E-cadherin (*CDH1*)	16q22.1	Cell adhesion regulator	Familial gastric cancer	Breast, colon, skin, lung
TSC2	16	Cell cycle regulator	Tuberous sclerosis	Renal, brain
PMS1	2q31	Mismatch repair (DNA)	Hereditary non-polyposis colorectal cancer	Colorectal
APC	5q21	Binds and regulates B-catenin activity (regulation of stem cells).	Familial adenomatous polyposis	Colon
NKX3.1	8p21	Homeobox protein (transcriptional regulator of whole organ development)	Familial prostate carcinomas	Prostate

(continued)

Table 4.3 (*Continued*)

Tumour suppressor gene	Locus	Function	Predisposition syndrome	Type of cancer
MET	7q31	Receptor tyrosine kinase	Hereditary papillary renal cancer	Papillary renal
VHL	3p25	Regulates proteolysis (degradation of oncogenic proteins)	Von Hippel–Lindau	Kidney, haemangioma, phaeochromocytoma
SMAD4	18q21.2	Growth factor signalling	Juvenile polyposis coli	Gastrointestinal
LKB1	19p13.3	Serine/threonine kinase	Peutz–Jeghers	Gastrointestinal
FANCA, FANCC	16q24.3, 9q22.3	DNA repair (recessive)	Fanconi anaemia	Leukaemia
ATM	11q22.3	Serine/threonine kinase (recessive)	Ataxia telangiectasia	Lymphoma, chronic lymphocytic leukaemia
XPB, XPD	2q21, 19q13	Helicases, nucleotide excision repair (recessive)	Xeroderma pigmentosum	Basal cell and squamous cell carcinomas

Unless specified, inheritance is via dominantly expressed loss of function mutations of tumour suppressor genes. Recessive predisposition syndromes such as Fanconi anaemia, ataxia telangiectasia and xeroderma pigmentosum are disorders of DNA genes involved in DNA repair or genomic stability. Adapted from Guilford (2000).

with the disease. Individuals with FA show developmental abnormalities and suscept-ibility to leukaemia. Patients who have inherited XP, on the other hand, typically display UV sensitivity and as a result are susceptible to developing squamous cell and basal cell carcinomas, tumours affecting the skin. XP is caused by a germline mutation in genes that code for helicases, which unwind the DNA helix prior to the initiation of transcription; and nuclear excision repair enzymes, which remove damaged or mis-paired nucleotides. AT is so named for its non-malignant clinical effects, which include progressive neuromotor dysfunction leading to loss of co-ordination and unsteadiness (ataxia), alongside blood vessel dilatation, causing flushing of the skin and mucous membranes (telangiectasia). The condition is caused by a germ-line mutation of the gene coding for the ATM protein, a serine/threonine protein kinase that carries out critical phosphorylation and dephosphorylation steps on serine residues of p53. Nascent ATM therefore has two important effects on p53 functionality: protection from MDM2-dependent proteasomal degradation and the strengthening of its DNA-binding activity, which assist p53-mediated transcription and therefore promote chromosomal stability. Consequently, AT is associated with increased susceptibility to cancers such as T cell lymphoma, chronic lymphocytic leukaemia, medulloblastoma and tumours of the stomach, brain, uterus and breast.

5

Tumour metastasis: a convergence of many theories

5.1 Introduction

Metastasis is the process by which cells from a primary tumour disseminate to form tumour masses at distant sites. Tumour metastases may be detected as a relapse after remission has been achieved; that is, represents a stage of malignant progression which brings a poor prognosis. Therefore a major aim of anti-cancer therapy is to prevent metastatic spread. Metastases may occur in the regional lymph nodes, where tumour cells have migrated via the lymphatic vessels, or to distant organs, via blood vessels.

Traditionally, metastasis occurs in five stages, each determined by the expression of genes controlling the survival of cells within the tumour microenvironment and the production of signalling proteins. The level of gene expression may in turn be regulated by the physiological conditions within the tumour microenvironment, such as the level of oxygenation, nutrient availability and pH (see Chapter 12). The following sections describe the molecular and pathological changes taking place during metastatic progression, as summarised by Map 1.

5.2 Detachment and migration from the primary tumour

Within the primary tumour, only a small proportion of cells are capable of forming metastases; these tend to have a high replicative potential and show resistance to apoptosis. They are also capable of producing growth signals which promote processes such as angiogenesis; and although tumour cells may express tumour-associated antigens, they are able to evade circulating immune cells. The tumour mass is made up of tumour cells and the extracellular matrix (ECM) or stroma, which may include a range of associated cells such as carcinoma-associated stromal fibroblasts, macrophages, leukocytes, platelets, erythrocytes and vascular endothelial cells. Tumour cells initially must detach from the primary tumour mass and invade into the blood or lymph vessels, to be transported as micrometastases. Detachment itself depends upon the extent of cell

Cancer Chemotherapy   Rachel Airley
© 2009 John Wiley & Sons, Ltd.

adherence, brought about by plasma membrane-bound cell adhesion molecules (CAMs) that are expressed by specific cell types within the tumour mass, such as: the integrins, for example, fibronectin, collagen; the cadherins, for example, E-cadherin; the selectins, for example, P- and E-selectins; and the connexins, which are involved with the formation of gap junctions between cells. Migration of a tumour cell is amoeboid, or may be visualized by considering the movement of a slug or a snail, where the front regions propel the rest of the body forward by means of a pseudopodial appendage, the slimy substance acting as an adhesive. Similarly, in cells, migration is initiated by the formation of adhesion sites with actin fibres of the cytoskeleton; thus providing a toehold at the leading edge of the migrating cell, with the cell moving over the contraction site. Meanwhile, to complete detachment, the cell must break away from the extracellular matrix or cellular substratum, a process occurring at the rear of the cell. This depends upon the dissociation of linkages that bind adhesion complexes to both the cytoskeleton (intracellularly) and the ECM. The formation of leading edge adhesions is initiated by the binding of integrins to extracellular matrix ligands such as fibronectin, which induces integrin clustering and activation. This in turn activates a signal transduction cascade that induces catalytic proteins such as focal adhesion kinase (FAK), talin and vinculin. There are several mechanisms by which rear end release may occur. These include contractility-promoted release, where the front and rear coordination of contractile forces generated by actin–myosin complexes within the cytoskeleton directly brings about the breakage of adhesive contacts. Ca^{2+}-mediated release, where transient and local changes in Ca^{2+} levels influence actin–myosin contractility, is also thought to induce the production of calcineurin and calpain proteases. The calpains are cytosolic cysteine proteases that bind to the plasma membrane via phospholipids, inactivating important mediators of adhesion such as FAK, talin and integrins. Integrins may mediate rear end release, where activation of the oncogene *v-Src* causes the breakdown and rapid turnover of adhesion complexes by modulating integrin-dependent focal adhesion assembly, and integrins additionally bind proteolytic enzymes such as the matrix metalloproteinases and cathepsins, weakening their link with the extracellular matrix. Sheddases, including ADAM (a disintegrin and metalloprotease) are membrane-bound enzymes that have been found to influence the proteolytic shedding of cell surface proteins important for forming adhesive contacts, such as collagen XVII/BP 180, found on cells of epithelial origin; CD44, a membrane bound receptor on fibroblasts that binds the ECM glycosaminoglycan hyaluronan; as well as fibronectin and collagen IV. Rear end detachment results in the formation of migratory tracks, which are made up of cellular material such as the integrins. Tubular filaments are also observable at the rear end of the cell by electron microscopy, where the actin fibres of the cytoskeleton retract upon breakage of integrin–cytoskeleton linkages (Figure 5.1).

5.3 Intravasation

After detaching from the primary tumour, tumour cells will enter the blood or lymph supply. Initially, detached cells must invade and migrate first through the primary tumour cell stroma, or extracellular matrix, and then through the basement membrane

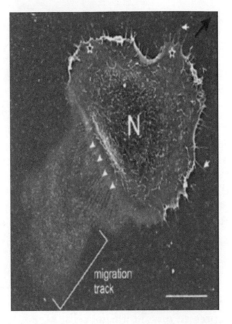

Figure 5.1 Experimental model of the detachment and migration of tumour cells from a primary tumour. This scanning electron micrograph of a migrating epidermal karatinocyte under EGF-induced chemotaxis shows the migration track resulting from rear cell detachment. Membrane protrusions for example, podosomes (arrows) can be clearly seen at the front of the polarized cell, whereas the dissociation of integrin linkages between the extracellular matrix and cellular cytoskeleton leads to the pattern of retracting actin/myosin contractile fibres at the rear of the cell. Reproduced with permission from Kirfel *et al.* (2004) *Eur. J. Cell Biol.* 83:717–724, Elsevier.

and endothelial cell layers of localized vasculature. Two mechanisms have been proposed, which may be described as passive, where cells shed from the primary tumour exposed to tumour microenvironmental conditions, such as hypoxia, gain a survival advantage. In time, the rapid proliferation of such cells in a limited space causes collapse of the fragile tumour blood and lymph vessels, forcing the cells to breach their walls and enter the vascular network. An active mechanism involves changes in the tumour cell phenotype, also brought about by the physiological conditions of the tumour microenvironment, which induce changes in the activity of proteins such as the integrins and the matrix metalloproteinases. These coordinate with cytoskeletal contraction machinery to engineer migration towards the blood or lymph vessel.

Invasion through tissue requires the expression of proteolytic enzymes, such as the matrix metalloproteinases, which degrade collagen fibres and allow passage through the cell matrix. Migration of the cells also requires morphological changes, where tumour cells form pseudopodia-like structures that polarize the cell and afford it with amoeboid motility. These structures are derived from the adhesion complexes found in plasma membrane protrusions which allow attachment to the extracellular matrix. The formation of membrane protrusions depends upon changes in cell volume that occur

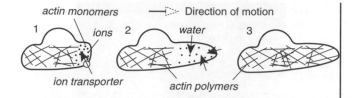

Figure 5.2   The role of aquaporins in the formation of membrane protrusions during migration. Actin depolymerization and ion flux increase the osmotic pressure at the front of the cell, allowing the entry of water and an increase in local hydrostatic pressure, leading to membrane expansion and protrusion. Water enters the cell through membrane-bound aquaporins, which become polarized at the leading edge, for example, AQP1, expressed in tumour vascular endothelium, and AQP3, in certain skin neoplasms. The membrane protrusion is stabilized as the actin repolymerizes. Reproduced with permission from Verkman *et al.* (2008) *J. Mol. Med.* 2008;86:523–9, Springer.

following the ingress of water at the leading edge of the cell. Water is transported into cells by tissue-specific water channels, or aquaporins (AQPs). There are several iso-forms, such as AQP1, expressed on endothelial cells, AQP3, found in skin neoplasms, and AQP4, in astrocytes within the brain. The process is initiated by the polarisation of cells under chemotaxis, forming leading and retracting edges. Actin depolymerization is accompanied by the movement of ions into the front end of the cell due to the activity of Na^+/H^+ and Cl^-/HCO_3^- ion exchange channels. The resulting increase in osmolality allows the entry of water at the leading edge through AQPs, which have polarized at this end of the cell. The resulting increase in hydrostatic pressure causes a localized swelling, giving rise to the membrane protrusion, which is stabilized when the actin repolymerizes (Figure 5.2). By anchoring the actin cytoskeleton to the plasma membrane via integrin clusters and laminins at the site of adhesion, these membrane protrusions induce matrix degradation of the substrate surface by proteases such as matrix metalloproteinases, invadolysin; and membrane remodelling proteins such as Dynamin-2 and Arf6. Podosomes and invadopodia contain organized actin cores which provide the contractile machinery, apparent as actin 'ruffles' at the leading edge of migrating cells, where cofilin-dependent actin polymerisation determines the direction of cell movement (Figure 5.3). Although morphologically similar, podosomes and invadopodia vary in their duration of activity: whereas podosomes are dynamic and short lived, persisting for only minutes, invadopodia are stable for up to 3 hours. There is also an element of tissue specificity (Figure 5.4), where invadopodia are formed by invading tumour cells and podosomes may be formed by monocytic cells such as macrophages. Ultrastructurally, invadopodia present on the ventral surface of cells, occupying a space that is central and close to the nucleus and Golgi body. Whilst podosomes show increased motility, 'sampling' surrounding tissue composition and providing a path for invasion by binding to collagen fibres and degrading ECM at the migration front, the increased stability of invadopodia is linked to decreased motility. This suggests that invadopodia are formed primarily to induce the focal degradation of highly dense collagen fibres, including those existing in the

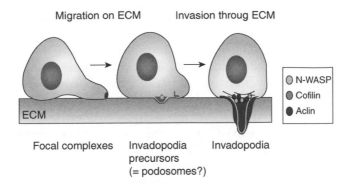

Migration on ECM   Invasion throug ECM

○ N-WASP
● Cofilin
● Aclin

ECM

Focal complexes   Invadopodia   Invadopodia
                   precursors
                   (= podosomes?)

Figure 5.3   Mechanism of cell motility and matrix degradation. Cell membrane potrusions attach to collagen fibres via focal adhesion complexes. Podosomes and invadopodia contain contractile machinery, arising from cofilin-dependent polymerisation of actin which is used to generate directional amoeboid movement. Podosomes tend to be dynamic, and may be precursors of invadopodia, which are stable, long-lived and have the capacity to degrade extracellular matrix. For this reason, invadopodia are typically observed on the surface of migrating tumour cells and play an important part in the dissemination of metastases. Reproduced from Yamaguchi *et al.* (2005) *Current Opinion in Cell Biology* 17:559–564, Elsevier.

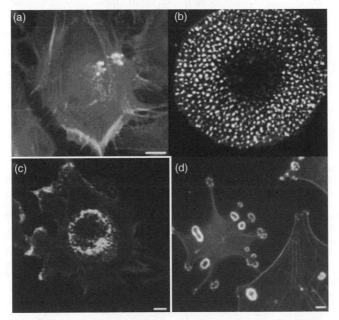

Figure 5.4   Different cell types within a tumour mass invade and migrate through surrounding tissue. The generation of actin-rich adhesions in the form of podosomes or invadopodia gives rise to the matrix degradation and amoeboid cell motility that facilitates processes integral to the formation of metastases such as intravasation and extravasation. (a) shows invadopodia in melanoma cells; (b) podosomes in human macrophages; (c) rosette formation of podosomes in endothelial (HUVEC) cells; and (d) podosome type adhesions in the form of numerous rosette structures in the transformed fibroblast cell line NIH-3T3. Reproduced with permission from Linder (2007) *Trends in Cell Biology* 17: 2007;17:107–17, Cell Press, Elsevier.

basement membranes of blood vessels; ultimately allowing rapid penetration through the endothelial cell layer during the intravasation process. Equilibrium may exist between podosome and invadopod formation, where signalling by cofilin, which is linked with epidermal growth factor (EGF)-induced chemotaxis, and growth factors such as vascular endothelial growth factor (VEGF), may determine their morphology and function. Additionally, there is evidence to indicate an element of cooperativity between cells forming podosomes and/or invadopodia, an interesting example being the macrophage-induced movement of tumour cells through blood vessels during intravasation. Here, macrophages secrete EGF, which acts as a chemoattractant for tumour cells. The tumour cells in turn release colony stimulating factor-1, which stimulates the production and chemotaxis of macrophages, leading to intravasation of both cell types into blood vessels via the formation of podosomes and invadopodia (Figure 5.5).

5.4 Transport

Transport of tumour cells or micrometastases may be haematogenous (via blood vessels) or lymphatic, although disseminating tumour cells may pass from the lymphatic vessels into the blood supply at the left and right lymphatic ducts, which drain into the subclavian veins. Travelling from the primary tumour site, tumour cells will pass through a succession of lymph nodes, initially passing through the nearest, or sentinel lymph node, which drains the organ carrying the tumour and is used as a biopsy site in cancer staging (sentinel lymph node biopsy).

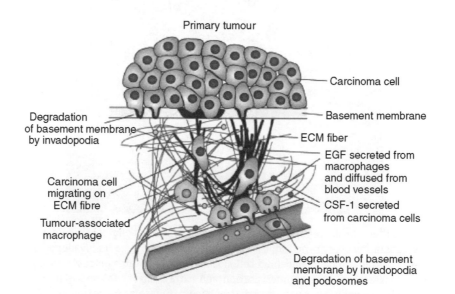

Figure 5.5 Cooperativity of macrophages and tumour cells forming podosomes and invadopodia during intravasation. Reproduced with permission from Yamaguchi *et al.* (2005) *Current Opinion in Cell Biology* 17:559–564, Elsevier.

Which route the metastasis takes depends to a certain extent on the primary site, where certain tumours, such as melanomas and carcinomas, are more likely to disseminate through the lymphatics, an observation believed to be linked with the increased rate of lymph node metastases in these tumours relative to sarcomas. The link between tumour angiogenesis and metastasis is well established, where the presence of tumour blood capillaries to a large extent determines the ease of haemato-genous dissemination. There is now additional evidence that lymphangiogenesis, or the generation of new lymph vessels by tumours increases the likelihood of lymphatic spread, where mobilisation of lymphatic endothelial cells is induced via binding of the angiogenic growth factor VEGFC to the membrane-bound receptor VEGFR3. The destination of disseminating tumour cells and therefore the eventual site of metastasis follows a characteristic pattern which is dependent upon identifying the 'first pass' organ of the primary tumour site. For example, cancers of the colon progress to liver metastases via spread through the hepatic portal vein. Metastasis has often been thought of as a passive process, forming when tumour cells get trapped within the capillaries of their first-pass organs (Figure 5.6). However, there have been several rethinks over the years as knowledge of the tumour microenvironment has increased, giving rise to such concepts as the 'seed and soil' hypothesis (Section 5.6.3).

5.5 Extravasation

Once tumour cells reach their target organ, they must traverse through the vascular endothelium and basement membrane and into the tissue parenchyma. To a certain

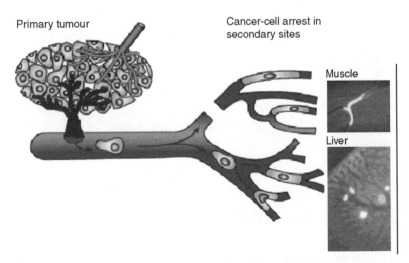

Figure 5.6 Transport of tumour cells from the primary tumour to sites of metastasis. Following intravasation from the primary tumour, cells are carried in the blood circulation (sometimes via the lymphatic vessels) to secondary sites where they become 'trapped' in small capillaries within the target organ. The size restriction imposed by the capillaries in the new organ may induce morphological changes to the cell, for example, in liver and muscle tissue. Reprinted with permission from Chambers *et al.* (2002) *Nat. Rev. Cancer* 2: 563–572, Nature Publishing Group.

extent, extravasation is similar to intravasation but in reverse, where receptor mediated binding of cellular adhesion proteins mediates migration through the tissue layers. However, the exact mechanism will vary according to the type of cell, where tumour cells are accompanied by other cell types of the tumour stroma, for example, macrophages. When a tumour cell becomes trapped or 'arrested', tentative and reversible adhesion or 'docking' takes place, a process mediated by cell adhesion molecules such as the endothelial cell surface E, P and L-selectins and glycoproteins expressed on the surface of the tumour cell, such as SLeA and SLeX. This is followed by more robust adhesion, or 'locking', brought about by binding of cell type-specific adhesion proteins which influence the pattern of metastatic dissemination from primary tumours derived from different tissues. For example, in experimental models, breast tumour cells bind bone marrow endothelium via the CD44 receptor, the β4 integrin subunit allows binding of colon cancer cell lines to endothelial cells, whereas extravasation of melanoma cells into the liver is mediated by integrin a6b1. This is described as 'homing', where the pattern of expression of chemokine and adhesion protein receptors in the target organ leads to the 'active arrest' of cells emanating from the primary tumour. Once 'locking' has taken place, transendothelial migration or diapedesis takes place. In leukocytes this happens without disruption of the endothelial cell barrier, where they are able to squeeze between cells or through non-junctional sites (transcellularly). Tumour cells are much larger, their passage inducing endothelial retraction and morphological changes to the endothelial cell layer. Endothelial retraction may be signalled by vascular permeability factor (VPF), an alternative name for VEGF that reflects its ability to reduce endothelial integrity via the redistribution of actin and production of stress fibres. Another mechanism by which tumour cells induce endothelial retraction is by the release of the lipid 12-(S)-hydroxyeicosatetraenoic acids (HETE), an effect that may be mediated by the redistribution of avb3 integrins (Figure 5.7).

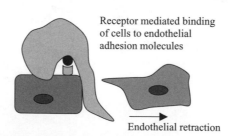

Receptor mediated binding of cells to endothelial adhesion molecules

Endothelial retraction

Figure 5.7 Extravasation of tumour cells by transendothelial migration or diapedesis. Site specific binding of tumour cells to endothelial cells by adhesion molecules induces cytoskeletal arrangements that allow transmigration through the endothelium. This is facilitated by endothelial retraction, where endothelial cells also undergo morphological changes to allow passage of tumour cells, a process that may be regulated by VEGF in the guise of the alternative name VPF (vascular permeability factor). Adapted from Miles *et al.* (2008) *Clin. Exp. Metastasis* 25:305–24.

5.6 Growth of the metastatic tumour mass

5.6.1 Cancer dormancy

Cancer dormancy describes the latent period between remission and the clinical diagnosis of relapse. Tumour recurrences are thought to be a consequence of *minimal residual disease*, where small undetectable numbers of tumour cells remain after treatment. Although these tumour cells persist within the patient, they do not have any clinical effects until, under certain circumstances, they are 'activated', leading to recurrences sometimes years later. The bone marrow, blood and lymph nodes are typical reservoirs for minimal residual disease, consisting of chemo- or radioresistant tumour cells that have gained the survival advantage during treatment with these therapies and have the potential to form a recurrence if the microenvironmental conditions provide sufficient selection pressure, for example, in hypoxic conditions (see Chapter 12).

Dormant tumour cells may exist singly (cellular dormancy) or as dormant micro-metastases (angiogenic dormancy), where both states are dependent upon microenvironmental factors. Cellular dormancy occurs when single cells become quiescent, or enter G0 arrest. This may be triggered by changes in the functionality of proteins such as the tumour suppressor p53. Cellular dormancy is also dependent upon the ability of tumour cells to resist immune attack by circulating CD8 T lymphocytes, achieved through downregulation of tumour antigens. Angiogenic dormancy refers to the need for micrometastases to develop a blood supply to form a clinically detectable metastasis, where the 'angiogenic switch' allows the tumour cell mass to remain viable and progress once its volume has increased beyond the diffusion distance of oxygen (around 100 μm), when the host-derived blood supply is no longer sufficient. At this point, vascular endothelial cells will be recruited into the body of the micrometastasis under the direction of angiogenic growth factors such as VEGF and basic fibroblast growth factor (bFGF), which are produced by tumour and stromal cells such as fibroblasts. This will coincide with suppression of endogenous angiogenic inhibitors such as endostatin and thrombospondin-1, which have themselves become the focus for therapeutic antiangiogenic strategies (see Chapter 13). The development of metastases is opposed by a high rate of apoptosis, or metastatic insufficiency, ensuring that only a very small proportion of cells migrating from the primary tumour have the ability to colonize a target organ. Apoptosis of tumour cells may be classed as two separate processes: *anoikis*, caused by loss of cell adhesion, for example, through loss of integrin signalling; and *amorphosis*, caused by loss of the cytoskeleton. Metastatic insufficiency is overcome by mutational events that lead to overexpression of anti-apoptotic or downregulation of pro-apoptotic signalling proteins, for example, overexpression of the oncogene *Bcl2* and downregulation of the pro-apoptotic CD95 'death receptor'. Hypoxic conditions in the tumour microenvironment may also inhibit apoptosis by decreasing the activity of the pro-apoptotic proteins Bid and Bax.

5.6.2 Cells of the extracellular matrix

The tumour stroma is a collection of mesenchymal cells consisting of fibroblasts, myofibroblasts, endothelial cells, pericytes, and cells of the innate immune system such as macrophages. Of these, the majority are fibroblasts and activated or actin-containing myofibroblasts, where the latter have been given the term carcinoma-associated fibroblasts (CAFs). As well as producing bFGF, CAFs also have a role in the recruitment of endothelial precursor cells (EPCs) for neovascularisation, possibly via the production of stromal-derived factor-1, which exerts a chemotactic effect by binding to the membrane-bound receptor CXCR4 on their surface. Although controversial, one hypothesis to explain the origin of CAFs in tumours is *endothelial to mesenchymal transition*, where cells undergo a de-differentiation process in order to gain a phenotype advantageous to malignant progression, such as loss of cell to cell adhesion and the ability to migrate and invade through basement membrane into neighbouring tissue. This process is believed to be fundamental to the transformation of non-malignant to malignant cells, for example, epithelial to carcinoma cells. CAFs may be derived from transition of epithelial or endothelial cells; although there remains a school of thought that they are derived from pre-existing stromal fibroblasts. Pericytes are vascular mural cells existing within the perivascular matrix, that is, the extracellular matrix and the vascular basement membrane lying adjacent to the blood vessels. In normal tissue, pericytes line up along the abluminal surface of the vascular endothelium, stabilizing newly formed blood vessels by extending cytoplasmic processes into the endothelial cells that act as tight contacts between cells. In contrast, pericytes are relatively scarce in tumour perivascular matrix, offering an explanation for the characteristic leakiness of tumour blood vessels that smooths the progress of tumour cells during intra- and extravasation and therefore encourages metastasis.

5.6.3 Seed and soil

The 'seed and soil' hypothesis was originally proposed by Stephen Paget in 1889 after observing that the typical pattern of metastatic spread in breast cancer patients was to the liver. In an attempt to explain why the liver was the preferred secondary site over equally highly perfused organs such as the spleen, he suggested that metastasis was selective, where the target organ provided the favourable conditions for the growth, survival and proliferation of cells arriving from a distant primary tumour. In a gardening analogy, tumour cells were described as the seeds, which are dispersed randomly and in all directions from the plant, but only germinate and put down roots when they land in fertile soil, which has the optimum nutrients and trace elements to support the growth of the new plant (Figure 5.8). In the case of tumours, the fertile soil is provided by the stromal microenvironment, which are able to express the chemotactic and adhesion protein receptors needed to capture tumour cells, and once captured, to support the establishment of a tumour-derived blood supply. It is now believed that this process also depends upon the formation of a premetastatic niche, where the stromal microenvironment at the secondary site is prepared for the arrival of primary tumour cells. The premetastatic niche sites in organs such as the lung, bone, lymph nodes and brain each show a specific pattern of gene expression directing the interactions taking place between the 'seeds' and 'soil' that will favour such site-specific metastasis. Bone metastasis is a particularly interesting example, due to both its clinical importance – it occurs in 70% of patients with prostate or breast cancer; and its biological complexity,

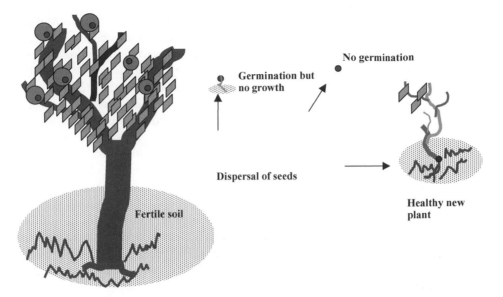

Figure 5.8 The 'seed and soil' hypothesis compares the selective targeting of tumour cells to the germination of seeds and the successful growth of a new plant when gardening. Although distribution may be random, new growth only takes place if the local environment matches specific requirements.

where metastases are generated by one of two prevailing mechanisms according to the cancer type. Osteoblastic metastasis, occurring in prostate cancer, hijacks the process by which new bone is deposited, where osteoblasts are mobilized by growth factors released from metastatic tumour cells. These include prostate-specific antigen (PSA), a serine protease that stimulates osteoblastic differentiation, and bone marrow morphogenic proteins (BMPs) such as BMP6, which stimulates oasteoblastic activity and skeletal invasion. The vasoconstrictor peptide endothelin-1 is also able to modulate osteoblast function as well as induce their production of VEGF to promote site-specific angiogenesis. Osteoblastic metastasis is believed to be regulated by the transcription factors osterix (osx) and runt-related transcription factor 2 (RUNX2). Osteolytic metastasis occurs in breast cancer and is linked to bone resorption. During osteolytic metastasis, a vicious circle arises, which involves interactions between tumour cells, osteoclasts, osteoblasts and bone matrix. Here, disseminated tumour cells trigger osteoclast activation and therefore bone degradation, which in turn upregulates mediators that increase the aggressiveness and encourage growth of the tumour. The vicious circle is initiated by the production of the vasoconstrictor peptide parathyroid hormone-related protein (PTHrP), which stimulates the production of RANK ligand and osteopontenegrin by osteoblasts, the balance of which in turn determines the activation of osteoclasts. Osteoclasts degrade bone matrix by releasing matrix metalloproteinases, and this degradation ultimately leads to the release of growth factors such as fibroblast growth factor (FGF), which stimulate tumour cells to release PTHrP, and so on. Mutations in genes coding for oestrogen receptors are also associated with bone metastasis in breast cancer, where oestrogen normally induces osteoclast apoptosis.

Further, osteopontin, which stimulates angiogenesis, is secreted by macrophages present in the extracellular matrix of bone and is overexpressed in breast cancer.

Another version of this hypothesis proposes that tumour cells mobilize bone marrow cells, which act as 'emissaries' and are able to migrate to the secondary site. These include haematopoietic progenitor cells (HPCs), which express the VEGF receptor VEGFR1. HPCs, along with tumour cells, are able to signal for the release of VEGF itself as well as other angiogenic growth factors such as angiopoietin, placental growth factor and platelet-derived growth factor (PDGF). The HPCs also express the cell surface integrin $\alpha 4\beta 1$, which favours site-specific adhesion to fibronectin produced by fibroblasts present in the parenchyma of the target organ tissue. This encourages clustering of the HPCs in advance of the arrival of tumour cells, where tumour cells are themselves believed to regulate the production of fibronectin, thus creating their own 'docking' site. The accumulation of VEGFR1-expressing HPCs promotes the influx of tumour cells. The presence of VEGFR1-expressing HPCs also supports the recruitment of VEGFR2-expressing endothelial progenitor cells (EPCs) for angiogenesis, where the stability of newly synthesized blood vessels is dependent upon their presence in the perivascular matrix.

6

Health professionals
in the treatment of cancer

6.1 Introduction

The treatment of cancer, that is, the detection, diagnosis, administration of therapy and monitoring of a patient, needs a multidisciplinary team. This team includes clinicians of several specialities, pharmacists, nurses and allied health professions such as radiographers, dieticians and their respective support staff. For many patients, the initial point of contact will be through their general practitioner, who can distinguish whether certain presenting signs or symptoms warrant further investigation. In many cases, the initial detection may result from routine screening, for example, the use of mobile mammography facilities and cervical screening in the community. Upon referral, diagnosis and characterization of the suspected cancer depend upon the union of pathology, radiology and surgical services.

6.2 Pathology

Using biopsy material, the pathologist can classify tumour malignancy and type, where pathologists may specialize in certain cancers, for example, those of the brain such as glioblastoma (Figure 6.1). The tumour biopsy may also be used for the detection of certain genes or proteins expressed in the tumour that may have value as biomarkers or prognostic indicators. These are used to predict the aggressiveness of the tumour, the likelihood of metastases and local recurrence, and the eventual response to treatment (see Section 7.3). Diagnosis may also be possible by examination of effusions, for example, from the pleural cavity and blood.

Cancer Chemotherapy   Rachel Airley
© 2009 John Wiley & Sons, Ltd.

TNM staging for breast cancer
Primary tumour (T)
T_{is} Carcinoma *in situ*, e.g. ductal carcinoma *in situ* (DCIS)
T_1 Tumour ≤ 2 cm in greatest dimension
$T1_{mic}$ microinvasion ≤ 0.1 cm
$T1_a$ tumour >0.1 cm but not >0.5 cm
$T1_b$ tumour >0.5 cm but not >1.0 cm
$T1_c$ tumour >1.0 cm but not >2.0 cm
T2 Tumour >2.0 cm but not >5.0 cm
T3 Tumour >5.0 cm
T4 Tumour of any size, including the following:
$T4_a$ Extension into chest wall
$T4_b$ Oedema, peau d'orange, or ulceration of the skin, or satellite skin nodules confined to the same breast
$T4_c$ Both $T4_a$ and $T4_b$
$T4_d$ Inflammatory carcinoma

Regional lymph nodes (N)
NO No regional lymph node metastasis
N1 Metastasis to moveable ipsilateral axillary lymph node(s)
N2 Metastasis to ipsilateral axillary lymph node(s) fixed to one another or to other structures
N3 Metastasis to ipsilateral internal mammary lymph node(s)

Distant metastasis (M)
MO No distant metastasis
M1 Distant metastasis, including ipsilateral supraventricular lymph node(s)

TNM-tumour/node/metastasis.

6.3 Radiology

The speciality of radiology involves diagnostic radiologists and radiotherapists, who design and oversee regimens that include the administration of ionizing radiation to

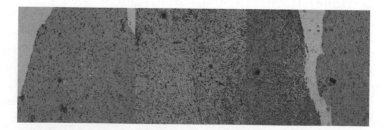

Figure 6.1 Pathology of glioblastoma: typical pathology shows a gradation between normal tissue, infiltrating border zones of hyperplasia and tumour tissue. These samples have been immunohistochemically stained for facilitative glucose transporter Glut-1 (brown). Reproduced with permission from an original photograph by Natalie Charnley, Academic Department of Radiation Oncology, University of Manchester. A colour reproduction of this figure can be viewed in the colour section towards the centre of the book.

a tumour. Diagnostic radiology provides information, through the use of procedures such as ultrasonography, magnetic resonance imaging (MRI) and positron emission tomography (PET) as to the extent and spread of the tumour. Radiotherapy may be curative, that is, delivered with the aim of eradicating the tumour and prolonging life; or palliative, where it is used to reduce symptoms such as pain, with the additional benefits to skeletal integrity and organ function. The most common form of radiotherapy is external beam radiotherapy, where X-rays or gamma-rays produced by a linear accelerator are used.

Pathological and radiological data is collated so that the cancer may be described in terms of grade and stage. Tumours may be graded 1, 2 or 3, according to the extent of differentiation of tumour cells. The transformation of normal cells to malignancy is accompanied by the gradual loss of specialization and functionality. Poorly differentiated tumour cells resemble the normal tissue from which it is derived much less than well differentiated tumour cells, and are of a higher grade. Grade 3 tumours are the least differentiated, the least cytologically normal, and the most aggressive. Staging of tumours is carried out to describe the extent of tumour spread. The definition of each tumour stage varies according to tumour site, but all are roughly defined according to TNM (tumour/lymph nodes/metastasis) classification (see box).

6.4 Role of the surgical oncologist

The initial role of the surgeon is to carry out diagnostic procedures. In a lot of cases this is primarily to obtain biopsy material, but procedures specific to a suspected tumour site such as cystoscopy, to investigate a suspected bladder tumour; endoscopy, to allow examination of the upper gastrointestinal tract or hysteroscopy, to investigate a possible gynaecological malignancy are also performed.

6.4.1 Biopsy

There are four types of biopsy. If possible, a fine needle aspiration, which is performed with a 22–25-gauge needle, will be carried out to collect a smear of cells for cytological analysis. Although the sample size is small, cells can be collected from a wide tumour area. A core biopsy may be used to collect larger tumour fragments, and is collected using a 14–16-gauge needle. This procedure requires a local anaesthetic and may cause bleeding. However, the procedure allows the examination of tumour architecture. A cutaneous punch biopsy uses 2–6 mm surgical blades to cut an area from a cutaneous lesion that includes a full-thickness sample of skin and subcutaneous fat. This procedure also requires local anaesthesia, and must be closed with a suture afterwards. It is typically used to investigate suspected melanoma or squamous cell carcinoma. Open biopsies are an option where there is insufficient access for a needle or where large amounts of tissue are necessary for effective diagnosis. These may be either incisional, which remove a sample of the lesion, or excisional, where the entire lesion is removed. The latter may be curative for small solid tumours for example, melanoma or breast cancer.

6.4.2 Staging

Non-radiological investigative procedures designed to stage the tumour and to decide if the tumour may be removed (surgical resection) as a treatment option may be performed by a surgical oncologist. Such procedures use a device which is inserted via a small incision at a convenient site. These include laparoscopy for abdominal malignancies (for example, ovarian cancer), and sentinel lymph node biopsy, which is used to diagnose metastatic spread to the lymph nodes.

6.4.3 Surgical treatment

Several modes of surgical treatment may be indicated. Surgical resection is the removal of the primary tumour along with a margin of surrounding normal tissue, which will help prevent local recurrence. Prophylactic surgery may be carried out in some circumstances, for example where there are premalignant lesions such as abnormal dysplasias of the cervix, detected by the Papanicolaou smear test, or non-invasive cancers such as basal cell carcinoma of the skin. Certain inherited conditions may also indicate prophylactic surgery in specific circumstances for example, thyroidectomy in patients expressing the *MENII/FMTC* gene, which is a genetic screen for medullary thyroid cancer. Palliative surgery may be carried out to alleviate symptoms and improve quality of life, and reconstructive surgery has developed and improved as the understanding of circulatory biology has advanced.

Other surgical techniques include cryotherapy, where small tumours can be controlled by freezing (for example, multiple liver lesions) and radiofrequency ablation, where an electrode emitting radio waves is inserted into a tumour, the resulting heat causing destruction of tumour tissue.

6.5 Oncology pharmacy

The role of the oncology pharmacist is to carry out and supervise the preparation of cancer chemotherapy within the cytotoxic dispensing unit (Figure 6.2). They also contribute clinical and pharmaceutical expertise to the design of chemotherapy treatment plans in individual patients and clinical trials. The oncology pharmacist will liaise with medical oncologists, oncology nurses and other oncology support staff to deliver evidence-based chemotherapy regimens to the patient, and will be in the position to provide information on the toxicology and pharmaceutical aspects of chemotherapy. An oncology pharmacist has clinical input in several areas. The use of anticancer agents is subject to local or national guidelines, data from clinical trials and tumour characteristics that may render the cancer more responsive or resistant to a particular drug. There may also be patient characteristics, such as age or organ function that determine the acceptability of a chemotherapy regimen. The administration of cytotoxic drugs may have associated complications, such as extravasation or thrombophlebitis. The oncology pharmacist will have access to, and will often be responsible for hospital guidelines covering the treatment of these complications. The formulation, reconstitution and preparation of chemotherapy is also subject to dose checks,

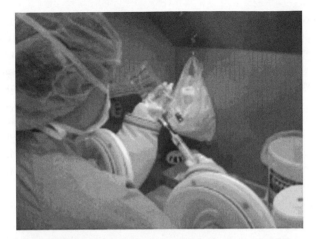

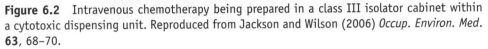

Figure 6.2 Intravenous chemotherapy being prepared in a class III isolator cabinet within a cytotoxic dispensing unit. Reproduced from Jackson and Wilson (2006) *Occup. Environ. Med.* **63**, 68–70.

compatibility checks, where a parenteral formulation contains more than one drug, and the addition of agent-specific ancillary formulations, such as mesna and hydration fluid to be administered alongside the bladder-toxic cytotoxic drug cyclophosphamide. The oncology pharmacist has an important role in ensuring the correct route of administration is used, for example, much publicity has been focused on the accidental administration of intrathecal vincristine; the correct wording on labels can help minimize the risk of this occurring. Chemotherapy is most often prepared in a hospital-based compounding unit. Whereas the oncology pharmacist will be responsible for the formulation of the chemotherapy, the preparation is most likely to be carried out by pharmacy technicians trained to work in the aseptic environment. The work is stringently supervised and documented, and the staff, because they are handling carcinogenic agents, is subject to health and safety regulations. With the increased use of oral chemotherapy, such as the recently adopted agent imatinib (Gleevec), it is recommended that these drugs should be treated with the same principles of safe oncology practice as parenteral chemotherapy. Several practice interest groups with an interest in oncology pharmacy exist, such as ISOPP (International Society for Oncology Pharmacy Practitioners and BOPA (British Oncology Pharmacy Association); web addresses are provided (see Chapter 23), which can provide more information on oncology pharmacy.

6.6 Oncology nursing

The oncology nurse contributes to cancer care by assessing, educating, monitoring and delivering treatment to the patient. Areas of practice include many settings, ranging from acute-care hospitals, to out-patient oncology clinics, home care and community care facilities. They are involved in direct care of the patient, which includes the administration of chemotherapy, assessment of physical and emotional status and the taking of detailed nursing histories. Their role is also to educate patients in order to assist them to cope with their diagnosis and long-term treatment and prevention goals. As with oncology pharmacists, oncology nurses also liaise with clinical oncologists to build an effective care plan for the cancer patient. To carry out their role, oncology nurses must be skilled in venipuncture technique and in the handling of the various venous access and drug administration devices used. They are also trained to recognize immediate side effects, such as hypersensitivity, and those that are delayed onset, such as pulmonary fibrosis. Nurses will triage patient issues such as chemotherapy-induced diarrhoea and emesis and assist in determining their management. A strategic plan for nursing, *The Nursing Contribution to Cancer Care*, was a Department of Health report launched in 2000, which describes a programme of action for cancer care nurses which defines how their role will be developed in the future.

6.7 The NHS Cancer Plan

The NHS Cancer Plan was published in July 2000 in recognition of the problems faced by those treating and being treated for cancer in the United Kingdom. Concerns had been registered at the poor survival rate in the United Kingdom relative to the rest of Europe, as well as the inconsistencies in cancer care that led to phenomena such as 'post code prescribing', inequality of treatment and recruitment and workforce issues. The plan was produced after consultation with oncology professionals and patients throughout the United Kingdom, and describes the strategies that will be used to overcome some of these problems. Among the aims of the plan are to save more lives, to ensure people with cancer get access to the correct professional support and best treatment, to tackle inequalities in cancer care and to invest in the future of the oncology workforce. The objectives that were set out to achieve these changes included initiatives to reduce the risk of cancer, such as smoking cessation and healthy eating, and through raising public awareness and extending cancer-screening services, promoting more efficient early detection. There is an intention to improve cancer services in the community, which includes a partnership between the NHS and Macmillan Cancer Relief to provide funding for a lead oncology clinician in every primary care group, and for training in cancer care for district nurses. There are also efforts in progress to achieve faster access to treatment and to combat waiting lists by investment in staff and equipment. NICE (National Association for Clinical Excellence) will play a part in publishing guidelines to ensure there is more equality in the prescribing of new anticancer drugs; and to promote and improve the standing of UK cancer medicine and research, the NCRI (National Cancer Research Institute) has been established.

7
Principles of cancer chemotherapy

7.1 Introduction

Cancer chemotherapy is the treatment of cancer using anticancer drugs. These drugs are often used as part of multimodality therapy, that is, along with surgery and/or radiotherapy, to achieve and maintain remission. The process is likely to be long term, where single agents or combination chemotherapy are given at intervals in pulsed doses or in cycles, and is highly dependent upon the tumour type and characteristics. Monitoring of the patient takes place throughout the process, so that tumour response to therapy or incidences of tumour progression can be tracked, and treatment aims adjusted accordingly. Traditionally, cancer chemotherapy is according to guidelines set by the appropriate clinical specialities, for example, the minimum clinical recommendations for diagnosis, treatment and follow-up described by the European Society for Medical Oncology (ESMO, see Boxes 7.1 and 7.2). However, it is now recognized that significant tumour heterogeneity exists between and within patients, so that efforts to individualize therapy according to tumour and patient characteristics are being investigated and put into practice. Molecular biology, and diagnostic techniques such as magnetic resonance imaging (MRI) and positron emission tomography (PET) have revealed a range of biomarkers that may be used as prognostic indicators (Figure 7.1). Prognostic indicators, which help predict the survival of a patient after a specific treatment, have considerable value in the rational selection of patients to receive both standard treatments and novel anticancer drugs that are in clinical trials. They also help determine the need for additional treatments such as radiotherapy (Figure 7.2).

7.2 Timing of chemotherapy

The aim of chemotherapy is to induce remission, that is, complete eradication of disease for at least 1 month. The challenge of anticancer treatment, though, is to prevent recurrence, which may occur locally or at a distance (metastasis) of the primary tumour site. To address this, additional strategies are adopted prior to or following the

Cancer Chemotherapy   Rachel Airley
© 2009 John Wiley & Sons, Ltd.

Box 7.1   Summary of ESMO minimum clinical recommendations for the treatment and follow-up of locally recurrent or metastatic breast cancer

Staging

- History of management of primary tumour and menopausal status

- X-ray, computerized tomography (CT) scan, MRI

- Biomarkers: oestrogen, progesterone and HER2 receptor status

Hormone receptor positive tumours

- Endocrine therapy: selective oestrogen receptor modulating agents (SERMs), e.g. tamoxifen, toremifene; aromatase inhibitors, e.g. anastrazole, letrozole; LHRH analogue, e.g. goserelin; progestins, e.g. megestrol; novel oestrogen receptor antagonist, e.g. fulvestrant.

- *Premenopausal*: no prior tamoxifen – tamoxifen plus ovarian ablation, otherwise use aromatase inhibitor plus ovarian ablation.

- *Postmenopausal*: tamoxifen or aromatase inhibitor.

Hormone receptor negative tumours
Cytotoxic chemotherapy:

- Cyclophosphamide/methotrexate/fluorouracil

- Adriamycin/cyclophosphamide

- Adriamycin/docetaxel

Metastatic breast cancer expressing HER2
Chemotherapy plus trastazumab.

Response evaluation: after 3 months endocrine therapy and two or three cycles of chemotherapy.

---

achievement of remission. Therefore, chemotherapy is classified, according to timing, as follows:

- *Induction chemotherapy*. This is initial therapy administered with the aim of achieving significant cytoreduction, and ideally, complete remission of the disease. The outcome of induction chemotherapy may be a complete response, where there is disappearance of the disease for one month; partial response, where there is a reduction in tumour volume of 50% or more; stable disease, which is defined as a

Box 7.2 Summary of ESMO minimum clinical recommendations for the treatment and follow-up of non-small cell lung cancer (NSCLC)

Staging

- Chest X-ray/CT scan/MRI of the brain to detect possible brain metastases

- Lymph node biopsy

- PET scan, bone scintigraphy to detect presence of bone metastases

Stage 1–2 disease: surgery plus adjuvant and/or neoadjuvant chemotherapy. For inoperable tumours: curative radiotherapy.

Stage 3 disease: induction chemotherapy plus surgical resection. For inoperable tumours, platinum-based (e.g. cisplatin) chemotherapy plus thoracic radiotherapy

Stage 4 disease: platinum-based combination chemotherapy prolongs survival, improves quality of life and controls symptoms.

Response evaluation: mandatory after two or three cycles of chemotherapy after repetition of diagnostic radiological tests.

Follow-up: history and physical examination every 4 months for 2 years and every 6 months thereafter.

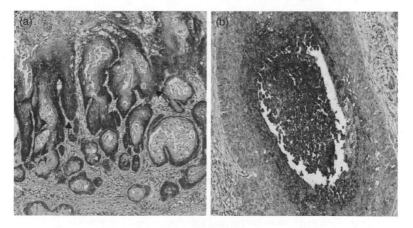

Figure 7.1 Facilitative glucose transporter Glut-1 expression (brown staining) detected by immunohistochemistry in samples of oral squamous cell carcinoma surgically removed from a patient. The highest level of expression was found in (a) invading tumour tissue (arrows) or (b) around necrosis, indicating a biological link with malignancy and hypoxia. Accordingly, Glut-1 may be used as a marker of malignancy, hypoxia and prognosis in a range of solid tumour types. Reproduced from Oliver *et al.* (2004) *Eur. J. Cancer*, 40, 503–7. A colour reproduction of this figure can be viewed in the colour section.

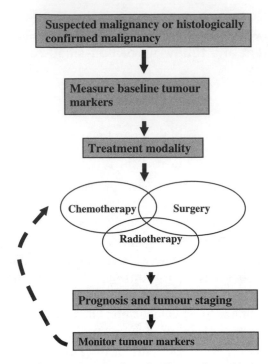

Figure 7.2   Clinical use of biomarkers in the selection and monitoring of cancer treatment.

decrease in tumour volume of less than 50% with no new disease sites for at least one month; or progression, where there is an increase in tumour volume of 25% or more, or evidence of new disease sites.

- *Consolidation/intensification chemotherapy.* This is administered remission after remission induction to prolong freedom from disease and overall survival. Whereas consolidation chemotherapy uses the same drugs as for induction of remission, intensification therapy uses drugs that are non-cross resistant to induction chemotherapy.

- *Adjuvant chemotherapy.* This is given following eradication of the disease with localized treatment such as surgery or radiotherapy, used to treat microscopic disease and prevent local recurrence.

- *Neoadjuvant chemotherapy.* Treatment is given prior to local therapy to maximize efficacy for example, to shrink a tumour before surgery.

- *Maintenance chemotherapy.* Prolonged, low-dose chemotherapy is issued on an outpatient or community basis to extend the duration of remission and achieve cure.

- *Salvage chemotherapy.* Drug treatment may be given after failure of other treatments to control the disease or provide palliation.

- *Combination chemotherapy.* Although single agent chemotherapy may be indicated in some situations, more than one agent, or combination chemotherapy, is often used (see examples in Section 8.6). The rationale of combination chemotherapy is to maximize tumour cell kill using drugs with different modes of action, and acting on different parts of the cell cycle. Combination chemotherapy may also decrease the potential for adverse toxic events, where lower doses of each agent may be used, and by selecting agents with dissimilar toxicity profiles.

7.3 Biomarkers and their uses

Biomarkers are biological characteristics or phenomena that may be used to provide information on the malignancy, aggressiveness, stage and extent of differentiation of a tumour. They may be used in the initial diagnosis of cancer, for example, prostate-specific antigen (PSA) is used in the detection of otherwise asymptomatic prostate cancer. Because they can reveal genotypical information that determines response to various anticancer agents, radiation and surgery, they are assuming increased importance as prognostic markers, that is, in the prediction and evaluation of treatment response, survival and in the rational selection of patients into treatment arms of clinical trials. Biomarkers are typically genes or their corresponding protein product that are expressed at varying levels within and between patients, detectable either in biopsy or resected tissue, by radiological means, or in the serum. Many tumour types have a specific biomarker that predicts prognosis in that tumour type, whereas there are some biomarkers that are widespread in a wide range of malignancies. Table 7.1 shows examples of biomarkers, the associated tumour types and their predictive value.

7.4 Clinical assessment of biomarkers

To gain acceptance in the clinic, a biomarker must be validated in human subjects. In general, a biomarker should be non-toxic, minimally invasive and the results precise, rapid, with low risk of false negativity. The method should not compromise treatment, and should minimize any further discomfort or inconvenience to the patient. For these reasons, the biomarkers ideally should be collected at the time of biopsy. A biomarker gains acceptance as a prognostic marker if it correlates specifically with treatment outcome independently of known parameters. To validate a prognostic marker, retrospective studies are carried out, in the first instance, using archival material from a series of patients with a specific tumour type that is large enough to maintain statistical significance of the emerging data. This series of patients will have been treated in the past within a speciality at one or several hospital sites over a period of time that is not critical. However, these patients should have received similar treatment, and adequate data describing clinical and pathological characteristics, treatment follow-up, disease progression and survival should be available, which is used to determine any statistical correlation with the prognostic marker being investigated. If the retrospective study ultimately shows the biomarker to be an independent predictor of adverse prognosis, it is followed up by a prospective study. Here, patients are recruited into a study as they receive treatment, and the prognostic relevance of the

Table 7.1 Biomarkers, associated tumour types and their predictive value

Biomarker	Tumour type	Molecular basis	Detection
Pathological characteristics			
Diagnostic criteria			
Stage	All		Diagnostic radiology
Lymph node status	All		Pathological/ cytological examination of biopsy material
Grade of differentiation	All		
Depth/anatomy of invasion	All, of particular importance for tumours of the gastrointestinal tract		
Markers of proliferation			
Ki67	All	Nuclear antigen associated with proliferation, not present in G0 phase	IHC
Cyclins	All	Regulation of cell cycle phase transition e.g. at check points	IHC
Chromosome abnormalities			
p53	All	Tumour suppressor gene which shows loss of function in ∼50% tumours	IHC, RT-PCR, FISH
bcl-2	Mixed – predicts poor prognosis in haematological malignancies but better prognosis in non-small cell lung cancer. May predict poor prognosis in some prostate cancers	Oncogene that inhibits cell death, overexpressed due to chromosomal translocation process	IHC, RT-PCR, FISH
H-ras, K-ras, N-ras	Colorectal, breast, pancreas and lung tumours, melanoma	Membrane-associated GTPase integral to signal transduction cascade, if mutated, causes increased cellular proliferation	IHC, RT-PCR, FISH

Table 7.1. (*Continued*)

Biomarker	Tumour type	Molecular basis	Detection
MYCN	Neuroblastoma	Amplification causes increased cellular proliferation via myc/max transcription factor	RT-PCR
BRCA1, BRCA2	Breast	Involved in the cellular response to DNA damage	RT-PCR
Bcr/Abl	Chronic myeloid leukaemia	Chromosomal translocation leading to increased tyrosine kinase activity and promotion of cellular proliferation	RT-PCR, FISH, IHC
Telomerase	Wide range of tumours: good predictive ability in pancreatic, uterine and lung cancers	Maintenance of telomeres and therefore chromosomal length enables progression through successive cell cycles	TRAP assay
Tumour microenvironment			
Hypoxia			
Bioreductive markers e.g. 2-nitro-imidazoles	Head and neck, cervix tumours	Nitroimidazole metabolites form intracellular addicts with cellular components in hypoxic cells	MRI, PET imaging, IHC
Hypoxia-regulated genes			
HIF-1		HIF-1 transcription factor complex stabilized in hypoxic conditions, leading to transcription of hypoxia-regulated genes	IHC
Glut-1	Cervix, head and neck, breast, colorectal, oesophageal, ovary, bladder tumours	Increased Glut-1 expression caused by malignant transformation and upregulated by hypoxia. Promotes switch to anaerobic glycolysis to support hypoxic tumour	IHC (see Figure 7.1)

(*continued*)

Table 7.1. (*Continued*)

Biomarker	Tumour type	Molecular basis	Detection
CAIX	Cervix, head and neck, breast, bladder tumours: predicts poor prognosis; renal clear cell carcinoma, may predict survival	Adaptation to low pH caused by production of lactate in hypoxic conditions; cell to cell adhesion	IHC
Angiogenesis			
VEGF		Angiogenic growth factor that binds VEGF receptor	IHC, FISH, immunoassay
PD-ECGF		Angiogenic growth factor with thymidine phosphorylase activity	IHC
Vascularity		New vasculature supports tumour growth. Vascular "hot spots" form in hypoxic areas, and large intercapillary distances may be causative of hypoxia	IHC staining for endothelial receptors e.g. CD31, CD34, von Willebrand (factor VIII) combined with measurement of ICD or MVD using digital image analysis techniques
Radiosensitivity			
SF2	Tumours treated using multi-modality therapy that includes radiation	Survival fraction of cells treated with 2Gy dose of ionizing radiation	Clonogenic assay-growth rate of tumour cells ex vivo post radiation
Multi-drug resistance MDR1 (p-glycoprotein), MRP, LRP, BRP	Lung, breast, leukaemias	Multi-drug resistance efflux transporters that prevent intracellular accumulation of anticancer agents	IHC, FISH

Table 7.1. (*Continued*)

Biomarker	Tumour type	Molecular basis	Detection
Serum/urinary metabolites/enzymes			
Catecholamines: VMA (vanillylmandelic acid)/ HVA (homovanillic acid)	Neuroblastoma	Neuroblastomas overproduce catecholamines,	HPLC
PSA	Approved by the US Food and Drug Administration for mass screening for early prostatic carcinoma	Serine protease specifically produced by prostate tumour cells, acts upon semenogelin I, semenogelin II and fibronectin in seminal fluid, causing liquefaction of the seminal plasma clot after ejaculation, regulates growth factors such as IGF-1, interferes with bone remodelling and may have role in formation of bone metastases	RIA

CAIX, carbonic anhydrase IX; FISH, fluorescent in-situ hybridization; HIF-1, hypoxia inducible factor-1; HPLC, high pressure liquid chromatography; ICD, intercapillary distance; IGF-1, insulin growth factor-1; IHC, immunohistochemistry; MVD, microvessel density; PD-ECGF, platelet-derived endothelial cell growth factor; RT-PCR, reverse transcription–polymerase chain reaction; RIA, radioimmunoassay; VEGF, vascular endothelial growth factor.

biomarker is assessed at the end of a time period, usually 5 years, upon completion of treatment and follow-up protocols. If the data show agreement with the retrospective study, the clinical application of a putative prognostic marker may be considered. The most likely application is in the rational selection of patients to receive certain treatment modalities based upon the level of expression of the biomarker (Figure 7.2). Here, baseline expression is measured upon diagnosis, treatment modality is selected and biomarker expression is monitored following each round of treatment. If a biomarker is a good predictor of chemosensitivity, for example, multidrug resistance efflux transporter expression; the dose, timing and type of chemotherapy regimen used may be individualized and adjusted to each patient according to the level of expression upon diagnosis and during the course of treatment. To establish the benefit of using a biomarker to select a specific treatment regimen, a phase III clinical trial is carried out which compares the outcome of patients treated according to or independently of biomarker status.

7.5 Pharmacogenetics and pharmacogenomics of cancer chemotherapy

Response to anticancer chemotherapy may be determined by the level of enzymes or drug transporter proteins expressed within a tumour that are essential for the uptake, activation and elimination of anticancer agents. Expression levels may show intra-patient (between tumours within the same patient) or inter-patient (between patients) variation, so that determination of expression levels at biopsy may offer a useful means of individualizing the clinical use of these agents by allowing the design of bespoke treatment regimens. Clinical response may refer to the efficacy of drug, that is, cytoxicity to the tumour or susceptibility to adverse drug reactions.

Pharmacogenetics may be defined as the study of how genes regulate the response to a drug. Genetic differences may exist within the tumour, where the expression of certain biomarkers (for example, oncogenes, tumour suppressor genes, drug-activating enzymes) is a manifestation of the molecular pathology of that specific tumour. Alternatively, pharmacogenetics may deal with genetic differences specific to the patient as a whole, described as genetic polymorphism, where certain patients show inherited differences in the expression of drug handling enzymes. Examples of genetic polymorphism that may determine the clinical response to anticancer agents include the enzymes cytochrome P4503A4 and 3A5 (CYP3A4/3A5), which determine the pharmacokinetics of the anticancer agents etoposide, paclitaxel and vincristine; 5,10- methylenetetrahydrofolate reductase, which maintains folate levels and therefore influences susceptibility to toxicity to the antifolate drugs such as methotrexate; and thiopurine methyltransferase, which catalyses the metabolic elimination of 6-mercaptopurine. Simplistically put, if a genetic polymorphism leads to either the expression of a mutant inactive form, or decreased levels of the active form of a drug-activating enzyme, upward dose adjustment may be necessary to obtain the optimum cytotoxic

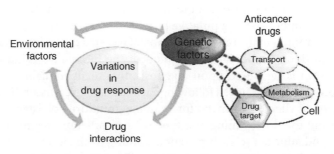

Figure 7.3 Factors affecting clinical response to anticancer agents. Reproduced from Lee, W. et al. The Oncologist **10** (2), 104–11. 2005 AlphaMed Press.

effect. Conversely, if a patient is affected by a genetic polymorphism such that the enzymes involved in a drug detoxification pathway are affected, downward dose adjustment may be necessary to avoid adverse drug toxicity.

The principals of pharmacogenetics may be applied to pharmacogenomics, which explores how therapy may be individualized to improve clinical outcome. Clinical response to anticancer agents is determined by a number of factors, shown in Figure 7.3. These include the level of expression of drug targets: for example, thymidylate synthase for 5-fluorouracil and dihydrofolate reductase for antifolate drugs; prodrug-activating enzymes, for example, the CYP450 family for etoposide, NADH cytochrome P450 reductase for tirapazamine and NQO1 for mitomycin C; and the presence of carrier proteins either for uptake of drug, for example, the reduced folate carrier transports antifolates such as methotrexate and pemetrexed into the tumour cell; and drug efflux transporters, for example, the multi-drug resistance efflux transporters MRP and p-glycoprotein transport methotrexate, paclitaxel, vincristine, etoposide and doxorubicin out of the cell, preventing intracellular accumulation at sufficient levels to achieve cytotoxicity. Pharmacogenomic studies may employ microarray technology (see Section 10.2.3) for the genotyping of patients, so that individual variation in gene expression may be correlated with drug response, providing data on their suitability for recruitment into clinical trials.

8

Classical anticancer agents

8.1 Introduction

Classical anticancer agents, summarized according to the point in the cell cycle at which they are most active (Figure 8.1), are represented by the following groups of drugs.

8.2 Alkylating agents

These include the nitrogen mustards (mustine, cyclophosphamide, ifosfamide, chlorambucil and melaphalan), alkyl sulphonates (busulphan), aziridines (thiotepa, triethyline melamine), nitrosoureas (carmustine, lomustine, semustine) and the platinum based alkylating agents (cisplatin, carboplatin, oxaliplatin). The general mode of action of alkylating agents centres around the formation of an ethyleneimonium ion intermediate, which is highly unstable and forms covalent bonds with DNA bases, the most vulnerable to attack being guanine. Guanine base alkylation is illustrated in Figure 8.2, which shows the effect of bifunctional alkylating agents such as cyclophosphamide. The generalized structure of bifunctional alkylating agents is shown in Figure 8.3. These drugs typically possess two reactive groups characterized by the presence of a lone pair of electrons on the nitrogen atom, donation of which giving rise to an unstable ethyleneimonium ion following loss of a negatively charged chloride radical. The ethyleneimonium ion may further destabilize to form a carbonium ion, both intermediates being capable of sequentially forming bonds with two guanine residues within the DNA double helix, ultimately allowing the formation of cross-links between DNA strands. Platinum-containing alkylating agents act in a similar way, where the reactive intermediate is formed upon exposure of the drug to water, which carries lone pairs of electrons on its oxygen atom. The redistribution of electrons towards the chlorine atoms leads to the loss of chlorine radicals from the drug molecules, which are replaced by OH_2 groups. This intermediate is unstable and forms covalent bonds with DNA bases leading to cross-linking of DNA. Dacarbazine and temazolamide are both prodrugs for the alkylating agent MTIC (3-methyl-(triazen-1-yl) imidazole-4-carboxamide) (Figure 8.4). Decomposition of MTIC yields methane diazohydroxide, which produces molecular nitrogen

Cancer Chemotherapy   Rachel Airley
© 2009 John Wiley & Sons, Ltd.

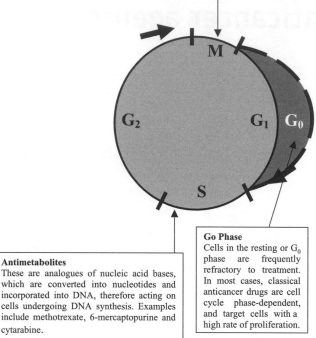

Mitotic Poisons/Tubulin Inhibitors
These prevent formation of the mitotic spindle by binding to tubulin subunits, therefore act on cells undergoing mitosis, e.g. vincristine, paclitaxel.

Cell cycle phase-independent Agents

Alkylating Agents
These act by alkylating guanine bases, leading to the formation of cross-links between opposite bases in double-stranded DNA. Because alkylating agents act on DNA that has already been synthesised, they are most likely to act at a point in the cycle other than S-phase. Examples include carmustine, cisplatin and cyclophosphamide.

Intercalating/Groove Binding Agents
These are planar compounds that intercalate between adjacent base pairs or slot into the external grooves of the DNA double helix. These agents include the antitumour antibiotics e.g. doxorubicin, bleomycin and mitomycin C.

Go Phase
Cells in the resting or G_0 phase are frequently refractory to treatment. In most cases, classical anticancer drugs are cell cycle phase-dependent, and target cells with a high rate of proliferation.

Antimetabolites
These are analogues of nucleic acid bases, which are converted into nucleotides and incorporated into DNA, therefore acting on cells undergoing DNA synthesis. Examples include methotrexate, 6-mercaptopurine and cytarabine.

Topoisomerase Inhibitors
These may be inhibitors of topoisomerase I, e.g. the camptothecins; or topoisomerase II, e.g. the epipodophyllotoxins. They are active during S-phase because they interfere with the activity of enzymes functioning during DNA replication

Figure 8.1 Summary of the mode of action and cell-cycle phase dependency of the classical anticancer agents.

and the alkylating species, a methyl cation that alkylates guanine at the O6 position. Activation of dacarbazine requires an oxidative N-demethylation step catalysed by the cytochrome P450 family of enzymes, whereas temozolomide undergoes a chemical degradation reaction consisting of decarboxylation and ring opening steps, in basic conditions. Temozolomide was developed to target the brain cancer glioblastoma multiforme, the major advantages over dacarbazine being that, first, the basic conditions found in this type of tumour relative to surrounding normal brain tissue targets MTIC activation to the malignant tissue; and second, it passes freely through the blood–brain barrier. Temozolomide has since been recommended by the National Institute for Clinical Excellence (NICE) for the second-line treatment of recurrent malignant glioma and is now undergoing clinical evaluation in other

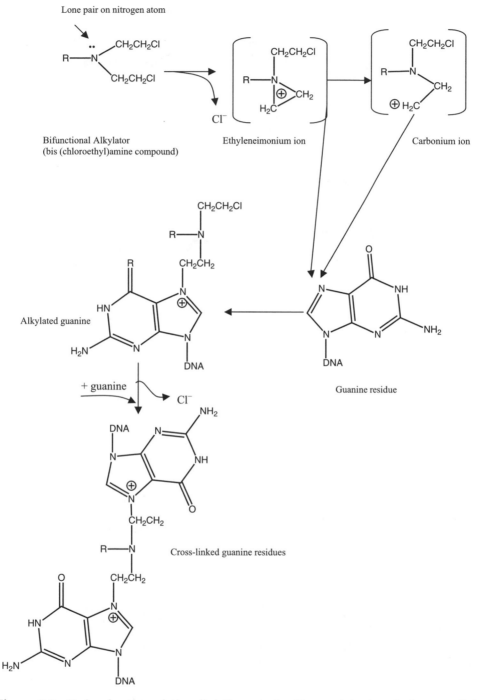

Figure 8.2 Mode of action of the alkylating agents. These act by transferring an alkyl group to the N7 of guanine residues in DNA, via production of reactive ethyleneimonium and carbonium ions.

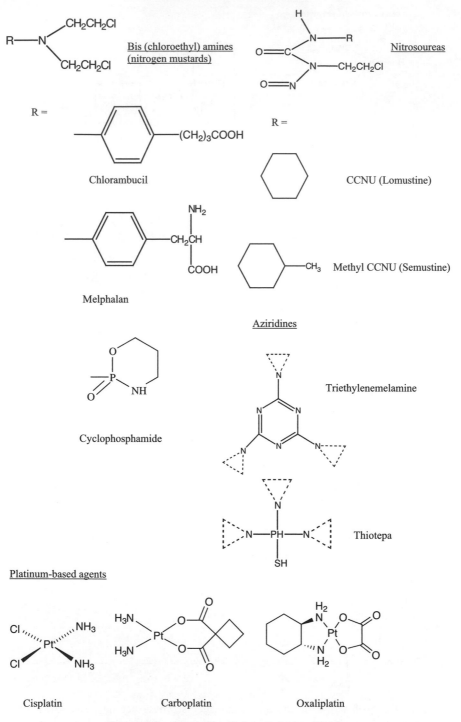

Figure 8.3 Structure of the alkylating agents.

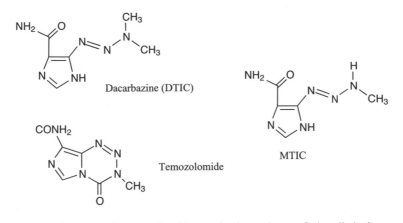

Figure 8.4 Dacarbazine and temozolomide are both prodrugs of the alkylating compound MTIC (3-methyl-(triazen-1-yl) imidazole-4-carboxamide). The conversion of dacarbazine to MTIC is via an N-demethylation step catalysed by cytochrome P450 oxidases. Decomposition of MTIC yields methane diazohydroxide, which produces molecular nitrogen and a methyl cation that alkylates guanine at the 06 position. Though structurally related to dacarbazine, temozolomide does not require metabolic activation by enzymes. Instead, the reaction is thought to be pH dependent, where MTIC is formed when temozolomide undergoes decarboxylation and ring opening in basic conditions.

cancer types such as malignant melanoma, non-small cell lung carcinoma and haematological malignancies.

8.3 Antimetabolites

8.3.1 Inhibitors of purine and pyrimidine biosynthesis

Antimetabolite anticancer agents have a similar molecular structure to substrates of enzymes involved in the synthesis of DNA, a process that eventually disrupts DNA structure and functionality and leads to tumour cell death. These drugs may interact with DNA in two ways – either by acting as structural analogues of precursors and intermediates along the synthetic chain and therefore interfering with the synthesis of purine and pyrimidine bases; or by behaving as 'false' bases in the assembly of the DNA double helix during replication and transcription. Folic acid is an important DNA precursor which undergoes reduction to first dihydrofolate and then tetrahydrofolate by the enzyme dihydrofolate reductase (DHFR), which is the primary target of the folic acid analogue methotrexate. Methotrexate and other folate analogues (Figure 8.5) such as raltitrexed and pemetrexed act as folate antagonists, in that they inhibit the de novo synthesis of purines. A further effect of DHFR inhibition is a decreased intracellular reduced folate pool. Reduced folate acts as a cofactor for thymidylate synthase, which catalyses the synthesis of pyrimidine nucleotides by converting deoxyuridine monophosphate (dUMP) to deoxythymidine monophosphate (dTMP) (Figure 8.6).

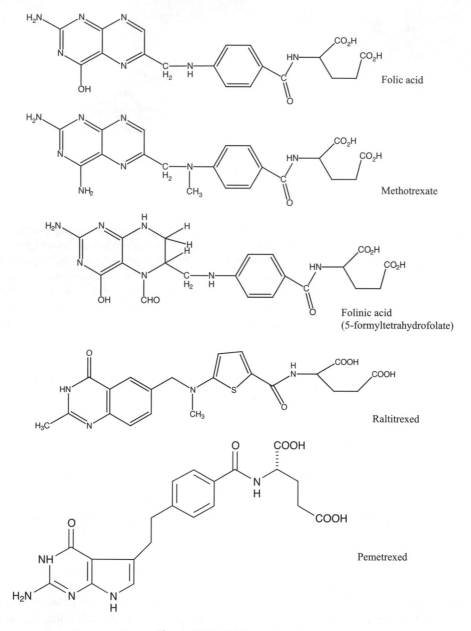

Figure 8.5 Folate analogues.

Consequently, folate analogues inhibit the synthesis of both purines and pyrimidines, although drugs within this class differ in their relative specificities as inhibitors of DHFR and thymidine synthase function.

The polyglutamination of folates increases their intracellular accumulation and retention. Methotrexate and other folate analogues enter cells through the

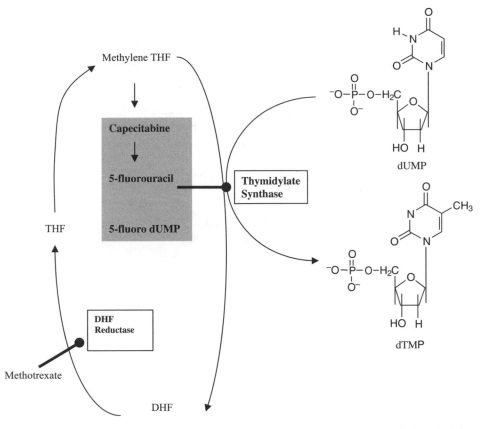

Figure 8.6 Integration of purine and pyrimidine metabolism. Inhibition of dihydrofolate reductase (DHFR) by antifolate agents such as methotrexate blocks the conversion of dihy-drofolate to tetrahydrofolate (THF), a purine precursor. This also interferes with the synthesis of pyrimidine nucleotides, as a metabolite of THF, methylene THF, acts as a co-factor for thymidylate synthase, which catalyses the conversion of deoxy uridinemonophosphate (dUMP) to deoxythymidine monophosphate. Thymidylate synthase in turn is blocked by the thymine analogue 5-fluorouracil.

membrane-bound reduced folate carrier (RFC-1), where sequential addition of glutamine residues by the enzyme folylpolyglutamate synthase (FPGS) leads to the formation of polyglutamates; for example, methotrexate polyglutamate (MTXPG) formed by the polyglutamination of methotrexate (Figure 8.7). The concentration of folate polyglutaminates, and ultimately the individual patient response to antifolate drugs, is determined by the relative expression and activity of FPGS and the opposing enzyme γ-glutamyl hydrolase (GGH), which catalyses the deconjugation of glutamine residues from folates. Polyglutaminated folates also have higher affinity for folate-metabolizing enzymes, thereby influencing their metabolism and down-stream incorporation into nucleotides. The other major folate transport systems are the folate receptors FR a, b and g, which are membrane-bound folate-binding proteins; and a low pH RFC-independent transport pathway has also been discovered.

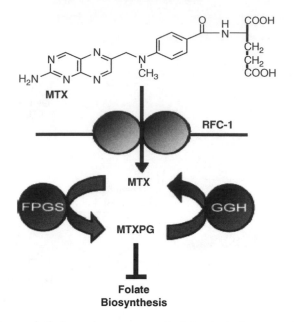

Figure 8.7 Folates and their analogues are polyglutaminated upon entry into the cell, therefore the action of folate antimetabolite agents such as methotrexate are dependent upon tumour levels of membrane-bound folate carriers such as the reduced folate carrier RFC-1 and the enzyme folylpolyglutamate synthase. Reproduced from Dervieux *et al.* (2005) *Mutation Research* 573:180–194, Elsevier.

8.3.2 Purine analogues – 6-thiopurines

The 6-thiopurines (Figure 8.8) are purine analogues with a single substitution of a thiol group in place of the ketone group on carbon 6 of the purine ring. Two examples of 6-thiopurines are 6-mercaptopurine, which is a structural analogue of the purine precursor hypoxanthine, and 6-thioguanine, an analogue of guanine. These drugs are activated by the enzyme hypoxanthine: guanine phosphoribosyl transferase (HGPRT). This enzyme ordinarily transfers phosphoribosyl pyrophosphate (PRPP), which consists of a ribose and phosphate group, to a free purine base to form a nucleotide. This process, known as the purine nucleotide salvage pathway, maintains the intracellular purine nucleotide pool necessary for various cellular functions (Figure 8.9). However,

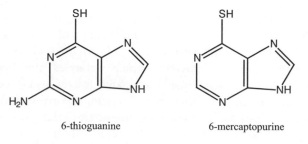

Figure 8.8 The 6-thiopurines as analogues of purine bases.

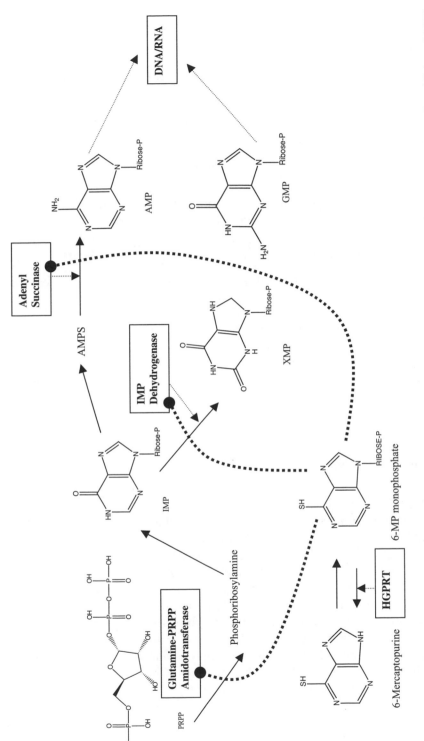

Figure 8.9 Activation of the 6-thiopurines by the enzyme HGPRT. In normal purine nucleotide synthesis, HGPRT catalyses the addition of PRPP (a complex of ribose and phosphate) to free purine bases. However, in the presence of 6-mercaptopurine, this antimetabolite is incorporated into a nucleotide in place of hypoxanthine, therefore inhibiting the synthesis of XMP (xanthine monophosphate).

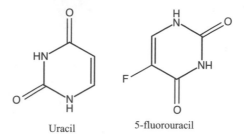

Uracil   5-fluorouracil

Figure 8.10 The pyrimidine analogue 5-fluorouracil.

the structural similarity of the 6-thiopurines means they also show substrate specificity for HGPRT and are consequently incorporated into nucleotides.

8.3.3 Pyrimidine analogues

The most widely used pyrimidine analogue is 5-fluorouracil, a fluorine-substituted analogue of uracil (Figure 8.10). Capecitabine is a prodrug of 5-fluorouracil activated in tumour tissue via the enzymes cytidine deaminase and thymidine phosphorylase (Figure 8.11). Activation of 5-fluorouracil takes place in tumour cells, where it is converted to the nucleotide 5-fluoro-2′-deoxyuridine 5′ phosphate (FdUMP). During normal DNA synthesis, deoxyuridine monophosphate (dUMP) is converted to deoxythymidine monophosphate by thymidylate synthase. In the presence of 5-fluorouracil, however, FdUMP will bind covalently to thymidylate synthase and its methylene tetrahydrofolate cofactor, blocking the synthesis and incorporation of thymine nucleotides.

8.3.4 Nucleoside analogues

Though free nucleobase antimetabolites such as 5-fluorouracil have been in clinical use since the 1950s, there has been significant progress with the development and use of purine and pyrimidine nucleosides, leading on from the FDA approval of cytosine arabinoside (Ara-C, cytarabine) in 1969. Nucleoside analogues have a generalized structure consisting of a purine or pyrimidine base linked to a deoxyribose sugar (Figure 8.12). Purine nucleosides include the deoxyadenosine derivatives cladribine, fludarabine and clofarabine; and examples of pyrimidine nucleoside analogues include the deoxycytidine analogues cytarabine (Ara-C), gemcitabine and 4-thio-Ara-C. Nelarabine is a prodrug that is demethylated to its active form, the deoxyguanosine analogue Ara-G (9-β-D-arabinofuranosylguanine), by adenosine deaminase. The nucleoside analogues are phosphorylated intracellularly by deoxycytidine kinase to the triphosphate form, which is incorporated into DNA. This interferes with DNA chain elongation via inhibition of DNA polymerase and also reduces the pool of deoxynucleotide triphosphates (dNTPs) available for DNA replication by inhibiting the enzyme ribonucleotide reductase. Fludarabine is approved for the treatment of B-cell chronic lymphocytic leukaemia, whilst cladribine is used to treat hairy cell leukaemia. Clofarabine and nelarabine are new generation purine nucleoside analogues – clofarabine was approved

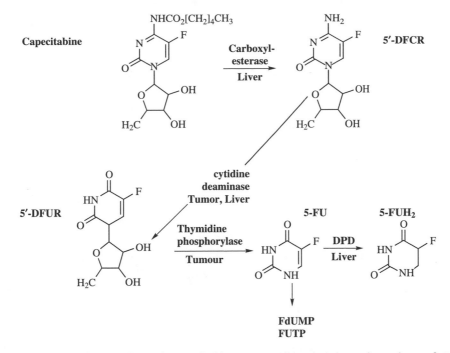

Figure 8.11 The activation of capecitabine, an orally administered prodrug of 5-FU (5-fluorouracil). Capecitabine is converted by the liver enzyme carboxyl esterase to 5-DFCR (5-deoxy-5-fluorocytidine) and then to 5-DFUR (5-deoxy-5-fluorouridine) by cytidine deaminase, an enzyme expressed in both the liver and in the tumour. 5-DFUR is then converted intracellularly to the antimetabolite 5-FU by thymidine phosphorylase, tumour specificity being achieved due to the high level of expression of this enzyme in malignant relative to normal tissue. Reproduced from Schellens, J.H.M., *The Oncologist* 2007;12:152–155, Alphamed Press.

in Europe in 2006 for use in children with acute lymphoblastic leukaemia and nelarabine in 2007 for T-cell acute lymphoblastic leukaemia (T-ALL) and T-cell lymphoblastic lymphoma (T-LBL). The novel pyrimidine nucleoside analogue 4-thio-Ara-C has shown promise in preclinical studies involving a range of human tumour xenografts and is now in phase I clinical trials.

8.4 Agents derived from natural or semisynthetic products

8.4.1 Antitumour antibiotics

These drugs are often referred to as antitumour antibiotics as the early examples were produced by microorganisms. These drugs tend to be cell-cycle non-specific and therefore are of use in the treatment of slow-growing tumours that have a low growth fraction.

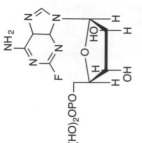

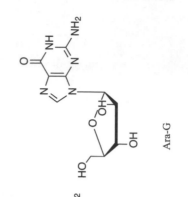

Fludarabine

Ara-G

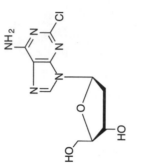

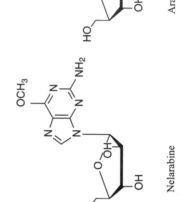

Cladribine

Nelarabine

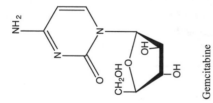
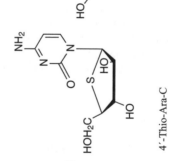
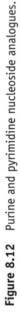

Gemcitabine

4'-Thio-Ara-C

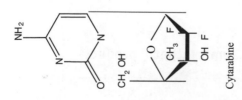
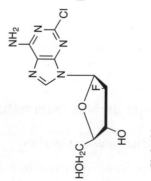

Cytarabine

Clofarabine

Figure 8.12 Purine and pyrimidine nucleoside analogues.

Anthracyclines

The anthracycline antibiotics are a major class of antitumour antibiotics that were originally isolated from *Streptomyces peucetius* var. *caesius.* This group includes doxorubicin and the closely related daunorubicin and epirubicin (Figure 8.13). The antitumour antibiotics as a group have complex pharmacodynamic effects, where studies that have in most cases looked at the anthracyclines, particularly doxorubicin, have revealed several modes of action. These are described in the following paragraphs.

Intercalation between DNA bases

Intercalating agents slot between adjacent DNA base pairs. This action disrupts the topology of the double helix structure, causing inhibition of both DNA polymerase and DNA-dependent RNA polymerase which interferes with DNA synthesis and transcription (Figure 8.14).

Production of free radicals

Anthracyclines are quinone derivatives that may undergo a one-or two-electron bioreductive reaction, catalysed by oxidoreductase enzymes such as NADPH cytochrome P450 reductase, NADH dehydrogenase and xanthine oxidase, to produce an unstable semiquinone radical. This radical auto-oxidizes to forms a C7-centred aglycone free radical intermediate that acts as an alkylating agent, leading to scission of DNA strands; or through DNA-intercalation (Figure 8.15). Interaction between the anthracycline and molecular oxygen also leads to the production of peroxides, superoxide and hydroxyl radicals that can cause further injury to cellular components. Free radicals are thought to be responsible for some of the adverse drug reactions specific to anthracyclines, such as cardiotoxicity, where they induce lipid peroxidation of the sarcolemma and interfere with mitochondrial function in cardiac muscle cells. Anthracyclines also behave as DNA cross-linking agents (Figure 8.16), by forming adducts with NH_2 residues in the guanine bases in both strands of the double helix. The drug is thought to be covalently linked to one strand (c-strand), while this complex is further stabilized by a strong but non-covalent bond to the opposite strand (n-strand).

Inhibition of topoisomerase II

The anthracyclines are inhibitors of topoisomerase II, a homodimeric enzyme (two identical subunits) enzyme that acts at the replication fork of DNA to prevent tangling of daughter DNA strands and maintain DNA topology (Figure 8.17). Usually, this is carried out by breakage and resealing of the DNA strands. However, in the presence of anthracycline, topoisomerase II remains bound to the 5' end of the DNA molecule after completing the cleavage reaction. The formation of this stable DNA-enzyme intermediate prevents rejoining of the DNA breaks.

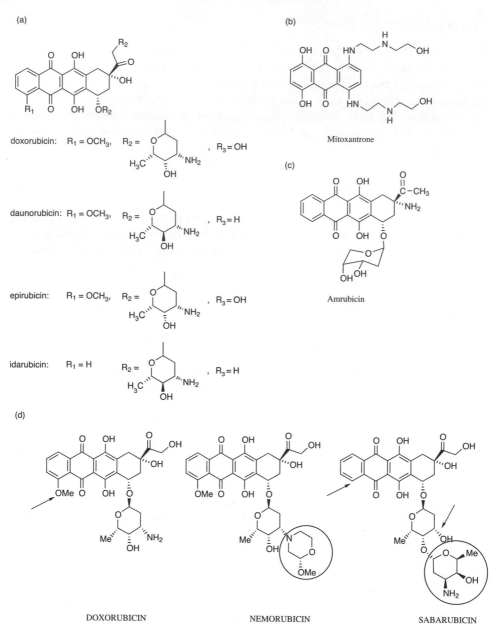

(a)

doxorubicin: $R_1 = OCH_3$, $R_2 =$, $R_3 = OH$

daunorubicin: $R_1 = OCH_3$, $R_2 =$, $R_3 = H$

epirubicin: $R_1 = OCH_3$, $R_2 =$, $R_3 = OH$

idarubicin: $R_1 = H$ $R_2 =$, $R_3 = H$

(b)

Mitoxantrone

(c)

Amrubicin

(d)

DOXORUBICIN   NEMORUBICIN   SABARUBICIN

Figure 8.13 (a) the classical anthracycline doxorubicin and its derivatives daunorubicin, epirubicin and idarubicin are all routinely used in the clinic, sharing a common four-ringed 7,8,9,10-tetrahydrotetracene-5,12-quinone structure with substitutions at the R1–4 groups. Reproduced with permission from Kratz *et al.* (2006) *Curr. Med. Chem.* 13:477–523, Bentham Science Publishers Ltd; (b) the second generation anthracycline derivative mitoxantrone; (c) the 9-amino-anthracycline amrubicin; (d) comparison of the chemical structures of doxorubicin with the newer third generation anthracyclines nemorubicin, a methoxy morpholinyl doxorubicin derivative; and sabarubicin, a disaccharide anthracycline. Reproduced from Sessa *et al.* (2007) *Cardiovasc. Toxicol.* 7:75–79, Springer.

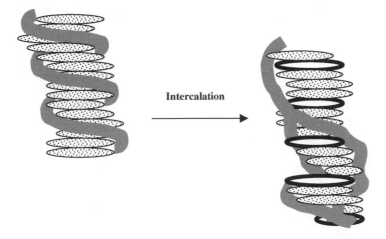

Figure 8.14 Intercalating agents slot into adjacent pairs of bases disrupting the topology of the DNA double helix.

Recent developments in anthracycline chemotherapy

There are currently ongoing phase I and II clinical trials involving novel anthracyclines with the aim of improving the side effect profile and tumour specificity of established agents either through the development of novel formulations or the design of semisynthetic analogues.

Doxorubicin analogues

Second-generation anthracyclines were developed following the observation that manipulation of the doxorubicin molecule at the C-3' position, that is, at the sugar group, improves binding and inhibition of topoisomerase II, as well as activity in resistant cells. This eventually led to the approval and introduction of epirubicin, idarubicin, pirarubicin, aclacinomycin A and mitoxantrone. Despite their widespread use in the clinic, their use still comes with the risk of cardiotoxicity. Therefore, third generation anthracyclines are currently being developed (Figure 8.13d), such as the disaccharide anthracycline analogues, for example, sabarubicin, where the amino group is displaced to a second sugar; and the morpholinyl derivatives, for example, nemorubicin, which has a methoxy morpholinyl group substitution on the 3' position of the doxorubicin amino sugar. Following promising preclinical studies which showed the drug to have reduced cardiotoxicity, sabarubicin has undergone phase I dose escalation studies and is currently being evaluated in phase II trials involving patients with sarcoma, ovary, breast and lung tumours. Nemorubicin showed good activity against liver metastases in preclinical and phase I studies, these data providing the rationale for phase II trials in patients with hepatocellular carcinoma. A totally synthetic novel anthracycline, the 9-amino-anthracycline amrubicin, is a prodrug converted by carbonyl reductase to the active compound amrubicinol by reduction of its C-13 ketone group to a hydroxy group (Figure 8.13C). A phase II clinical trial evaluating the use of amrubicin in non-small cell lung cancer was completed recently, following on from a phase I trial where amrubicin was given in combination with carboplatin in elderly patients with small-cell lung cancer.

Free radicals reactions of Adriamycin

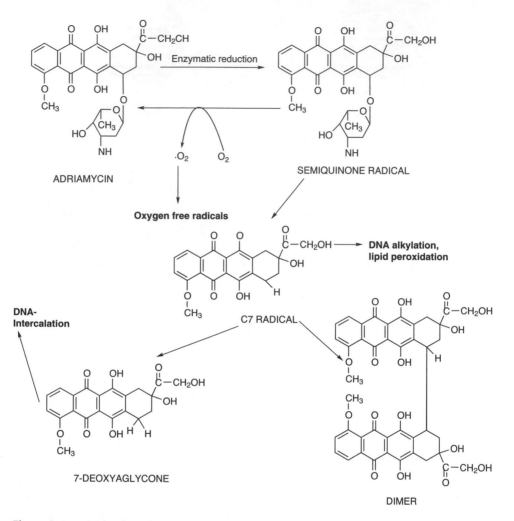

Figure 8.15 Activation of anthracyclines depends upon the production of superoxide radicals and an unstable semiquinone radical, which auto-oxidizes to forms a C7-centred aglycone free radical intermediate that acts as an alkylating agent leading to scission of DNA strands; or through DNA-intercalation. Free radical production is also thought to be a cause of cell membrane lipid peroxidation, which may be responsible for the cardiotoxic effects seen in patients receiving anthracycline chemotherapy. Reproduced from Jung and Reszka (2001) *Advanced Drug Delivery Reviews* 49:87–105, Elsevier.

Liposomal doxorubicin

Packaging of anthracyclines into liposomal formulations is a way of improving their safety profile by achieving more specific targeting to the tumour. Liposomes are composed of lipid molecules, usually phospholipids, which have hydrophobic and

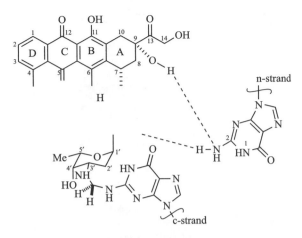

Figure 8.16 Adriamycin causes inter-strand DNA crosslinks by forming adducts with NH_2 residues in guanine bases in both DNA strands of the double helix. The drug is thought to be covalently linked to one strand (c-strand), this complex being stabilized by a strong but non-covalent bond to the opposite strand (n-strand). Reproduced with permission from Zeman *et al.* (1998) *Proc. Natl. Acad. Sci. USA* 95: 11561–11565, National Academy of Sciences.

hydrophilic groups. Analogous to cell membranes, they are able to form lipid bilayers, and when dispersed in an aqueous medium they form vesicles. These vesicles may be used to entrap and carry drug constituents either in the internal aqueous environment or within the hydrophobic compartment of the outer membrane, depending upon the lipophilicity of the drug. By manipulation of its chemical constituents, the pharmacokinetic properties of the liposome, such as half-life, can be manipulated. For instance, to avoid capture by macrophages and uptake by the liver and spleen (the reticuloendothelial system) liposomes may be surface coated with polyethyleneglycol (pegylation), to produce 'stealth' liposomes which show decreased clearance and increased circulation time. The use of 'stealth' liposomes takes advantage of the poorly organized vasculature of tumours occurring as a result of a high rate of angiogenesis (see Chapter 13), where passive tumour targeting is achieved through extravasation of the drug through leaky blood vessels into the tumour microenvironment (Figure 8.18). At present, there are three liposomal formulations of anthracycline (Figure 8.19). Liposomal daunorubicin (DaunoXome) is licensed for acquired immune deficiency syndrome-related Kaposi's sarcoma, as is pegylated liposomal doxorubicin (Caelyx), but more specifically in patients with low CD4 count and extensive mucocutaneous or visceral disease. Caelyx is also licensed for advanced ovarian cancer that is refractory to or allergic to platinum-based chemotherapy and as monotherapy in the treatment of metastatic breast cancer in patients with increased cardiac risk. Myocet, or D-99, is a doxorubicin-citrate complex encapsulated in liposomes used with cyclophosphamide in metastatic breast cancer. Liposomal anthracyclines are now undergoing evaluation in clinical trials along with novel anticancer agents such as the proteasomal inhibitor bortezomib. There are also novel liposomal formulations currently in development, including one formulation where

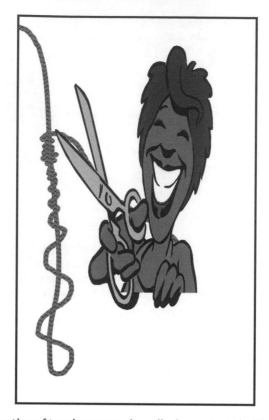

Figure 8.17 The function of topoisomerases is easily demonstrated with a rope. When twisted in a manner similar to the double helix formation seen in DNA, it is extremely difficult to pull apart. In fact, the more it is pulled the tighter it gets. The easiest way to unwind the rope is to cut one or both of the strands.

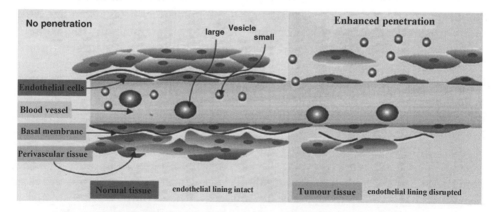

Figure 8.18 Accumulation of stealth liposomes in solid tumours occurs by extravasation from the poorly organized tumour vasculature into the extracellular space following intravenous administration. Reproduced with kind permission from Professor Uchegbu Ijeoma, Ijeoma *et al.* (1999) *Pharm. J.* 263:309–318.

Liposomal formulation	$t_{1/2}$ (h)	Avoids immune uptake	Tumor targeting	Diameter	
Liposomal daunorubicin	4.4	No	No		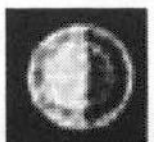 45 nm
Pegylated liposomal doxorubicin	>55*	Yes*	Yes*		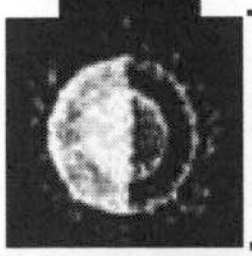 100 nm
Liposomal doxorubicin (D-99)	2-3	No	No		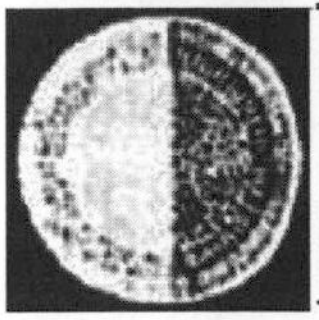 180 nm

Figure 8.19 Comparison of size, tumour specificity and immunogenicity of liposomal formulations of doxorubicin; including liposomal daunorubicin (DaunoXome), pegylated or 'stealth' liposomal doxorubicin (Caelyx), and D-99 (Myocet), a doxorubicin-citrate complex encapsulated in liposomes. Reproduced from Rivera, E. *Oncologist*. 2003; 8(Suppl. 2):3–9. Alphamed Press.

doxorubicin is packaged in immunoliposomes that target HER2, where small unilamellar liposomes (70–100 nm) are covalently conjugated with the HER2 monoclonal antibody (mAb) trastuzumab (Herceptin).

Anthracycline prodrugs

There are several strategies employed in the design of prodrugs that are less toxic than the anthracyclines and are specifically activated intracellularly in tumours. Prodrugs may be synthesized through manipulation at the 3′-amino group of the sugar moiety or at the C-13-keto position (Figure 8.20a). The mechanism of activation of the prodrug is through intracellular cleavage of these bonds, which may occur via tumour-specific enzymes, or through the use of acid-sensitive bonds, a device which exploits the low pH microenvironment of tumours. Prodrugs may be sugar derivatives, where glucuronic acid, galactose and glucose are linked to the 3′-amino position of the drug. For example, the B-glucuronide prodrug HMR-1826 (Figure 8.20b) is a prodrug of doxorubicin activated by B-glucuronidase, a lysosomal enzyme that is released into sites of inflammation and necrosis in tumours. HMR-1826 has been evaluated preclinically in human tumour xenografts, although there have been concerns about its lack of specificity due to the high level of B-glucuronidase in normal tissue such as the liver. An alternative strategy has been designed, where HMR-1826 is co-administered with a B-glucuronidase fusion protein that binds specifically to tumour antigens. This enzyme–antibody conjugate consequently targets B-glucuronidase-mediated prodrug activation to tumour cells, where high concentrations of the active drug are achieved. Anthracycline–albumin conjugates, where doxorubicin is bound to the cysteine-34 residue of human serum albumin via a maleimide peptide spacer, have been synthesized for activation by tumour specific proteases (Figure 8.20c). The peptide spacer is designed according to the protease being targeted, where a sequence from the protease is incorporated into the spacer. One such conjugate, evaluated

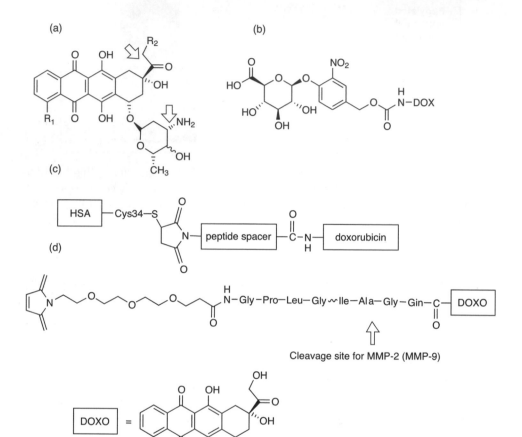

Figure 8.20 (a) prodrugs of doxorubicin may be may be acid-sensitive or have bonds that are cleaved by tumour specific enzymes. They are derived by chemical modification of the 3'-amino group of the sugar moiety or at the C-13-keto position, as indicated by the arrows. A promising prodrug developed using this strategy is HMR 1826, which is activated by B-glucuronidase (b). (c) albumin:doxorubicin conjugates, which contain peptide spacers cleavable by tumour-specific proteases have also been synthesized, a system that may be used to target the matrix metalloproteinases MMP-2 and MMP-9, which are important in angiogenesis and overexpressed in tumours (d). Reproduced with permission from Kratz *et al.* (2006) *Curr. Med. Chem.* 13:477–523, Bentham Science Publishers Ltd.

preclinically in human melanoma xenografts, includes a peptide sequence specific to the matrix metalloproteinases MMP-2 and MMP-9 (Figure 8.20d), which are over-expressed in this tumour model and in a range of tumours where they play a part in angiogenesis. The MMPs are therefore able to cleave the prodrug at the site of the tumour, releasing a doxorubicin tetrapeptide that is degraded to doxorubicin in tumour tissue.

Other antitumour antibiotics

There are other clinically established antitumour antibiotics that have a similar mechanism of action to the anthracyclines as well as some additional specific effects (Figure 8.21). The actinomycins, the best example being actinomycin D (dactinomycin), are polypeptide antitumour antibiotics derived from the *Streptomyces* species, for example, *S. parvullus*. Bleomycin is a glycopeptide antibiotic that was first isolated from *S. verticillus*, where the clinically used anticancer agent is composed of a mixture of bleomycins, the major components being bleomycins A2 and B2. Bleomycin is converted to its active form in the presence of oxygen, a reducing agent and a reduced transition metal (Fe (II) or Cu (I)), which is obtained systemically from the blood. The mechanism of bleomycin activation is described in Figure 8.22, where the bleomycin initially binds Cu (II) ions, and the resulting bleomycin–Cu(II) complex is reduced intracellularly to bleomycin–Cu(I), which reacts with molecular oxygen to exert DNA damage. In the presence of Fe (II) ions, the bleomycin–Cu (I) complex is also able to exchange the copper ion for Fe (II), forming the bleomycin–Fe (III)–OOH complex. The resulting activated metallobleomycins induce single or double DNA strand breaks, initiated by cleavage of pyrimidine bases. Bleomycin has the unpredictable adverse effect of interstitial pneumonitis and a small percentage of patients go on to develop pulmonary fibrosis. Although the mechanism of this effect is largely unknown, it has been suggested that it is due to endothelial cell damage in lung vasculature that elicits an inflammatory response.

Mitomycin C, like the anthracyclines, is a bioreductive drug preferentially activated by tumour-specific reductase enzymes such as NADPH cytochrome P450 reductase and/or DT-diaphorase (NQ01), which to a certain extent determine their mechanism of activation. Structurally, mitomycin C is a quinone-based drug that also contains carbamate and aziridine groups. Although the large numbers of studies investigating the mechanism of mitomycin C activation have not consistently revealed it to be hypoxia dependent, this drug is widely thought to be the prototype hypoxia-activated bioreductive agent (discussed in more depth in Section 12.2). Bioreductive activation occurs by different mechanisms in normoxic versus hypoxic conditions. In a similar fashion to the bioreductive activation of anthracyclines, a one-electron reduction catalysed by NADPH cytochrome P450 reductase produces a semiquinone free radical intermediate that alkylates DNA, leading to the generation of cross-links. Although this mode of activation occurs in hypoxic conditions, the presence of oxygen causes the semiquinone intermediate to enter a redox cycle to produce reactive oxygen species, which have limited antitumour activity but will impede the production of the semiquinone. The one-electron reduction is therefore hypoxia selective. Alternatively,

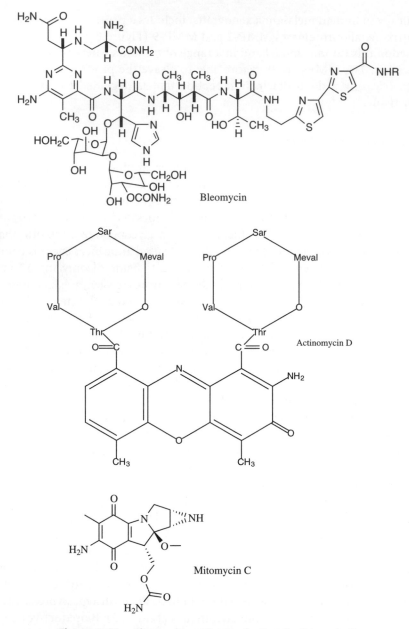

Figure 8.21 Bleomycin, actinomycin D and mitomycin C.

where there are high levels of DT-diaphorase, a 2-electron reduction will take place, producing a hydroquinone intermediate that will ultimately give rise to a quinone methide that induces DNA cross-linking. The 2-electron reduction is unimpeded by the presence of oxygen and therefore occurs in both normoxic and hypoxic conditions. DT-diaphorase, however, is an oxygen-dependent enzyme; therefore the

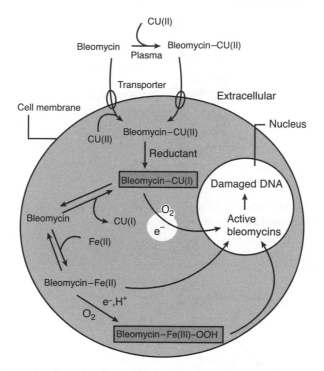

Figure 8.22 The systemic activation of bleomycin depends upon the binding of transition metal ions (Fe(II) or Cu(I)) in the presence of O_2 and a reducing agent to form a metallo-bleomycin complex which induces single or double DNA strand breaks at the site of pyrimidine bases. Reproduced from Chen and Stubbe (2005) *Nat. Rev. Cancer.* 5: 102–112, Nature Publishing Group.

2-electron reduction is more likely to occur in normoxic conditions. Mitomycin C is derived from *S. caespitosus*, its major clinical use being the intravesical treatment of bladder tumours, where the drug is instilled via a catheter directly into the bladder and acts locally.

8.4.2 Groove-binding agents

Intercalating agents may slot between adjacent base pairs, as discussed in Section 8.4.1, or alternatively, they may bind to the minor groove of the double helix (Figure 8.23). Such minor-groove binding agents may also show specificity to either AT (adenine/thymine) or GC (guanine/cytosine) rich regions. Agents such as 4'-6-diamidine-2-phenyl indole (DAPI) and the bis (benzimidazole) Hoechst 33 342 (Figures 8.24 and 8.25) target AT-rich regions and are established experimental tools with which to observe nuclear material when it is necessary to detect proliferative changes in tumour tissue.

The minor groove-binding agent trabectedin (Yondelis, ecteinascidin 743 (ET-743), was approved for use in Europe in autumn 2007 for the treatment of advanced

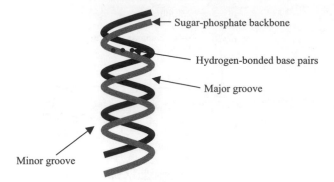

Figure 8.23 Schematic view of double stranded DNA structure, where the minor groove is a target binding site for novel anticancer agents.

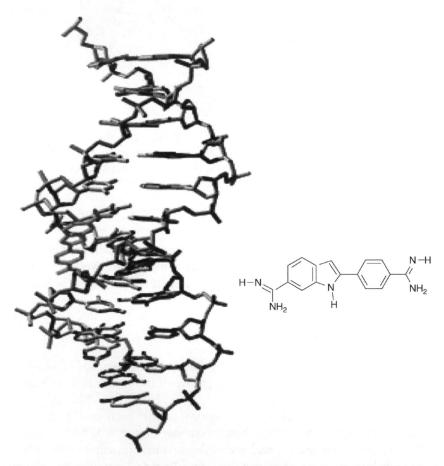

Figure 8.24 Binding of the experimentally used DNA fluorochrome 4'-6-diamidine-2-phenyl indole (DAPI), chemical structure pictured right, at AT clusters in the minor groove of DNA. Reproduced from Invitrogen, http://probes.invitrogen.com/handbook/figures/1558.html August 2008.

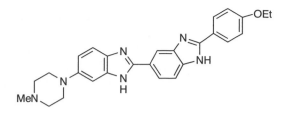

Figure 8.25   Hoechst 33 342.

soft tissue sarcoma, for use in patients refractory or unsuitable for treatment with anthracyclines and ifosfamide. Structural studies of the agent, a tetrahydro-isoquinoline alkaloid isolated from the Caribbean tunicate *Ecteinascidia turbinata*, which grows on mangrove roots, have revealed three subunits (Figure 8.26). Subunits A and B recognize and bind DNA, the most stable adducts formed by alkylation of guanine bases situated within certain sequences (5′-A/G G C-3′ or 5′-C/T G G-3′), whereas subunit C remains unbound, protruding from the minor groove. Trabectedin binding disrupts the DNA helix, bending it towards the major groove and widening the minor groove. Such structural change inhibits DNA function, preventing binding of transcription factors and DNA repair enzymes. Further clinical trials are underway to explore its use in other cancers. These include investigations of its use in combination with liposomal doxorubicin in advanced malignancies, and more specifically for the treatment of ovarian cancer. Other trials currently in progress are evaluating its efficacy in osteosarcoma, breast, prostate and paediatric cancers such as Ewing's sarcoma. Trabectedin is an interesting example of an anticancer agent developed after being given orphan drug status, where certain incentives such as regulatory assistance are given to pharmaceutical companies wishing to develop drugs to treat rare diseases that might otherwise be neglected due to the risk of not recouping research and development costs and poor profitability. In this case, orphan drug status was granted in the United States and Europe for the treatment of ovarian cancer.

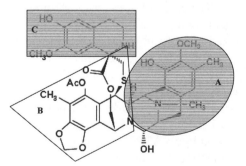

Figure 8.26   Structure of the minor groove binding agent trabectedin (showing A, B and C subunits), a natural product originally isolated from the Caribbean tunicate *Ecteinascidia turbinata*. This agent was approved in 2007 for the treatment of advanced soft tissue sarcoma.

There are several strategies being used to develop novel minor groove binding agents. The polypyrroles, for example, distamycin A, are a group of antitumour antibiotics known as 'shape-selective' binders, by virtue of their curved topology, which matches that of the minor groove. Here, efforts to determine binding characteristics and define their mode of action have shown them to be AT-specific, where binding to the minor groove leads to inhibition of enzymes such as helicases, topoisomerases I and II and RNA polymerase II. Semisynthetic derivatives have been developed to varying degrees of success (Figure 8.27). For example, tallimustine, a benzoyl nitrogen mustard-substituted distamycin derivative, showed initial promise in mouse tumour models though clinical development was halted due to severe myelotoxicity in clinical trials. To this end, further examples of 'combilexins', or polypyrrole analogues with substituted alkylating groups, are in the process of being investigated. The cyclopropylpyrroloindole (CPI) family, which includes compounds such as bizelesin, are also highly AT- specific, targeting AT 'islands' in the minor groove. Bizelecin has been evaluated in a phase I trials in patients with advanced solid malignancies, where it has proven to be relatively well tolerated in terms of myelotoxicity. Agents that bind specifically to GC-rich regions in the minor groove have also been studied, such as the aureolic acid antibiotics for example, mithramycin (plicamycin), a chromomycin antibiotic isolated from *S. plicatus*.

8.4.3 Inhibitors of topoisomerase

Both topoisomerase I and II are valid targets for anticancer agents. The two topoisomerases have little sequence similarity and differ in their molecular mass and function. Although these enzymes both induce DNA strand breaks to facilitate correct unwinding and supercoiling, topoisomerase I catalyses a single DNA strand break and is ATP-independent, while topoisomerase II catalyses cleavage of both strands and is ATP-dependent. Topoisomerase I catalyses a 'nicking–closing reaction' (Figure 8.28), where a single strand of DNA is nicked and rotated around the intact strand by the enzyme, this being followed by realignment and religation of the broken ends. The transient topoisomerase I cleavage complex formed by the topoisomerase I and the nicked end of the DNA is unstable, and only exists until DNA religation. However, in the presence of topoisomerase I inhibitors, there is misalignment of the broken DNA ends resulting in stabilization of the cleavage complex and inhibition of the enzyme.

Topoisomerase II, on the other hand, works at the point of a DNA cross-over along the supercoiled DNA, where binding of the enzyme induces a double-stranded DNA break. This is followed by an ATP-dependent conformational change, enabling the passage of the second DNA helix sited at the DNA cross-over through the double-stranded DNA break. After religation of the DNA strands, hydrolysis of the bound ATP releases the DNA, allowing the enzyme to return to its original conformation for recycling (Figure 8.29).

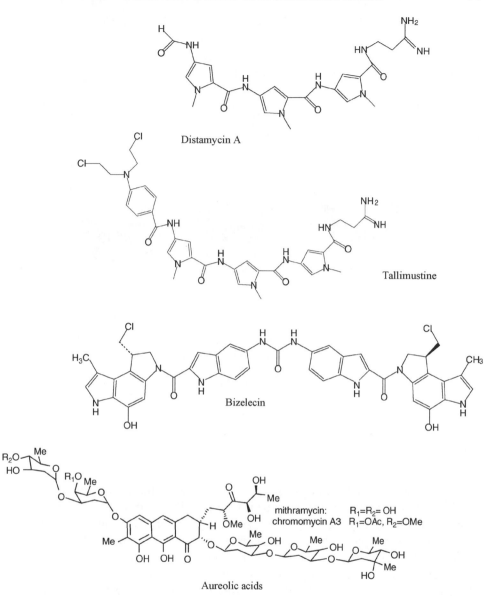

Figure 8.27 Minor groove binding agents in preclinical development. Reproduced from Nelson SM, Ferguson LR, Denny WA. Non-covalent ligand/DNA interactions: minor groove binding agents. *Mutat Res.* 2007;623:24–40, Elsevier.

Topoisomerase I inhibitors

Camptothecin is a plant alkaloid derived from the wood, bark and fruit of the Asian tree *Camptotheca acuminata*, which was observed to have cytotoxic activity as far back as 1966. However, its mode of action was not fully understood until significant

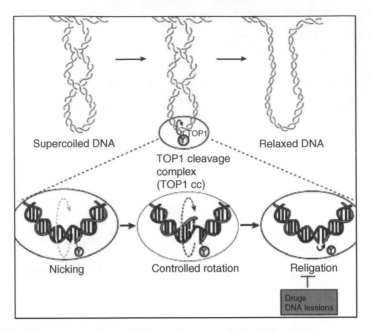

Figure 8.28 Cleavage and unwinding of supercoiled DNA by topoisomerase I is a 'nicking–closing reaction'. This takes place in three steps upon formation of the TOPO I cleavage complex: firstly, one strand of DNA is nicked, followed by rotation of the 5' end of the nicked DNA around the intact strand. 5' end of the nicked DNA is then realigned with the corresponding 3' end, enabling DNA religation, or closing of the DNA. The TOPO I cleavage complex is normally transient, only existing until religation. However, TOPO I inhibitors such as the camptothecins cause misalignment of the broken ends of the DNA and stabilization of the TOPO I complex. Reproduced from Pommier (2006) *Nat. Rev. Cancer.* 6:789–802, Nature Publishing Group.

advances had been made in the recognition of the role of the enzyme topoisomerase I in DNA replication, where this enzyme is its only cellular target. The camptothecins induce single-strand breaks in DNA by stabilizing the normally transient topoisomerase I cleavage complex. These strand breaks are reversible and non-lethal until the cleavage complex comes into contact with a DNA replication fork, when the single-strand breaks are converted to irreversible double-strand breaks. By interfering with DNA replication, the camptothecins are therefore most active against cells in the S-phase of the cell cycle. The camptothecin analogues topotecan (9-[(dimethylamino) methyl]-10-hydroxycamptothecin) and irinotecan (7-ethyl-10-[4-(1-piperidino)-1-piperidino] carbonyloxycamptothecin) (Figure 8.30) are currently approved for use in the clinic. Topotecan is licensed for the treatment of metastatic ovarian cancer where first-line or subsequent therapy has failed; and irinotecan is licensed for metastatic colorectal cancer in combination with 5-fluorouracil in patients that have not responded to other regimens containing 5-fluorouracil. In 2005, however, NICE guidance recommended irinotecan in combination chemotherapy as an option for first line chemotherapy. Novel topoisomerase I inhibitors in development include the homocamptothecins, for example, diflomotecan, gimatecan and the indolocarbazole

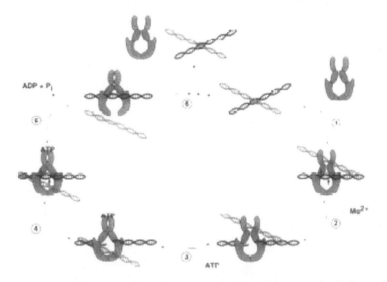

Figure 8.29   The catalytic cycle of topoisomerase II, where (1) a complex is formed between the enzyme and supercoiled DNA at the site of a DNA cross-over, preferentially at specific DNA sequences; (2) prestrand passage, where a double stranded DNA break is created in the presence of Mg^{2+} ions; (3) DNA strand passage, where ATP binding induces a conformational change in topoisomerase II, triggering passage of a second double helix through the double stranded DNA break; (4) poststrand passage, where religation of DNA takes place; (5) ATP is hydrolysed, releasing the DNA; and (6) topoisomerase II returns to its original conformation and is recycled. Reproduced from Fortune and Osheroff (2000) *Prog. Nucl. Acid Res. Mol. Biol.* 64:221–53, Elsevier.

edotecarin (Figure 8.31), which are all at the time of writing being evaluated in phase II clinical trials.

Topoisomerase II inhibitors

As discussed in Section 8.4.1, the anthracycline antibiotics and derivatives such as mitoxantrone are able to inhibit topoisomerase II along with other effects. Another class of agents able to target topoisomerase II activity is the epipodophyllotoxin derivatives, which include etoposide (VP-16) and teniposide (Figure 8.32). Epipodophyllotoxin itself was isolated from the root of the plant *Podophyllum peltatum* (mandrake); however, its derivatives are used in the clinic. Analogous to the mechanism of action of topoisomerase I inhibitors, the epipodophyllotoxin derivatives prevent religation of DNA strand breaks by stabilizing the transient topoisomerase II–DNA cleavage complex.

8.4.4 Mitotic inhibitors

Mitotic inhibitors target tubulins and so interfere with the dynamics of the mitotic spindle. For this reason, they are cell cycle-dependent, acting at M-phase. Mitosis, summarized in Figure 8.33, is an integral part of the cell cycle, where nuclear

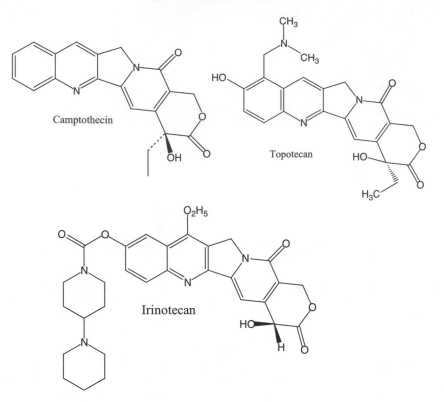

Figure 8.30 Topoisomerase I inhibitors camptothecin and its derivatives topotecan and irinotecan.

material that has replicated in S phase, effectively doubling the number of chromosomes, are segregated and passed to each daughter cell. These cells, like the parental cell, are diploid (2n), containing homologous pairs of chromosomes that each carry one copy (allele) of the genetic sequences at specific loci along the length of the chromosome. During metaphase, chromosomes are aligned on the mitotic spindle, which contract during anaphase to transfer each chromosome of a homologous pair to the poles of the cell, where they are positioned at telophase. This allows cytokinesis, where division of the rest of the cellular components including the plasma membrane takes place. The mitotic spindle is composed of microtubules formed by the polymerization of tubulins (Figure 8.34). The tubulin heterodimer is composed of α and β tubulin subunits (8 nm), which initially gather to form a short microtubule nucleus. The nucleus is then elongated by rapid addition and polymerization of further tubulin heterodimers, successive tubulin heterodimers being regularly arranged head-to tail, resulting in a microtubule consisting of 13 protofilaments arranged in a cylinder 24 nm in diameter. The head to tail arrangement of the tubulin heterodimers give the microtubules a plus (+) end, with β-tubulin facing the solvent, and a minus (−) end, with α-tubulin facing the solvent. Tubulin polymerization is non-covalent and reversible, where the length of the microtubule is determined by the relative rates of growth and shortening at either end (Figure 8.35), which is kept in balance by the

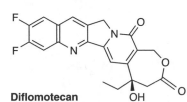

Diflomotecan

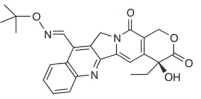

Gimatecan

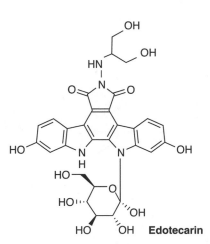

Edotecarin

Figure 8.31 Novel topoisomerase I inhibitors undergoing clinical evaluation. Reproduced from Teicher (2007) *Biochem. Pharmacol.*, Elsevier.

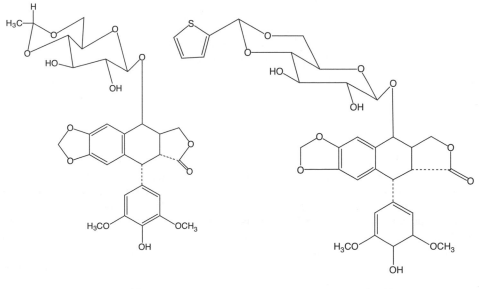

Etoposide

Teniposide

Figure 8.32 The epipodophyllotoxin derivative topoisomerase II inhibitors etoposide (VP-16) and teniposide.

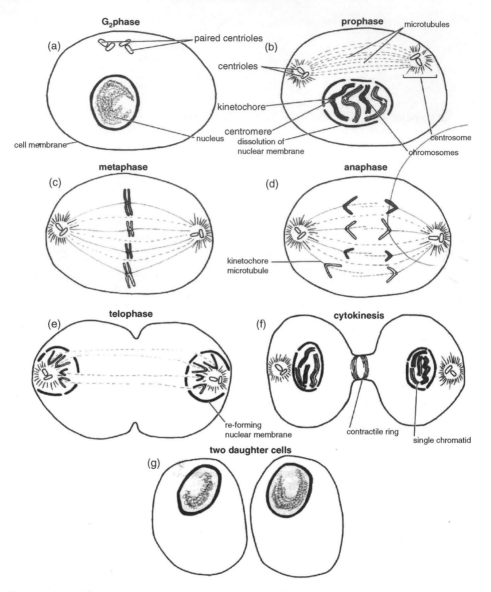

Figure 8.33   Mitosis takes place in four stages during the M-phase of the cell cycle- prophase, metaphase, anaphase and telophase. During mitosis, homologous chromosomes formed by replication of nuclear material during the S-phase of the cell cycle become segregated at the poles of the cell via contraction of the mitotic spindle fibres. Mitosis is followed by 'cytokinesis, where the nuclear material is transferred to two daughter cells. Before mitosis can take place, cellular components such as enzymes and structural proteins, as well as DNA replication, must take place. This occurs in interphase, which corresponds to G1, S and G2 phases of the cell cycle. Reproduced with permission from McGeady, Quinn, Fitzpatrick and Ryan (2006) *Veterinary Embryology*. Blackwell Publishing Ltd

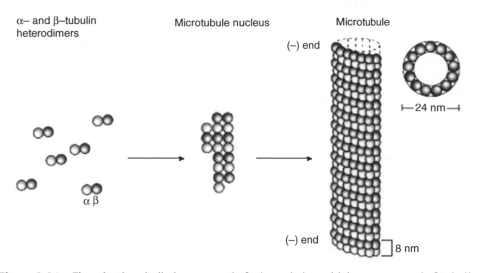

α– and β–tubulin heterodimers

Microtubule nucleus

Microtubule

(−) end

├─24 nm─┤

αβ

(−) end

8 nm

Figure 8.34 The mitotic spindle is composed of microtubules, which are composed of tubulin heterodimers of α and β subunits. During tubulin polymerization these are arranged head-to tail around a short microtubule nucleus to form a microtubule consisting of 13 protofilaments arranged in a cylinder 25 nm in diameter, with a plus (+) end, where β-tubulin faces the solvent, and a minus end (−), where α-tubulin faces the solvent. Reproduced from Jordan and Wilson (2004) *Nat. Rev. Cancer* 4:253–265, Nature Publishing Group.

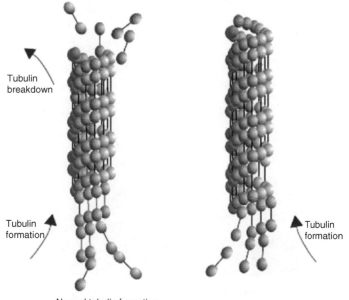

Tubulin breakdown

Tubulin formation

Tubulin formation

Normal tubulin formation

Figure 8.35 The length of the microtubule is determined by the balance between tubulin polymerization (lengthening) and breakdown or depolymerization of tubulin (shortening) occuring at each end. Reproduced from Montero *et al.* (2005) *Lancet Oncol.* 2005; 6: 229–39, Elsevier.

transfer of tubulin from the plus to the minus end. The length of the microtubule is further influenced by the presence or absence of a layer of tubulin bound to GTP or a 'GTP cap', where its presence stabilizes the microtubule and allows it to grow; and its absence leaves an unstable microtubule core that rapidly shortens. Microtubule dynamics, that is, the capacity for controlled microtubule degradation and shortening, is essential for mitotic spindle function. Tubulin inhibitors are used as anticancer agents by virtue of two major effects: their ability to change the rate of polymerization or depolymerization; and their ability to suppress microtubule dynamics. Preclinically, this may be observed *in vitro* in tumour cell lines by using time-lapse photography to observe changes in microtubule length over time in the presence or absence of the drug (Figure 8.36). The different types of tubulin inhibitor exert these effects in various ways according to where along the microtubule length they bind, binding affinity and the ability to bind the tubulin subunit precursors (Figure 8.37). The common result, however, is to prevent progression from metaphase to anaphase, eventually leading to apoptotic cell death.

Vinca alkaloids

The first vinca alkaloids, vincristine, vinblastine and vindesine (Figure 8.38) were derived from the plant *Vinca rosea*, or periwinkle. Since then, semisynthetic derivatives, such as vinorelbine and more recently, vinflunine have been developed, where

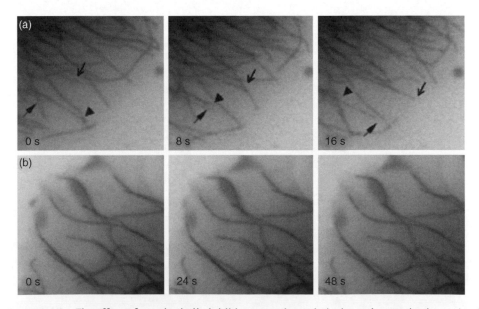

Figure 8.36   The effect of novel tubulin inhibitors on microtubule dynamics may be determined *in vitro* by using time-lapse photography to observe changes in microtubule length over time in the presence or absence of the drug. Here, in breast tumour MCF7 cells in the presence (a) of epothilone B, it is possible to see microtubules changing length over the course of 16 seconds (shown by arrows). However, in the absence (b) of epothilone B, no changes in length are apparent over the 48 seconds shown here. Reproduced with permission from Kamath *et al.* (2003) *Cancer Res.* 63, 6026–6031, American Association for Cancer Research.

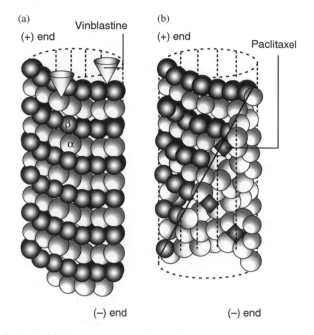

Figure 8.37 Tubulin inhibitors suppress microtubule dynamics and therefore the function of the mitotic spindle. The vinca alkaloids, colchicine and the taxanes bind microtubules at different points, where (a) the vinca alkaloids such as vinblastine bind at the ($+$) end to prevent the polymerization and depolymerization necessary for lengthening and shortening the microtubules; and (b) the taxanes bind the interior surface of the microtubule cylinder. Reproduced from Goodin *et al.* (2004) *J. Clin. Oncol.* 22:2015–2025, High Wire Press Stanford University Libraries – US.

vinflunine has been evaluated in phase II clinical trials involving patients with advanced breast, non-small cell lung, bladder and renal and skin cancers; and has now entered phase II trials for the treatment of non-small cell lung and bladder cancers. Vinca alkaloids induce depolymerization of microtubules. They have a high affinity to soluble tubulin, binding the B-subunit at the vinca-binding domain, which induces a conformational change that may increase the tendency for tubulin self-association and lead to dynamic stabilization of the microtubule. The vinca alkaloids also interfere with microtubule dynamics by directly binding to the microtubule filament at the ($+$) end, which inhibits depolymerization and prevents the transfer of tubulins to the ($-$) end. Overall, vinca alkaloids exert their effect by reducing the rate of microtubule growth and shortening, leading to a pause in microtubule dynamics that prevents normal mitotic spindle assembly and therefore the central alignment of the chromosomes at metaphase. This also reduces the ability of the spindle fibres to pull the chromosomes to the poles of the cell, accordingly preventing progression from metaphase to anaphase.

Taxanes

The first generation taxane to enter routine clinical use was paclitaxel, a plant alkaloid derived from the Western yew, *Taxus brevifolia*. This was followed by docetaxel,

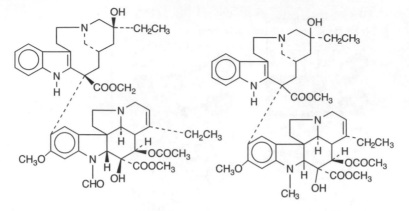

Vincristine   Vinblastine

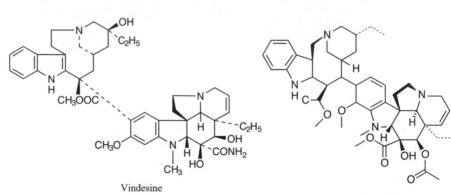

Vindesine

Vinorelbine

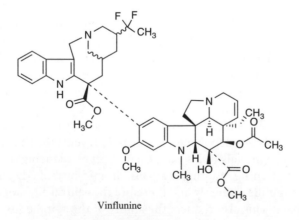

Vinflunine

Figure 8.38   vinca alkaloids vincristine, vinblastine and vindesine, and their semi-synthetic derivatives vinorelbine and vinflunine.

a semisynthetic taxane, and there are currently several third-generation taxanes in development (Figure 8.39). These include MAC-321 (milataxel), which has undergone phase I pharmacokinetic studies in solid malignancies, although limited clinical activity was observed in a recently reported phase II trial that evaluated its use for the treatment of advanced, refractory colorectal cancer. The clinical activity of newer versus older taxanes has also been compared, such as in the phase III ERASME 3 study, which compared the efficacy of doxorubicin and docetaxel versus doxorubicin and paclitaxel in patients with metastatic breast cancer. Taxanes, in contrast to the vinca alkaloids, increase the rate of tubulin polymerization. They do not bind with high affinity to soluble tubulin, although they bind tightly to the B subunit of tubulin residues at a site on the interior surface of the microtubule cylinder. This, as with the vinca alkaloids, leads to a conformational change in tubulin structure that increases their affinity to surrounding tubulin molecules and so facilitates their self-association. In doing so, taxanes are able to stabilize the microtubule and therefore increase the rate of tubulin polymerization. Further observations have also shown that lower doses

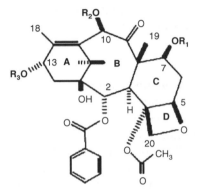

Compound	$R_1=$	$R_2=$	$R_3=$
Paclitaxel	H	$CH_3\overset{O}{\overset{\|}{C}}-$	
Docetaxel	H	H	
MAC-321	$CH_3CH_2\overset{O}{\overset{\|}{C}}-$	H	

Figure 8.39 Comparison of the chemical structures of the taxanes paclitaxel and the semisynthetic derivatives docetaxel and milataxel (MAC-31). Reproduced with permission from Sampath *et al.* (2003) *Mol. Cancer Ther.* 2003;2:873–884, American Association for Cancer Research.

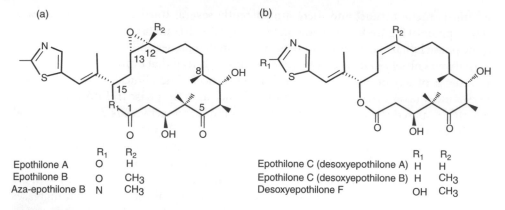

(a)

(b)

	R₁	R₂
Epothilone A	O	H
Epothilone B	O	CH₃
Aza-epothilone B	N	CH₃

	R₁	R₂
Epothilone C (desoxyepothilone A)	H	H
Epothilone C (desoxyepothilone B)	H	CH₃
Desoxyepothilone F	OH	CH₃

Figure 8.40 Structures of epothilone (a) and desoxyepothilone (b) and their analogs. Reproduced from Goodin *et al.* (2004) *J. Clin. Oncol.* 22:2015–2025, High Wire Press Stanford University Libraries – US.

of taxanes inhibit microtubule dynamics, interfering with microtubule shortening and consequently, progression from metaphase to anaphase.

Epothilones

The epothilones are newly emerging macrolide tubulin inhibitors that are produced by the myxobacterium *Sorangium cellulosum*, and include the epothilones, for example, epothilone B; and the desoxyepothilones, for example, desoxyepothilone B (epothilone D) (Figure 8.40). Like the taxanes, they induce tubulin polymerization by binding B-tubulin at a similar site on the microtubule. In preclinical studies, however, tumour cell lines resistant to taxanes by virtue of a mutation in the gene coding for B-tubulin remained sensitive to the epothilones. Epothilone sensitivity was also less susceptible to p-glycoprotein-mediated multi-drug resistance than the taxanes, suggesting a clinical application in patients with taxane resistant cancers. Fittingly, a derivative of epothilone B, ixabepilone (aza-epothilone B) (Figure 8.41), has been evaluated in phase II trials for the treatment of metastatic and locally advanced breast cancer, in patients previously treated with taxanes as neoadjuvant chemotherapy. Following on from this, a phase III trial has now been carried out in patients with anthracycline or taxane-resistant metastatic and locally advanced breast

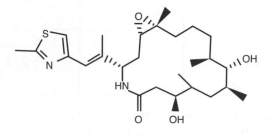

Figure 8.41 The epothilone B derivative ixabepilone.

cancer, to compare treatment with ixapepilone plus capecitabine versus capecitabine alone, where the ixabepilone group showed significant improvement in progression-free survival. Ixapepilone has also been evaluated in preclinical studies in models of paediatric cancers, such as neuroblastoma and rhabdomyosarcoma.

8.4.5 Asparaginase

Asparaginase (crisantaspase) is an enzyme derived from the bacterium *Erwinia chrysanthemi* that converts the amino acid L-asparagine to aspartate, producing an ammonium ion (Figure 8.42). In normal cells, L-asparagine is synthesized intracellularly by the enzyme L-asparagine synthetase. Leukaemic lymphoblasts, however, affectively lack this enzyme, L-asparagine becoming an essential amino acid, where the tumour cells rely on L-asparagine present in the serum. They are therefore extremely sensitive to the depletion of serum L-asparagine by asparaginase, which induces cell death by inhibiting tumour protein synthesis whilst leaving adjacent normal cells unaffected. Pegasparaginase is a preparation consisting of asparaginase conjugated to polyethylene glycol, which has been developed for use in patients showing hypersensitivity to standard preparations of asparaginase.

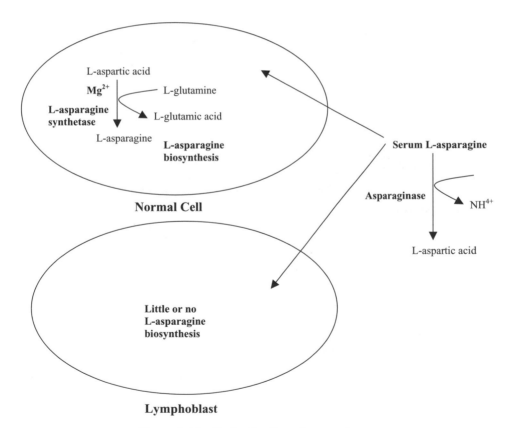

Figure 8.42 Mode of action of asparaginase.

8.5 Hormonal anticancer agents

Hormone-dependent cancers include those of the breast and prostate, as well as the ovary, uterus and testicles. Oestrogens and androgens are steroidal sex hormones derived from cholesterol via production of the intermediate androstenedione, which is used to synthesize the androgens dihydrotestosterone and testosterone. The enzyme aromatase has an important role in the synthesis of the oestrogen 17β-oestradiol, either from testosterone iteself, or from androstenedione via the production of the intermediate oestrone (Figure 8.43). The link between exposure to the male and female steroidal sex hormones and the risk of hormone-dependent cancers is well established. Two major discoveries in this area included that of Beatson in 1896, who demonstrated that oophorectomy, or removal of the ovaries, improved prognosis in women with advanced breast cancer; and Huggins and Hodges in 1935, who showed the analogous effect of testosterone in prostate cancer by investigating the effects of orchiectomy, or removal of the testicles, in effected male patients. The oestrogens and androgens regulate the growth and differentiation of their target tissues via binding to their respective receptor. The androgen dihydrotestosterone binds to the androgen receptor (AR) present in the cytoplasm, whereas oestradiol

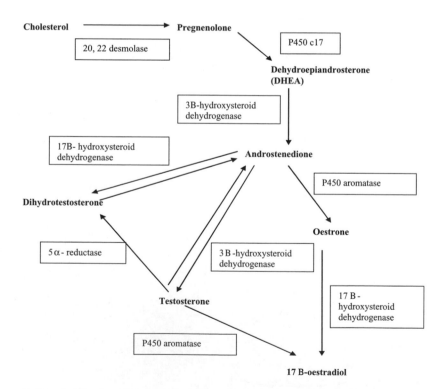

Figure 8.43 Synthesis of androgens and oestrogens from cholesterol. The conversion of androgens (dihydrotestosterone and testosterone) to oestrogens is via the enzyme aromatase, the target of aromatase inhibitors such as anastrozole, letrozole and exemestane.

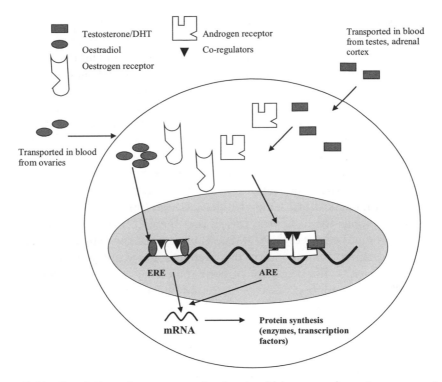

Figure 8.44 Regulation of gene expression by steroid hormones in oestrogen receptor or androgen receptor positive tumours. Oestrogen binds to the nuclear oestrogen receptor (ER), whereas the androgens, predominantly dihydrotestosterone, bind cytoplasmic androgen receptor (AR). This allows complexation of ER or AR dimer to hormone response elements (oestrogen response element ERE, or androgen response element ARE), which are specific DNA sequences found in the promotor of hormone-regulated genes.

binds to the nuclear oestrogen receptor (ER) (Figure 8.44). Binding of the respective ligands induces dimerization of the receptors, and in the case of the AR, nuclear translocation. The ER and AR dimers then complex with the hormone response elements (the androgen response element and the oestrogen response element), which are DNA sequences contained in the promotor region of hormone-inducible genes. Co-regulators that either activate or repress hormone induced gene expression bind at additional sites on the ER and AR. In breast tumours, ER status is routinely determined at biopsy. Oestrogen regulates the expression of genes involved in the proliferation of breast epithelium, where microarray studies have demonstrated both a stimulatory effect on proliferative genes such as those controlling progression through the cell cycle or synthesis of growth factors; and an inhibitory effect on antiproliferative genes such as the pro-apoptotic protein caspase 9.

8.5.1 Oestrogen antagonists

The first significant advance in the development of oestrogen receptor blocking agents was the introduction of tamoxifen, a non-steroidal triphenylethylene, which is acknowledged as the first selective oestrogen receptor modulating agent (SERM) (Figure 8.45). Although tamoxifen is an effective ER antagonist in breast tumours, a pronounced partial agonist effect is evident in the endometrium and bone. Efforts to develop second generation ER antagonists with reduced partial agonist effects have resulted in the introduction of fulvestrant, which is licensed for ER positive advanced breast cancer in postmenopausal women. Like the SERMs, fulvestrant binds the ER. The fulvestrant–ER complex, however, is rapidly degraded, reducing the level of ER protein. ER dimerization and the recruitment of co-regulatory factors are also impaired by fulvestrant binding, leading to an overall suppression of oestrogen signalling and any downstream stimulatory and inhibitory effects on gene expression (Figure 8.46). Unlike SERMs such as tamoxifen, fulvestrant has no partial agonist effects – in fact experimental observations show that tamoxifen may be used to reverse its effects. This has positive ramifications for its clinical use, in that the uterotrophic (increased endometrial proliferation) effects of the SERMs is eliminated, along with any increased risk of endometrial cancer. Initial concerns that such unopposed antagonism of oestrogen signalling might be to the detriment of bone maintenance have also proved to be unfounded in terms of bone density data and the frequency of bone disorders experienced in human patients.

8.5.2 The aromatase inhibitors and inactivators

Aromatase inhibitors and inactivators (Figure 8.45) block the aromatization of androgens. This is the final step in oestrogen synthesis, mostly brought about by conversion of androstenedione to oestrone, though aromatase may also catalyse the direct conversion of testosterone to oestradiol. Aromatase inhibitors are non-steroidal, reversibly binding to the P450 site of aromatase. These include the first generation compound aminoglutethimide. This agent is not specific to aromatase, however, where it effectively causes total ablation of adrenal steroids by also inhibiting the conversion of cholesterol to pregnenolone. Subsequent efforts have turned to targeting the activity of aromatase produced in malignant tissue rather than total body oestrogen synthesis, leading to the design of the second-generation fadrozole and the third-generation compounds anastrazole and letrozole. Aromatase inactivators are steroidal compounds that are analogues of androstenedione and so are able to bind to the substrate binding site. Binding is irreversible, leading to degradation of the enzyme. This group of agents includes formestane and exemestane, where exemestane has proved to be useful in patients with showing disease progression after treatment with tamoxifen. For this reason, it is currently approved as adjuvant hormonal therapy for postmenopausal women with ER-positive early breast cancer who have 2 to 3 years of tamoxifen, and may now be switched to exemestane to complete the standard 5 consecutive years of anti-oestrogen therapy. Aromatase inhibitors and inactivators are contraindicated in premenopausal women in the absence of ovarian blockade with gonadotropin releasing hormone (GnRH) analogues, which are used to mop up any aromatase produced by functioning ovaries.

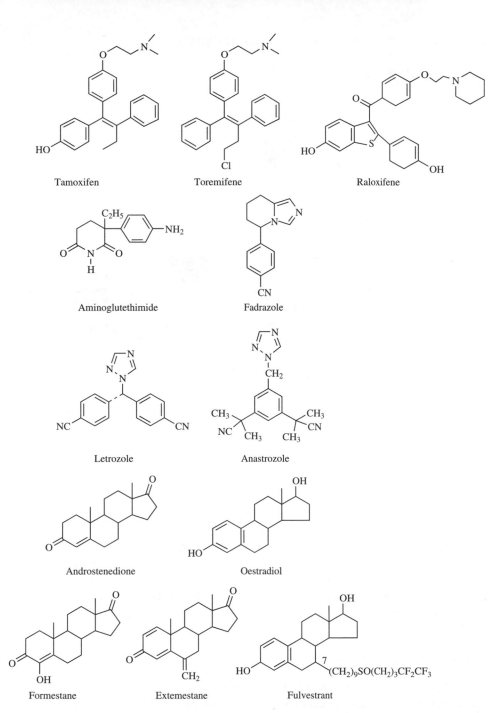

Figure 8.45 Structure of the selective oestrogen modulators (SERMs) tamoxifen, toremifene and raloxifene; the non-steroidal aromatase inhibitors aminoglutethimide, fadrozole, letrozole and anastrazole; the steroidal aromatase activtors formestane and exemestane, which are analogues of the natural aromatase substrate androstenedione; and fulvestrant, which represents a new class of high affinity oestrogen receptor antagonist that impairs ER dimerization as well as preventing binding of oestrogen and co-regulator recruitment.

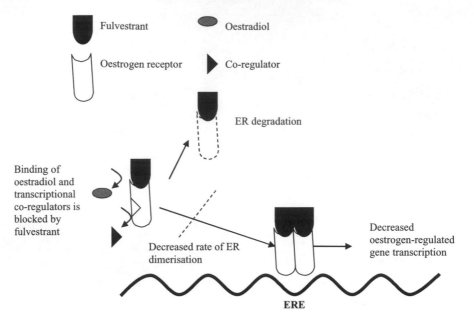

Figure 8.46 Mode of action of fulvestrant, a high affinity oestrogen receptor antagonist that does not exhibit the partial agonist effects of the SERMs. As well as blocking the binding of oestradiol and transcriptional co-regulators, it also induces ER degradation and inhibits dimerization.

8.5.3 Anti-androgens

Anti-androgens inhibit the AR and include the steroidal androgen analogue cyproterone acetate and the non-steroidal compounds bicalutamide, flutamide and nilutamide (Figure 8.47). Their major application, like endocrine therapy, is in the treatment of locally advanced prostate cancer. The more modern non-steroidal anti-androgens show more specificity to the androgen receptor expressed in prostate tumour cells. This is in contrast to cyproterone acetate, which due to its progesterogenic effect suppresses whole body testosterone leading to loss of sexual function.

8.5.4 Endocrine therapy

Endocrine therapy manipulates the hypothalamus–pituitary axis – the stimulatory, inhibitory and feedback processes involved in the production of the gonadotropins leutinizing hormone (LH) and follicle-stimulating hormone (FSH), which bring about a decrease in the production of testicular-derived testosterone. This group of therapies includes oestrogen agonists, GnRH agonists and the GnRH antagonists. The oestrogen agonists such as diethylstilboestrol are still used rarely but are administered parenterally to avoid cardiovascular toxicity. The GnRH (gonadorelin)

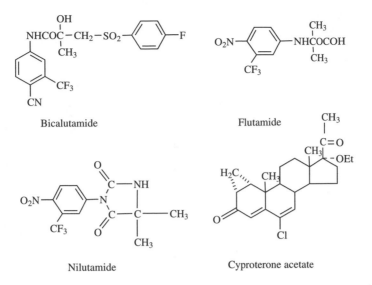

Figure 8.47 Structures of the steroidal antiandrogen cyproterone acetate and the non-steroidal antiandrogens bicalutamide, flutamide and nilutamide.

agonists, which include goserelin, leuprorelin, buserelin and triptorelin, stimulate the production of LH and FSH, initially increasing the production of testosterone. Long-term treatment with high concentrations, however, leads to downregulation of the GnRH-receptors and inhibition of LH release, consequently inhibiting further production of testosterone. The initial rise in testosterone levels may give rise to the tumour flare effect, where a testosterone surge at the start of treatment stimulates tumour growth. In those effected, increased growth of bone metastases can cause bone pain, compression of the spine and obstruction of the ureters. This effect is therefore countered by concurrent administration of anti-androgens, which are given from 3 days before the start of gonadorelin therapy and continued for 3 weeks. GnRH antagonists are undergoing development as a means of achieving a rapid fall in LH and FSH, and therefore androgen production, but without the risk of tumour flare. The first of this novel class of agents is abarelix, which was granted FDA approval in 2004 for the treatment of advanced symptomatic prostate cancer. Phase III clinical trials showed it capable of reducing testosterone levels more rapidly than GnRH agonists, and because it is a pure antagonist with no GnRH agonist activity, its use was not associated with tumour flare.

8.6 Clinically used chemotherapy regimens

Chemotherapy regimens are given standard abbreviations, such as those shown in Table 8.1.

Table 8.1 Standard chemotherapy regimens

Drug class	Regimen	Cancer treated
Alkylating agents		
Regimens including:		
Cyclophosphamide	CMF	Breast
	Cyclophosphamide, PO, 100 mg/m^2, days 1–14 or 600 mg/m^2, IV, days 1 and 8	
	Methotrexate, IV, 40 mg/m^2, days 1 and 8	
	5-Fluorouracil, IV, 600 mg/m^2, days 1 and 8; cycle repeated every 28 days	
	CAP	Head and neck
	Cyclophosphamide, IV, 500 mg/m^2, day 1	
	Doxorubicin, IV, 50 mg/m^2, day 1	
	Cisplatin, IV, 50 mg/m^2, day 1; cycle repeated every 28 days	
	CHOP	Non-Hodgkin's lymphoma
	Cyclophosphamide, IV, 750 mg/m^2, day 1	
	Mitoxantrone, IV, 10 mg/m^2, day 1	
	Vincristine, IV, 1.4 mg/m^2, day 1	
	Prednisolone, PO, 50 mg/m^2, days 1–5; cycle repeated every 21 days	
Melphalan	MP	Multiple myeloma
	Melphalan, PO, 8–10 mg/m^2, days 1–4	
	Prednisolone, PO, 40–60 mg/m^2/day, days 1–4; cycle repeated every 28–42 days	
Cisplatin	CVD	Malignant melanoma
	Cisplatin, IV, 20 mg/m^2, days 1–5	
	Vinblastine, IV, 1.6 mg/m^2, days 1–5	
	Dacarbazine, IV, 800 mg/m^2, day 1; cycle repeated every 21 days	

(continued)

CCNU	POC	Brain
	Prednisolone, PO, 40 mg/m², days 1–14	
	CCNU, PO, 100 mg/m², day 1	
	Vincristine, @IV, 1.5 mg/m², days 1, 8, 15	

Antimetabolites
Regimens including:

Methotrexate	MTX/6-MP/VP	Paediatric acute lymphoblastic leukaemia, maintenance therapy
	Methotrexate, PO, 20 mg/m²/week	
	Mercaptopurine, PO, 75 mg/m²/day	
	Vincristine, IV, 1.5 mg/m² moly	
	Prednisolone, PO, 40 mg/m² for 5 days each	

5-Fluorouracil	FAM	Gastric
	5-Fluorouracil, IV, 600 mg/m², days 1, 8. 29, 36	
	Doxorubicin, IV, 30 mg/m², days 1 and 29	
	Mitomycin C, IV, 10 mg/m², day 1; cycle repeated every 8 weeks	

Gemcitabine	Gemcitabine-Cis	Non-small cell lung cancer
	Gemcitabine, IV, 1000 mg/m², days 1,8,15	
	Cisplatin, IV, 100 mg/m², days 2 or 15; cycle repeated every 28 days	

Intercalating agents and DNA topology
Regimens including:

Bleomycin	MOBP	Cervix
	Bleomycin, IV, 30 units/day continuous infusion, days 1 and 4	
	Vincristine, IV, 0.5 mg/m², days 1 and 4	
	Mitomycin C, IV, 10 mg/m², day 1	
	Cisplatin, IV, 50 mg/m², days 1–22; cycle repeated every 28 days	

Table 8.1 (Continued)

Drug class	Regimen	Cancer treated
Doxorubicin	AC	Breast
	Doxorubicin, IV, 60 mg/m^2, day 1	
	Cyclophosphamide, IV, 400–600 mg/m^2, day 1; cycle repeated every 21 days	
Etoposide	EP	Testicular
	Etoposide, IV, 100 mg/m^2, days 1–5	
	Cisplatin, IV, 20 mg/m^2, days 1–5; cycle repeated every 21 days	
Irinotecan	Single agent therapy: Irinotecan, IV, 125 mg/m^2/week over 90 min, once a week for 4 weeks, or 350 mg/m^2 over 30 min; cycle repeated every 21 days	Colon
Microtubule binding agents Regimens including:		
Vincristine	PVD	Paediatric acute lymphoblastic leukaemia, induction therapy
	Prednisolone, PO, 40 mg/m^2/day for 28 days	
	Vincristine, IV, 1.5 mg/m^2/week for 4 weeks	
	Asparaginase, IM, 5000 int. units/m^2 on days	
Paclitaxel	CT	Epithelial tumours of the ovary
	Paclitaxel, IV, 135 mg/m^2 over 24 h, day 1 or 175 mg/m^2 over 3 h, day 1, followed by	
	Cisplatin, IV, 75 mg/m^2; cycle repeated every 21 days	

(continued)

Hormonal/antihormonal agents		
Regimens including:		
Flutamide	FL	Prostate
	Flutamide. PO, 250 mg tds, days 1–28	
	Leuprolide acetate, SC, 1 mg qds, days 1–28; cycle repeated every 28 d	
Goserelin	Single agent therapy: Goserelin acetate implant, SC, 3.6 mg every 28 days or 10.8 mg every 12 weeks	Prostate
Tamoxifen	CFPT	Oestrogen receptor positive breast cancer
	Cyclophosphamide, IV, 150 mg/m^2, days 1–5	
	5-Fluorouracil, IV, 300 mg/m^2, days 1–5	
	Prednisolone, PO, 10 mg tds, days 1–7	
	Tamoxifen, PO, 10 mg tds, days 1–42; cycle repeated every 42 days	
Anastrazole	Single agent therapy: Anastrazole, PO, 1 mg qds	Oestrogen receptor positive breast cancer
Biological agents		
Regimens including:		
Interferon α	Single agent therapy: interferon α, SC, 3–5 million units/day	Chronic myeloid leukaemia

Based on data from Solimando, D.A. *et al. Drug Information Handbook for Oncology* 1999–2000, Lexi-Comp Inc. Ohio, USA. IV, intravenous; IM, intramuscular; PO, per oram; SC, subcutaneous; tds, three times a day; qds. four times a day.

9

The philosophy of cancer research

9.1 Introduction

A question often asked of cancer research scientists is 'Will they ever find a cure?' The answer is very complex, and arguably, there are already cures for cancer being used every day in the clinic. However, cancer research is still a high profile and extremely competitive area of science, as the search for new therapies that improve upon those currently available continues. In 2006 a study was carried out by the UK Clinical Research Collaboration (UKCRC), the organization that coordinates clinical research across a range of disease areas including cancer, in an effort to analyse how the research funding provided by the nine largest medical and clinical research grant awarding bodies was spent. According to the report, which is available on the UKCRC web site (www.ukcrc.org), cancer research groups received the largest share (27%) of more than £700 million of health-specific funding analysed from the 2004–2005 financial year. Figure 9.1 shows how this funding was distributed according to the defined objectives of basic and translational research.

At present, many anticancer agents work by targeting DNA; either its synthesis, function or the mechanics of cell replication. Biochemical selectivity is poor, side effects are severe and drug resistance is common. The major goal of developing new anticancer agents is to find innovative treatments for solid tumours and leukaemias that bring about significant improvement in effectiveness and tolerability. In doing so, there is a benefit to patients, with decreased morbidity and mortality, but also a health economic benefit, where the cost of treatment failure and extended treatment due to adverse drug reactions is reduced.

Medical research may be broadly divided into two areas: basic and translational. Basic cancer research aims to increase the understanding of the structure and function of tumour cells, and how a tumour interacts with the host environment. Translational cancer research applies that knowledge to develop new cancer treatments. Therefore, whilst the discovery and the characterization of the function of the oncogene *H-ras* can be described as basic research, the subsequent studies relating to its use as a prognostic marker in patients, its validation as a target for novel anticancer strategies, and ultimately clinical trials of new therapies are appropriately described as translational

Cancer Chemotherapy   Rachel Airley
© 2009 John Wiley & Sons, Ltd.

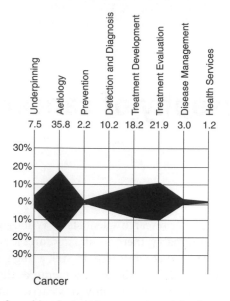

Figure 9.1   Proportion of combined spend by research activity for cancer research. The largest shares were received by research groups carrying out research into the aetiology of cancer, that is, basic research into the endogenous and physical factors, epidemiology, psychological and social factors causing cancer; and translational research intended for the development and evaluation of cancer treatment. Reproduced with permission from the UKCRC UK Health Research Analysis (2006) available at www.UKCRC.org August 2008.

research. There have been organizational developments in cancer research that reflect the priority that is now given to the advancement of translational research. Cancer research is sometimes called experimental oncology, which is distinct from clinical oncology, the medical speciality related to the treatment of cancer patients. Experimental oncology gathers knowledge from a wide range of disciplines, such as molecular biology, cell biology, histology, medicinal and pharmaceutical chemistry, pharmaceutics and the clinical sciences.

9.2 Structure of cancer research organizations in the United Kingdom

9.2.1 National Cancer Research Institute (NCRI) www.ncri.org.uk

The NCRI, set up in 2001, is a partnership between the Government, cancer charities and the pharmaceutical industry, coordinates the activity and collaborative partnerships of 20 member organizations. These organizations represent a broad range of government agencies, research councils and charities raising funds to provide research grants to academic and research institutions or for care of the cancer patient.

• Association of the British Pharmaceutical Industry www.abpi.org.uk;

• Association for International Cancer Research www.aicr.org.uk;

- Breakthrough Breast Cancer www.breakthrough.org.uk;

- Biotechnology and Biological Sciences Research Council www.bbsrc.ac.uk;

- Breast Cancer Campaign www.breastcancercampaign.org;

- Cancer Research UK www.cancerresearchuk.org;

- Scottish Executive- Chief Scientist Office www.sehd.scot.nhs.uk/cso;

- Department of Health www.dh.gov.uk;

- Economic and Social Research Council www.esrc.ac.uk;

- Leukaemia Research Fund www.lrf.org.uk;

- Ludwig Institute for Cancer Research www.ludwig.ucl.ac.uk;

- MacMillan Cancer Support www.macmillan.org.uk;

- Marie Curie Cancer Care www.mariecurie.org.uk;

- Medical Research Council www.mrc.ac.uk;

- Northern Ireland Research and Development Office www.centralservicesagency. com;

- Roy Castle Lung Cancer Foundation www.roycastle.org;

- Tenovus Cancer Charity www.tenovus.com;

- Wales Office of Research and Development www.new.wales.gov.uk;

- The Wellcome Trust www.wellcome.ac.uk;

- Yorkshire Cancer Research www.ycr.org.uk.

The NCRI has a number of national and international research partners, including the International Cancer Research Partners (ICRP), made up of organizations such as The American Cancer Society (www.cancer.org) and the National Cancer Institute (NCI; www.cancer.gov), which is part of the United States National Institutes of Health (NIH) (www.nih.gov).

The function of the NCRI is to maintain a cancer research database, which is built from data submitted by cancer research groups covering seven areas:

- Biology;

- Aetiology;

- Prevention;

- Early detection, diagnosis and prognosis;

- Treatment;

- Cancer control, survival and outcomes research;

- Scientific model systems.

The NCRI also develop research initiatives in specific areas. At the time of going to press, the three current research initiatives underway are the Prostate Cancer Collaborative, the Supportive and Palliative Care and the National Prevention Research Initiatives. They also help coordinate clinical trials and experimental cancer research programmes by overseeing the National Cancer Research Network (NCRN) (www.ncrn.org.uk). The NCRN superseded the National Translational Cancer Research Network (NTRAC) in 2006, and is made up of regional research networks around the United Kingdom and special interest clinical study groups. The stated aim of the network is to provide a clinical trials infrastructure to the NHS by bringing together individuals and organizations able to contribute funding, expertise and technology. There are a series of NCRI-accredited clinical trials units, for example, at the MRC clinical trials unit in London and the Bristol Randomised Trials Collaboration. Research groups may apply for a study to be included in the NCRI clinical trials portfolio, a process which involves peer review. Such studies will be included in the NCRI database of cancer research and will have access to the infrastructure resource within the NCRN. There are 21 NCRI clinical studies groups, designated by cancer site or speciality (Figure 9.2).

The NCRI aims to develop facilities and resources by pooling data and biosamples from clinical studies taking place within the network, so that they can be made available to other cancer research groups. These include the NCRI Informatics Initiative, which collates data, and biobanking initiatives such as onCore UK, the Wales Cancer Bank and the Confederation of Cancer Banks, which archive tumour material (biopsy samples, secretions or cell preparations) collected from patients enrolled in clinical studies. Pooling data and biosamples from patients already enrolled in a trial entered into the NCRI database helps cancer research groups avoid the problems associated with patient recruitment and collection of data, particularly the administrative procedures, time scales and the expense incurred enrolling a statistically significant number of patients that fit the inclusion criteria of a clinical study within the catchment area of a region or hospital.

9.3 Cancer research in the United States

The setup in the United Kingdom is seemingly modelled on that of the United States, where the NCI is an offshoot of the NIH, and is responsible for providing funding, networking and research resources for cancer research. There are several programmes providing resources such as tissue samples, *in vitro* and *in vivo* drug screening based on in-house protocols (Figure 9.3) and clinical trials networking. The Developmental Therapeutics Program provides drug screening services such as the hollow fibre assay, an *in vivo* assay based on the implantation of fibres containing tumour cell lines into mice (see Section 13.5). They also provide data handling services, for example, the

National Cancer Research Institute ←→ **CR-UK** ←→ **Dept of Health** ←→ **MRC** ←→ Cancer charities/ academic institutions/ pharmaceutical industry

The National Cancer Research Network clinical studies groups

- Bladder Cancer Group
- Brain Tumour Group
- Breast Cancer Group
- Colorectal Cancer Group
- Complementary Therapies Development Group
- Consumer Liaison Group
- Gynaecological Cancer Group
- Haematological Oncology Group
- Head and Neck Cancer Group
- Lung Cancer Group
- Lymphoma Group
- Melanoma Group
- Palliative Care Group
- Primary Care Development Group
- Prostate Cancer Group
- Psychosocial Oncology Group
- Radiotherapy Group
- Renal Cancer Group
- Sarcoma Group
- Teenage and Young Adults Clinical Studies Development Group
- Testis Cancer Group
- Translational Clinical Studies Group
- Upper Gastro-Intestinal Cancer Group

Experimental cancer medicine centres

ECMC status and funding awarded to "centres of scientific and clinical excellence"

Barts and the London
Birmingham, Belfast, Cambridge, Cardiff, Edinburgh, Glasgow, Imperial College, Institute of Cancer Research, King's College London, Leeds-Bradford-Hull-York, Leicester, Manchester, Newcastle, Oxford, Southampton and University College London. Two further centres in development- Liverpool and Sheffield

Academic clinical oncology and radiobiology research network (ACORRN)

National Cancer Intelligence Network
Cancer Epidemiology research

Cancer clinical trials units:
- NCRI-accredited clinical trials units (Bristol Randomised Trials Collaboration, CACTUS (Cancer Clinical Trials Unit Scotland) (Glasgow and Edinburgh), Cancer Research UK Clinical Trials Unit (University of Birmingham), Children's Cancer and Leukaemia Group, CR-UK & UCL Cancer Trials Centre, CTRU at Leeds University, ICR CTSU, MRC Clinical Trials Unit, Wales Cancer Trials Unit,
- Other clinical trials units (Basic and Clinical Virology IDG, Birmingham Clinical Trials Unit, Cancer Research UK Medical Oncology Unit (Southampton), Cancer Research UK Trials Office (Liverpool), Centre for Health Services Research (Newcastle), Department of Social Medicine (Bristol), European Group for Blood and Marrow Transplantation Central Office, International Collaborative Cancer Group, Medical Statistics Department (Christie Hospital), Medical Statistics Unit (Edinburgh), Northern Ireland Cancer Clinical Trials Unit, Oncology Clinical Trials Office (Oxford), Royal Marsden: Breast Cancer Trials, Scotland and Newcastle Lymphoma Group

Research resources and facilities: cancer informatics, cancer biobanking (onCORE UK, Wales Cancer Bank, Confederation of Cancer Biobanks)

Figure 9.2 How cancer research is organized in the United Kingdom.

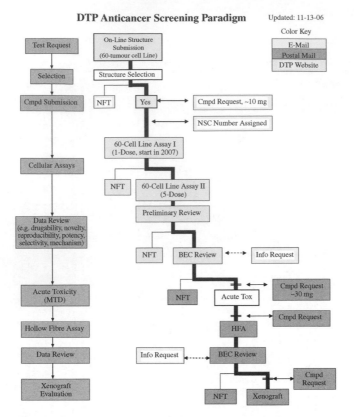

Figure 9.3 The NCI Developmental Therapeutics Program drug screening protocol showing the preclinical evaluation process for an anticancer drug candidate. *In vitro* testing is carried out using cellular assays involving the NCI-60 panel of tumour cell lines, followed by *in vivo* testing using the hollow fibre assay. After data review, the drug candidate is evaluated using xenograft models. Reproduced with permission from Developmental Therapeutics Program www.dtp.nci.nih.gov August 2008.

COMPARE analysis, where cytotoxicity data from drug screens are used to reveal trends that might predict anticancer activity of novel drug compounds. Core laboratories offer services in specific areas of research or in assay development. These are described on the web site and include biosampling programmes such as the tissue array research programme (TARP) which acts as a biosampling resource, the angiogenesis resource centre, which offers tumour endothelial cell line-based assays for screening agents that target tumour angiogenesis, and the laboratory animal production programme. There are also several genomics resources, such as the Cancer Genome Anatomy Project and the Cancer Chromosome Aberration Project, which aim to provide a searchable database of genes and chromosomal changes associated with the development, progression and treatment response of cancer. Facilities and resources for clinical trials are wide ranging, where the Cancer Therapy Evaluation Program (CTEP) coordinates and provides assistance for clinical trials, by overseeing programmes such as the Clinical Trials Cooperative Group Program, which support the development of multi-centre phase III clinical trials amongst research groups in receipt of CTEP sponsorship.

The National Cancer Institute, like the NCRI in the United Kingdom, has a cancer research portfolio of NIH-funded research, as well as their own research institutes (for example, at Bethesda/Frederick, Maryland). There are also NCI comprehensive cancers centres carrying out centre-focused NIH-funded research programmes, which are entitled to the use of shared resources to support epidemiological studies, basic laboratory science and clinical trials.

There are several well-known cancer charities in the United States, which provide funding and serve as a source of information to scientists, the health professions and members of the public, the largest organization being the American Cancer Society www.cancer.org, which occupies a scientific and political niche closely analogous to that of Cancer Research UK in the United Kingdom.

International collaboration in cancer research www.cancerportfolio.com is well established and encouraged by the respective key national organizations. The International Cancer Research Portfolio (ICRP) are a partnership of cancer research funding organizations, currently from the United States and the United Kingdom, that work together to compile a database of cancer research taking place under the seven common scientific outlines as used by the NCRI. ICRP partners include the NCI, the NCRI (and its constituent partner organizations), the American Cancer Society, the US Congressionally Directed Medical Research Programs, Department of Defense, the US cancer nursing charity the Oncology Nursing Society Foundation and other high profile US-based cancer charities.

10

Novel anticancer agents

10.1 Introduction

Table 10.1 shows the novel anticancer agents that were approved in the 1990s and the first decade of the twenty first century. Although the approval of the more traditionally DNA-targeting cytotoxic agents such as the taxanes and the topoisomerase I inhibitors represented a significant breakthrough in the treatment of therapeutically challenging cancers such as ovarian carcinoma, the start of the twenty first century heralded a trend for developing anticancer agents that looked beyond the differential in proliferative activity between normal and tumour cells. Therefore, rather than focusing solely on inhibiting the increased rate of DNA synthesis and replication, or aiming to destroy DNA in tumour cells, the aim was to discover and specifically target the genes, proteins, receptors and molecular pathways that regulate the growth, survival and malignant progression determining treatment outcome and prognosis in the cancer patient.

10.2 Target validation

Map 2 summarizes the processes used for the identification, optimization and validation of new anti-cancer agents. Chapters 2–5 covered some of the molecular changes that occur in the transformed cell that may lead to the up- or downregulation of biological pathways important in malignant progression, sensitivity to treatment and ultimately survival. This chapter will highlight some of the techniques and disciplines involved in the discovery and development of anticancer drugs. To identify and validate a new drug target, studies are carried out at the cellular and tissue level, using material derived from tumour cell lines, experimental animals and human or veterinary patients. Tumour cell lines are obtained from human or mammalian tumours, and may be primary cultures, that is, *ex vivo* samples taken from a growing tumour and placed into culture, or they may be established tumour cell lines that have undergone many passages. These have become immortalized or stabilized, having been harvested and sub-cultured many times in culture conditions. The advantage of stable cell lines is that they can be cultured indefinitely without undergoing any observable ageing effects. They are also usually fully characterized and therefore have established and predictable gene expression

Cancer Chemotherapy   Rachel Airley
© 2009 John Wiley & Sons, Ltd.

Table 10.1 Novel anticancer agents approved in the 1990s and the first decade of the twenty-first century

Proprietary/generic name	Approval	Target	Classification
Alimta/pemetrexed	2004	DNA (enzymes involved in purine and pyrimidine synthesis)	Cytotoxic
Avastin/bevacizumab	2004	VEGF	Antiangiogenic
Erbitux/cetuximab	2004	EGFR	Semi-selective
Bexxar/tositumomab	2003	CD20	Tissue-selective
Velcade/bortezomib	2003	Proteasome	Cytotoxic
Iressa/gefitinib	2003	EGFR	Semi-selective
Eloxatin/oxaliplatin	2002	DNA (alkylating agent)	Cytotoxic
Zevalin/ibritumomab tiuxetan	2002	CD20	Tissue-selective
Gleevec/imatinib mesylate	2001	Bcr-Abl/c-kit	Semi-selective
Campath/alemtuzumab	2001	CD52	Tissue-selective
Trisenox/arsenic trioxide	2000	Multiple	Cytotoxic
Mylotarg/gemtuzumab	2000	CD33	Tissue-selective
Temodar/temozolomide	1999	DNA (alkylating agent)	Cytotoxic
Valstar/valrubicin	1998	DNA (topoisomerase II)	Cytotoxic
Herceptin/trastuzumab	1998	erbB2/HER2	Semi-selective
Xeloda/capecitabine	1998	DNA (enzymes involved in pyrimidine nucleotide synthesis)	Cytotoxic
Rituxan/rituximab	1997	CD20	Tissue-selective
Intron A/interferon α	1997	IFN receptor	Tissue-selective
Camptosar/irinotecan	1996	DNA (topoisomerase I)	Cytotoxic
Hycamptin/topotecan	1996	DNA (toposiomerase I)	Cytotoxic
Gemzar (gemcitabine)	1996	DNA (incorporation of pyrimidine nucleotides)	Cytotoxic
Taxotere/docetaxel	1996	Microtubules of mitotic spindle	Cytotoxic
Vesanoid/tretinoin	1995	Differentiatiating agent (RAR)	Cytotoxic
Navelbine/vinorelbine	1994	Microtubules of mitotic spindle	Cytotoxic
Leustatin/cladribine	1993	DNA (incorporation of pyrimidine nucleotides)	Cytotoxic
Taxol/paclitaxel	1992	Microtubules of mitotic spindle	Cytotoxic

Adapted from Blagosklonny (2004). IFN, interferon; VEGF, vascular endothelial growth factor; EGFR, epidermal growth factor receptor.

profiles. They may be selected for use according to their individual biological characteristics, such as basal expression of a putative novel drug target, rate of growth, or compatibility with a particular assay. A primary tumour cell line is more difficult to work with, as they tend to cease proliferation after a few generations. However, where a line of research requires a cell culture model to closely resemble the characteristics of a specific tumour type existing in a host, for example, from a cohort of patients in a clinical study, or where the established cell lines available for a particular cancer subtype are limited, a primary cell line may be more appropriate. When a cell line is isolated or developed, it may be submitted to a repository and made available for use by other cancer research groups. In Europe, a major repository is the European Collection of Cell Cultures (ECACC), and in the United States, tumour cell lines may be obtained from a variety of sources, including the American Type Culture Collection (ATCC), and the National Cancer Institute. Figure 10.1 shows a range of tumour cell lines commonly used in *in vitro* cancer research, including the National Cancer Institutes NCI-60 tumour cell line panel.

10.2.1 Determining the role of a novel target in malignancy and tumour progression in vitro

A molecular or cellular mechanism will gain interest and status as a putative drug target in cancer if there is a differential in its expression between normal and malignant tissue. Evidence of this may accumulate from a number of sources. For instance, there may be observations of increased expression of a certain gene in studies involving the analysis of biopsy material from human patients, or transgenic mouse model developed specifically to study that cancer type. An essential part of anticancer drug discovery involves the validation of a target using mechanistic studies that determine its biological function and if it plays a critical role in either the formation and progression, or the inhibition of tumours. *In vitro* assays using tumour cell lines make up a significant portion of the target validation techniques in use. The objectives of these *in vitro* studies will be firstly, to characterize the relative constitutive (baseline) expression and activity of a putative target in a range of tumour cell lines relative to each other and the corresponding non-malignant cell line. This way, any observed differential offer insight into both the importance of the target and subsequent targeted anticancer agents in the treatment of cancers at specific sites, and the likelihood of toxicity of any targeted antitumour agents to normal tissue. Once constitutive expression has been characterized across the tumour cell lines, genetic manipulation techniques may be used to either increase, decrease or knock out the expression of the target. This involves transfection of the cell line with a vector, or a bacterial plasmid construct that either carries the gene of expression, or a sequence which will oppose or inhibit the transcription or translation of the target.

Characterization of constitutive expression may be carried out using immunological techniques that detect proteins such as enzyme-linked immunosorbent assay, immunoprecipitation or Western blotting. These techniques all broadly encompass the use of a primary antibody that specifically binds to the protein of interest within cells or tissue material. The antibody may be raised in a number of animals, but are most commonly derived from mice (monoclonal) or rabbits (polyclonal). A secondary antibody, which is an immunoglobulin that has been raised against antigens of the primary antibody species, for example, anti-rabbit or anti-mouse, is then applied, which binds and therefore amplifies the primary antibody step. A third step is then carried out which couples enzymes such as horseradish peroxidase or alkaline phosphatase to the secondary antibody. Therefore, where a protein target is expressed within a tissue, there will be large amounts of physically linked detection enzyme. The enzyme is then used to drive a chemical visualization reaction such as chromogen staining or chemo-illuminescence, so that the amount of protein can be easily

	Human (NCI-60 panel)	Doubling time
Leukemia	CCRF-CEM	26.7
	HL-60	28.6
	K-562	19.6
	MOLT-4	27.9
	RPMI-8226	33.5
	SR	28.7
Non-Small Cell Lung	A549/ATCC	22.9
	EKVX	43.6
	HOP-62	39
	HOP-92	79.5
	NCI-H226	61
	NCI-H23	33.4
	NCI-H322M	35.3
	NCI-H460	17.8
	NCI-H522	38.2
Colon	COLO 205	23.8
	HCC-2998	31.5
	HCT-116	17.4
	HCT-15	20.6
	HT29	19.5
	KM12	23.7
	SW-620	20.4
CNS	SF-268	33.1
	SF-295	29.5
	SF-539	35.4
	SNB-19	34.6
	SNB-75	62.8
	U251	23.8
Melanoma	LOX IMVI	20.5
	MALME-3M	46.2
	M14	26.3
	SK-MEL-2	45.5
	SK-MEL-28	35.1
	SK-MEL-5	25.2
	UACC-257	38.5
	UACC-62	31.3
Ovarian	IGR-OV1	31
	OVCAR-3	34.7
	OVCAR-4	41.4
	OVCAR-5	48.8
	OVCAR-8	26.1
	SK-OV-3	48.7
Renal	786-0	22.4
	A498	66.8
	ACHN	27.5
	CAKI-1	39
	RXF 393	62.9
	SN12C	29.5
	TK-10	51.3
	UO-31	41.7
Prostate	PC-3	27.1
	DU-145	32.3
Breast	MCF7	25.4
	NCI/ADR-RES	34
	MDA-MB-231	41.9
	HS 578T	53.8
	MDA-MB-435	25.8
	MDA-N	22.5
	BT-549	53.9
	T-47D	45.5

Rodent Cell Lines

b.End3 SV129	Brain endothelioma
BC3H1	Brain tumour
Hepa 1-6	Hepatoma
Hepa-1c1c7	Hepatoma
AC2	Lymphoblast
BCL1	B cell leukaemia
P388/ADR	Leukaemia
LL/2(LLc1)	C57BL Lewis lung carcinoma
Meta	Lung metastases
C127I	Mammary tumour
CNC 127I	Mammary tumour
MMT-060562	Mammary tumour
EMT6	Mammary tumour, drug-resistant
B16	Melanoma
TGP 49	Pancreatic acinar carcinoma
AtT-20/D16v-F2	Pituitary tumour
I-10 BALB/c	Leydig cell testicular tumour

Paediatric Tumours

N1E-115	neuroblastoma (mouse)
A673	rhabdomyosarcoma (human)
RD	Caucasian embryo rhabdomyosarcoma (human)
MOLT-3 and 4	Acute T lymphoblastic leukaemia (human)
RB247C	Retinoblastoma (human)
Y79	Caucasian retinoblastoma (human)

Other tumour cell lines

	Comment
Human	
Bladder	
EJ138	Bladder carcinoma
HT 1197	Caucasian bladder carcinoma
RT4	Caucasian bladder transitional-cell carcinoma
Cervix	
C-4I	Caucasian Cervical carcinoma
HeLa	Negroid cervix epitheloid carcinoma
Colon	
CACO-2	Caucasian colon adenocarcinoma
DLD-1	
KM20L2	
Fibrosarcoma HT 1080	
Oral squamous cell carcinoma PE/CA	
Squamous carcinoma A431	
Kidney	
CAKI-2	Caucasian kidney carcinoma
RXF-631	
SN12K1	
Leukaemia	
HL60	Caucasian promyelocytic leukaemia
Jurkat	Leukaemic T cell lymphoblast
P388	
Liver	
Hep 3B	Negroid hepatocyte carcinoma
Hep G2	Caucasian hepatocyte carcinoma
Lung	
LXFL 529	Non-Small Cell
DMS 114	Small Cell
SHP-77	Small Cell

Figure 10.1 Tumour cell line collections such as the NCI-60 panel of tumour cell lines used to screen drugs for antitumour activity. Cell lines may also be sourced from repositories such as ECACC (Europe) or ATCC (United States) and may originate from human, mouse or other mammalian tumours.

quantified and its ultrastructural location within a cell or tissue microenvironment may be determined.

If the putative target is a gene, or if it is necessary to determine the role of a protein relative to its rate or timing of transcription or translation, it may be necessary to use techniques that quantify DNA or RNA. These techniques are extremely sensitive, and can be used to measure extremely small amounts of nucleic acid. For instance, they may be based upon the polymerase chain reaction (PCR), which is used to amplify small amounts of specific DNA sequences. A variant of this technique, real-time (RT) PCR is often used for the quantitative analysis of gene sequences in biopsy or surgically resected tumour material in studies involving human patients in order to detect changes such as gene copy number or specific mutations. This is not to be confused with reverse-transcriptase PCR, where reverse-transcriptase is used in an additional step during the PCR process to amplify and therefore detect mRNA transcripts. However, the two techniques may be combined in order to quantify the level of transcription of a target gene occurring in different tumour cell or tissue types relative to non-malignant controls. PCR may also be used to amplify a signature DNA sequence of a target gene in order to develop fluorescent probes that bind the corresponding messenger RNA and therefore allow assessment of the level of gene transcription (fluorescence *in situ* hybridization).

To enable rapid analysis of a large number of tumour cell types tissue microarrays may be used, where cores of cell pellets or tissue material are arranged in a grid pattern on a microscope slide. These are prepared by taking cores of samples that have been routinely formalin-fixed and embedded into individual paraffin blocks for retention and future use in clinical diagnosis or research. Multiple cores are then arranged on a single master paraffin block, from which ultra thin sections (4–5 μm) may be cut and set on slides in a similar fashion to the histological preparation of slides from blocks containing individual samples (Figures 10.2 and 10.3). These arrays may be used for the detection of target at protein or nucleic acid level and have the advantage of allowing simultaneous evaluation of a large number of cell lines, therefore reducing the potential for experimental or intraobserver variation. Tissue microarrays obtained from the TARP laboratory are shown in Figure 10.4. These are prepared from cores of approximately 600 tumour samples from a range of sites. In this case, basic immunohistochemistry has been used to stain for the facilitative glucose transporter Glut-1, where observation using light microscopy showed distinct variation between normal and malignant tissue samples and between tumour types. Cell cultures may also be used to make microarrays (Figure 10.5), where cells are harvested, formalin-fixed and embedded into agarose. Cores of agarose-embedded cells are then used to prepare single master paraffin blocks from which microarrays are prepared in a similar fashion to those containing human tissue samples.

10.2.2 Genetic manipulation of cell lines

Genetic manipulation may be carried out in order to generate cell lines, or clones, with deregulated expression of a cellular component, which can be used as *in vitro* models to determine its function in the development, progression and treatment of malignancy,

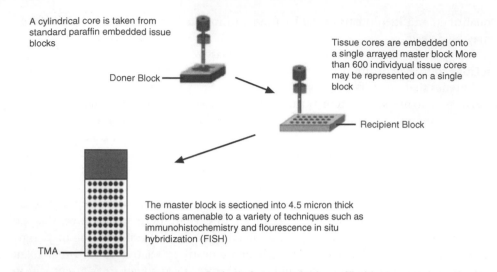

A cylindrical core is taken from standard paraffin embedded issue blocks

Doner Block

Tissue cores are embedded onto a single arrayed master block More than 600 individyual tissue cores may be represented on a single block

Recipient Block

The master block is sectioned into 4.5 micron thick sections amenable to a variety of techniques such as immunohistochemistry and flourescence in situ hybridization (FISH)

TMA

Figure 10.2 Tissue microarrays may be built from standard paraffin blocks containing human biopsy or resected tumour material that has been routinely retained and formalin-fixed for diagnostic and research use. Multiple cores from individual blocks are embedded onto a master block in a grid pattern, from which 4–5 μm sections are prepared and set onto slides. The tissue microarrays are suitable for analysis at protein or nucleic acid level, by a range of techniques such as immunohistochemistry, which measures protein expression; and fluorescence *in situ* hybridization, which allows the characterization of gene transcription by detecting messenger RNA. Reproduced from Manning A.T. *et al.*, *EJSO* (2006), doi:10.1016/j.ejso.2006.09.002, Elsevier.

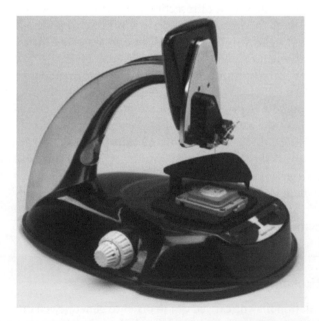

Figure 10.3 A Beecher MTA-2 manual tissue microarrayer (reproduced with permission from Beecher Instruments.)

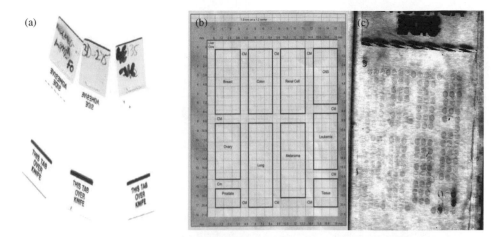

Figure 10.4 Tissue microarrays obtained from the National Cancer Institute TARP laboratory (a), consisting of cores of tumour samples taken from human patients, covering a range of tumour types including breast, colon, renal, central nervous system, ovarian, lung, skin, prostate and leukaemia (b). (c) basic immunohistochemistry was carried out to determine the variation of facilitative glucose transporter Glut-1 expression between normal tissue and across the different tumour types. The circular structures are tissue cores highlighted here by the blue haematoxylin counterstain, which stains cellular components such as nuclei and plasma membranes and provides structural context for immunohistochemical staining when observed by light microscopy.

and therefore its status as a candidate drug target. Such cellular components may be a gene, a DNA or RNA fragment that controls the expression of a gene, or a protein which may be structural or metabolic, such as an enzyme. Depending upon the constitutive expression of the 'target', genetic manipulation strategies aim to upregulate (over-express) or downregulate or functionally inactivate the cellular component. Once these cell lines are developed and expression validated, they may be fully characterized for a wide range of parameters used in experimental oncology. Specific evidence that might stimulate scientific interest in a candidate target might be, for example, changes in growth characteristics, such as rate of proliferation, or decreased rate of apoptosis, in the genetically manipulated cell lines relative to wild type controls. Such data would therefore support the hypothesis that targeting this gene or protein would either slow tumour cell proliferation or induce apoptosis, leading to a net decrease in tumour mass. On the other hand, if it is suspected that a gene or protein expressed in tumours is causing poor clinical response to treatment because it is linked with a cellular drug resistance pathway, genetically manipulated cell lines might be used in drug toxicity assays to assess *in vitro* response to anticancer agents. Some of the experimental applications of genetically manipulated cell lines are described in Figure 10.6. There are a range of molecular biology techniques available, which vary in complexity and efficacy, as well as the extent of gene deregulation that they offer. There are several highly reputable laboratory manuals, widely used by experimental biologists, which describe scientific rationale and provide precise instruction in the methodology necessary to carry out these techniques; the best known being the well-thumbed and usually

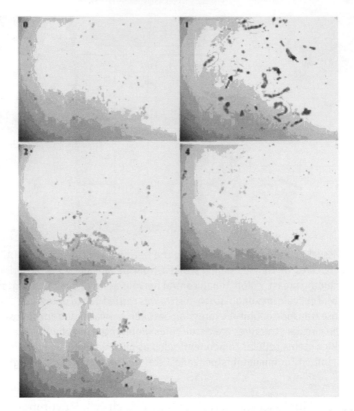

Figure 10.5 Microarrays may also be prepared using cores of agarose embedded pellets of formalin-fixed cell cultures. Pictured here are microarrays obtained from the National Cancer Institute TARP laboratory carrying the NCI-60 panel of tumour cell lines. These were stained for Glut-1 using immunohistochemistry and placed under ×400 magnification. The extent of Glut-1 expression was graded according to the area and intensity of staining (BT549 = 0; MCF7 = 1, OVCAR = 2; HCC2998 = 3, IGROV1 = 4; SNB19 = 5). Reproduced from Evans *et al.* (2007) *Cancer Chemother. Pharmacol.*, Springer. A colour reproduction of this Figure can be viewed in the colour section towards the centre of the book.

extremely dog-eared three-volume 'Maniatis', or *Molecular Cloning: A Laboratory Manual* (edited by Sambrook and Russell, Cold Spring Harbor Laboratory Press), also available at www.protocol-online.org and www.MolecularCloning.com.

Gain of function or upregulation of gene expression

To determine how the *presence* of or the amplification of a candidate target gene affects tumour pathology, techniques are used that lead to upregulation or gain of function. This is achieved through insertion of a vector, or a construct derived from a bacterial resistance plasmid (Figure 10.7). A plasmid is a circular, double-stranded piece of DNA which can be replicate independently of the bacterial chromosome. The biological function of plasmids is to enable exchange of genetic information between individual bacteria within a colony as a means of spreading advantageous characteristics such as drug resistance. In molecular biology, plasmids are usually taken up into bacterial cells by *transformation*, where exogenous DNA is introduced from the environment using a

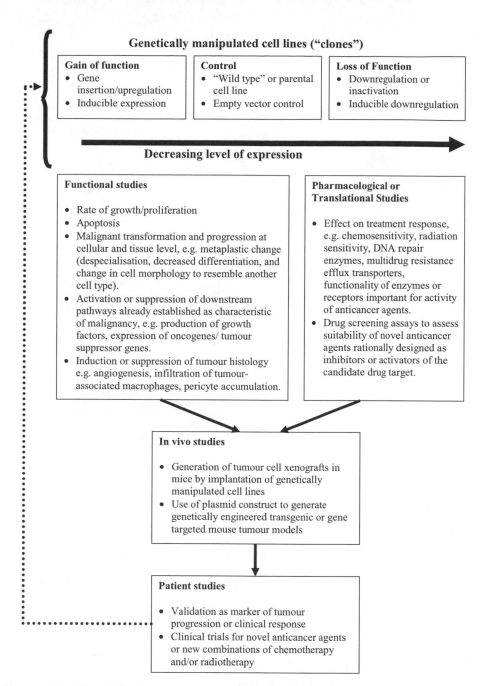

Figure 10.6 The application of genetically manipulated cell lines in experimental oncology and anticancer drug development. 'Clones' with deregulated expression of a candidate drug target may be used to determine how gain or loss of function of the target affect both the basic biology of malignancy and clinical response. Promising data obtained *in vitro* using genetically manipulated cell lines often provides the proof of principle necessary to progress to *in vivo* studies using mouse tumour models, and ultimately, to studies involving patients. Observations in translational studies involving patients will sometimes reveal new avenues for exploration involving further candidate tumour markers and possible novel drug targets, providing the focus for further *in vitro* studies involving the generation of genetically manipulated cell lines.

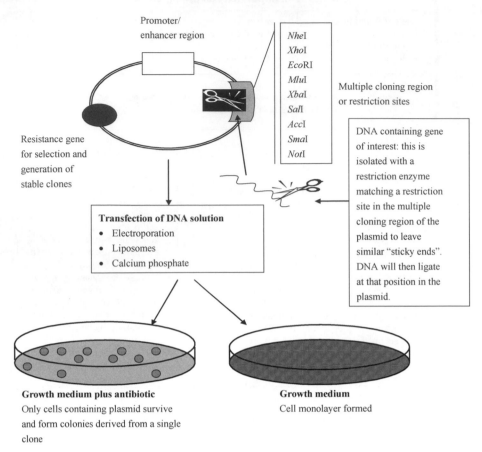

Figure 10.7 Genetic manipulation or transfection of cell lines with a bacterial plasmid that acts as an expression vector to induce or suppress expression of a candidate drug target. Stably transfected cell lines are generated using a vector that contains a DNA sequence marker for resistance to antibiotics such as neomycin or G418 (Geneticin). Following transfection, culture in medium supplemented with antibiotic provides the selection conditions necessary to promote survival of resistant colonies of cells or 'clones' that carry the expression vector and show stable expression of the gene of interest.

prepared solution of purified DNA. However, naturally occurring plasmid uptake may also occur by *conjugation*, which involves direct cell to cell contact between by bacteria, or *transduction*, where the plasmid is carried from one bacterium to another by a *bacteriophage*, a type of virus that infects bacteria. To achieve transformation in the laboratory, a bacterial strain must be *competent*, that is, permeable to DNA. Such bacterial strains may be prepared in the laboratory and are available commercially. Bacteria express many types of *restriction enzyme*, which are used to cut and paste specific DNA sequences, and thereby bring about stable changes in the overall DNA sequence of a plasmid. There are several proprietary preparations of bacterial plasmids available for genetic manipulation studies, which contain *multiple cloning regions*, or a set of DNA sequences that act as sites where one of the many naturally occurring bacterial restriction enzymes may be used to introduce the DNA sequence representative of the gene which codes for the candidate drug target. Commercially available bacterial plasmids also contain DNA cassettes which code for a promoter, which might contain DNA sequence that enhances the expression of the inserted gene, such as the lacZ promoter, found in the pGEM plasmid (Promega); the SV40 promoter, in the pGL3 plasmid (Promega) and the CMV promoter, found in the pcDNA3.1 plasmid (Invitrogen).

Once the gene of interest has been inserted at the multiple cloning region, the plasmid is introduced into the mammalian cell line by *transfection*. The three methods most widely used are electroporation, where an electric field applied to a suspension of the mammalian cells will increase plasma membrane permeability via the formation of temporary pores that will enable uptake of the plasmid construct into the cell. The other two methods are chemical, where plasmid uptake is achieved through conjugation with liposomes (*lipofection*), which are derived from phospholipid and are therefore easily carried into the cell though the plasma membrane; and calcium phosphate transfection, where calcium phosphate precipitates DNA into large aggregates which are taken up by the cell by a process that is reliable but, as yet, poorly understood.

At this stage, the resulting transfectants will be *transient*, where a proportion of cells in subsequent generations, depending upon the *transfection efficiency*, will not contain the plasmid and will therefore not show the change in target gene expression. To generate *stable* transfectants, that is, clones that express the target gene in subsequent generations, it is necessary to use a plasmid that contains a *selection marker*. These are usually DNA cassettes that confer resistance to antibiotics such as the aminoglycoside antibiotics neomycin or G418 (Geneticin (Invitrogen)). Thus, culture of transfected cell lines in media supplemented with these constituents will favour survival and proliferation of cells containing the plasmid vector, leading to a clonal population of cells showing stable target gene expression.

Loss of function or downregulation of gene expression

To determine how the *absence* of a gene may affect tumour pathology, or to model the therapeutic consequences of pharmacologically inhibiting a candidate target gene or the protein it encodes, molecular biology techniques are used that lead to downregulation and/or loss of function at transcriptional, post transcriptional or post-translational level.

RNA interference

RNA interference (RNAi) is based upon the use of RNA oligonucleotides to activate gene silencing processes within the cell. To a certain extent, RNAi is superseding the use of antisense techniques, where RNA oligonucleotides complementary to the 'sense' strand of the target gene sequence[1] compete with and sterically inhibit the action of messenger RNA, downregulating translation into the protein. RNAi is a naturally occurring immune response used to inactivate viruses that infect the cell and

---

[1]Antisense oligonucleotides are therefore themselves RNA versions of the 'antisense' strand of the double stranded gene and complementary to 'sense' mRNA transcripts manufactured using the 'antisense' strand as a template.

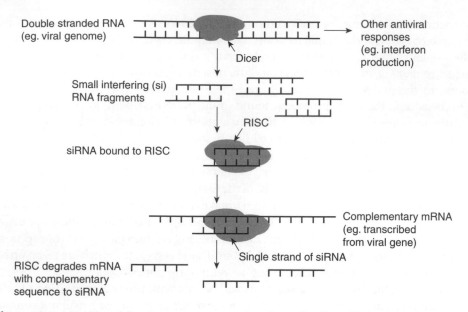

Figure 10.8   RNAi is a defensive response targeting the replication of infecting viruses. Dicer enzymes cut double stranded viral RNA (dsRNA) into 20 base pair fragments, which are used as templates by the RISC (RNA induced silencing complex) enzyme complex to recognize and destroy (via the ribonuclease Ago2) homologous mRNA sequences synthesized by viruses to direct the manufacture of viral DNA and proteins. Reproduced from Downward, J. *BMJ.* 2004;328:1245–8, BMJ Publishing Group Ltd.

appropriate cellular machinery for the replication of viral DNA/RNA. As part of the viral replication process, viruses usually manufacture double-stranded RNA (dsRNA) sequences. However, in response to viral infection, cells produce *dicer* enzymes (RNase III) that cut viral dsRNA into small interfering RNA fragments (siRNA) which are around 20 base pairs in length. The cellular enzyme complex RISC (RNA induced silencing complex) enlist the siRNA fragments as templates to recognize any homologous viral mRNA being used to direct the manufacture of viral DNA and proteins needed for viral replication (Figure 10.8). Viral mRNA is then degraded via the RISC catalytic unit ribonuclease Ago2.

In a research setting, complementary siRNA oligonucleotide sequences may be synthesized and applied to mammalian cell lines to trigger an RNAi response to a target gene. Initially, whole dsRNA sequences were used; however, non-specific sequence-independent gene silencing occurring in mammalian somatic cells, via an interferon-mediated pathway, reduced the efficacy of the technique and lead to cellular toxicity. Since then, siRNA's have been used successfully to target genes without mounting a non-specific response. These can be introduced directly by transfection into cells in culture or alternatively, via genetic manipulation techniques, where constructs encoding shRNA's (short hairpin RNAs) are inserted, which after processing of shRNA's by cellular nucleases, are incorporated into RISC. These may be stably expressed using plasmids in the generation of genetically manipulated *in vitro* and *in vivo* tumour models. Further, shRNA libraries are now available, providing sequence data with which to carry out screening assays in the search for new therapeutic targets.

The dominant negative gene

Dominant negative genes occur either naturally or can be generated in the laboratory by selective deletion of DNA sequences coding for specific peptide sequences integral to the structure or function of the resulting protein. One of the most well characterized naturally occurring dominant negative genes in tumour biology is the tumour suppressor gene *p53*. Germ-line mutation of wild type *p53* is known to cause familial predisposition to cancer, possibly due to its involvement in many protective cellular processes such as DNA repair. Mutated *p53* has been found in around 50% of human tumours. In its wild type state, *p53* encodes a transcription factor that functions as a tetramer. Point mutation in the gene for one of the subunits of the tetramer that retains the ability to bind to the rest of the p53 protein complex leads to the formation of a non-functional tetramer. This gives rise to a mutated p53 protein complex that has no DNA binding activity and has lost its tumour suppressor function. The mutated p53 protein is described as dominant negative because in individuals with a heterozygous genotype, the allele coding for mutated, that is, non-functional p53 protein is expressed. Accordingly, genetically manipulated cell lines and transgenic mouse models expressing dominant negative p53 protein have been used to establish the role of p53 protein as a transcription factor in tumorigenesis, and the generation of dominant negative gene expression systems is now a useful technique used to knock out or downregulate a gene in the validation of candidate target genes. For instance, dominant negative hypoxia-inducible factor-1(HIF-1) has been engineered to explore the potential for therapeutic inhibition of HIF-1 and its downstream hypoxia-regulated genes. As discussed in Chapter 12, HIF-1 has a multi-factorial role in the physiological adaptation of cells to the oxygen and nutrient deprived tumour microenvironment, targeting major groups of genes controlling glucose metabolism, tissue pH, angiogenesis and metastasis. HIF-1 functions as a dimer, where HIF-1α is stabilized and accumulates in hypoxic conditions and HIF-1β, its binding partner, is expressed constitutively. The dimeric structure of HIF-1 facilitates the experimental production of a dominant negative version, for instance as shown by Figure 10.9a. Here, dominant negative HIF-1α is derived from in tact HIF-1α lacking the DNA-binding, transactivation and oxygen-dependent degradation (ODD) domains that are essential to its functionality. When cell lines transfected to express dominant negative HIF-1α were transplanted into mice, the resulting xenografts showed a decreased rate of glucose metabolism and overall, tumour formation was suppressed.

The proto-oncogene *erbB2*, (*HER2*, *neu*) forms a heterodimer with various partners belonging to the ErbB or epidermal growth factor receptor (EGFR) family of ATP-binding tyrosine kinases in order to upregulate EGFR function. The exploitation of the erBB2/EGFR signal transduction pathway has been of particular interest in the diagnosis and treatment of breast cancer, where amplification of the gene leads to poor prognosis and changes in treatment response. This has led to the development of HER2/EGFR targeted anticancer agents such as trastuzumab (Herceptin), gefitinib (Iressa) and more recently, the dual EGFR/erbB2 inhibitor lapatinib (Chapter 14). Development of these

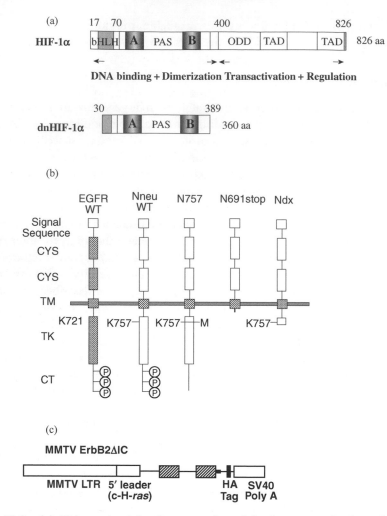

Figure 10.9 (a) DNA construct for the expression of dominant negative hypoxia-inducible factor HIF-1α (dn (HIF-1α)), consisting of a deletion mutant of in tact HIF-1α lacking the DNA-binding, transactivation and oxygen-dependent degradation (ODD) domains. Dominant negative HIF-1α inhibited the formation of functional HIF-1 by forming a non-functional heterodimer with HIF-1β, in turn leading to decreased expression of hypoxia-regulated glucose metabolism and tumour formation. Reprinted from *Am. J. Pathol.* 2003, 162:1283–1291 with permission from the American Society for Investigative Pathology. (b): Dominant negative versions of the plasma membrane spanning oncogene erbB2/HER2/neu, comparing the positions of cysteine-rich ectodomains (CYS), the transmembrane region (TM), and the tyrosine kinase endodomain (TK) for EGFR, Nneu (a rat wild type neu) and the erbB2 dominant negatives generated by point mutation at position K757M in the TK of Nneu (N757); through a stop codon at position Thr-691 of Nneu, causing deletion of the TK-containing endodomain (N691stop); or by deletion of the *Xba*I fragment from WT c-neu, leading to a partial deletion of the TK-containing endodomain, and a mutant protein 50 amino acids longer than N691stop (Ndx). Reprinted from Qian *et al.* (1994) *Proc. Natl. Acad. Sci. USA* 91:1500–1504, with permission from National Academy of Sciences. (c) ErbB2ΔIC, which was placed under the control of the mammary tissue specific promoter MMTV to facilitate tumour-specific expression of dominant negative erbB2 in transgenic mouse models of breast cancer. Reproduced from Jones and Stern (1999) *Oncogene* 18: 3481–3490, Nature Publishing Group.

novel agents followed earlier work first carried out by Qian *et al.* (1994), where dominant negative versions of erbB2 lacking kinase activity were co-expressed with the EGFR *in vitro*. The dominant negative versions of erbB2, shown in Figure 10.9b, were generated via point mutation at sites corresponding to different elements of the plasma membrane-spanning protein: either its tyrosine kinase activity (mutation of the tyrosine-kinase containing endodomain at the N757 ATP-binding site), or the ability to bind dimerization partners (by total or partial deletion of the endodomain through truncation at the transmembrane domain (N691stop) or 50 amino acids downstream (NdX)). Through this work, it was possible to determine the crucial role of the tyrosine kinase element erbB2 in the activation of EGFR and to gain insight into how each structural component within the molecule influences dimerization activity with members of the erbB family. Later work carried out in 1999 by Jones and Stern involved the formulation of a construct where dominant negative erbB2 was placed under the control of the mouse mammary tumour virus (MMTV) promoter. By inducing mammary gland-specific expression of mutated erbB2, it was possible to develop a transgenic mouse tumour model of breast cancer showing deregulated erbB2 activity. The dominant negative erbB2 used in this work, erbB2Δ1c, was derived from the wild type rat erbB2, where tyrosine kinase activity was abolished by replacement of the endodomain with sequences encoding an influenza virus haemagglutinin (HA) epitope-tag (Figure 10.9c). Such work no doubt contributed to the validation of the erbB2 tyrosine kinase as a therapeutic target and provided biochemical data potentially of use in the molecular modelling and design of targeted erbB2 inhibitors.

Inducible gene expression systems

Inducible or variable gene expression may be achieved using the bacterial protein synthesis inhibitor tetracycline or its derivatives such as doxycycline. This is achieved by transfection of mammalian cells with vectors containing tetracycline response element DNA sequences, giving rise to a dose-dependent inducible activation or repression of target gene transcription when cells are cultured in media containing a variable concentration of the appropriate inducing agent. Several types of inducing system have been developed, including TET-ON, where tetracycline induces a dose-dependent upregulation, and TET-OFF, a dose-dependent down-regulation of the target gene. The tetracycline-regulatable system, first described in 1992 by Gossen and Bujard, is based upon the generation of the tet transactivator protein, rTA, a fusion protein consisting of the *Escherichia coli tet repressor* and the activating domain of virion protein 16 (VP16) of the herpes simplex virus (Figure 10.10). In the absence of tetracycline, the fusion protein, because it contains the *E. coli* tet repressor, binds to tet resistance operator sequences

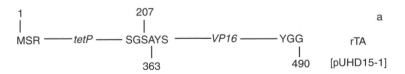

Figure 10.10 The rTA tet repressor-VP16 fusion protein developed by Gossen and Bujard. Reproduced from Gossen and Bujard (1992) *Proc. Natl. Acad. Sci. USA.* 89: 5547–5551, with permission from the National Academy of Sciences.

(*tetO*) that are found in a promoter sequence (*tetP*), that may be used to drive expression of a candidate target gene in an expression vector stably transfected into tumour cell lines. In the presence of tetracycline, however, a conformational change occurring in the tet repressor inhibits prevents binding of the rTA fusion protein to tetO, therefore inhibiting the function of the promoter tetP and consequently the target gene expression that it drives. This is a dose-dependent effect, where the concentration of tetracycline in cell culture medium influences the extent of promoter tetP inhibition, giving rise to a variable gene expression system. Some years later, the sytem was modified to produce the reverse transactivator (rtTA), which binds tetO *in the presence* of tetracyclines.

Since then, the ecdysone system has been developed, which uses the steroid insect moulting hormone ecdysone, a steroid hormone that induces metamorphosis into the adult stage in *Drosophila melanogaster*. The ecdysone-mediated inducible gene expression system, as described and validated by No *et al.* (1996), is achieved by transfection of cell lines with a vector where the gene of interest has been placed under the control of a promoter containing ecdysone response element (*EcRE*) enhancer sequences, which are transactivated through dose-dependent stimulation of the functional ecdysone receptor by the ecdysone agonist muristerone A. The functional ecdysone receptor is a product of the ecdysone receptor *EcR* and the ultraspiracle gene *USP*. Modifications have been described which have refined this system with the aim of producing improved sensitivity, increased specificity and decreased basal activity. This has been achieved through the use of various constructs, such as those shown by Figure 10.11, where the

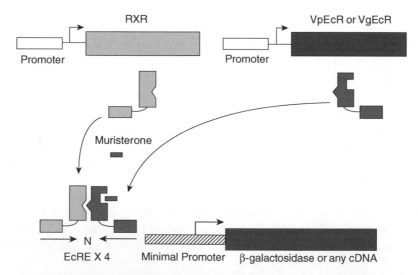

Figure 10.11 A modification of the ecdysone–inducible gene expression system allows improved sensitivity, specificity and decreased basal gene expression. Cell lines are transfected with a vector constructed with a heterodimer of the RXR and VpEcR, which transactivates the EcRE-containing promoter upon exposure to ecdysone or the ecdysone agonist muristerone A. The EcREs are placed upstream of a further minimal promoter, which drives the expression of the target gene. Reproduced from No *et al.* (1996) *Proc. Natl. Acad. Sci. USA.* 93: 3346–3351, with permission from the National Academy of Sciences.

EcRE promoter is transactivated by a heterodimer of the retinoid X receptor (*RxR*) and the VpEcR, itself a fusion protein derived from the EcR and VP-16.

The advantage of the ecdysone-inducible system is that, owing to the improved pharmacokinetic properties of muristerone over the tetracyclines, it allows effective transfer of this system to *in vivo* tumour models. Whereas tetracyclines show slow clearance from bone, muristerone/ecdysone, being lipophilic, rapidly penetrates all tissues and clears effectively. This short half life consequently allows swift response times when inducing changes in target gene expression in experimental conditions.

10.2.3 Molecular genetics and microarray technology

Microarray technology was developed to enable rapid and simultaneous expression profiling of a wide range of genes (in the order of thousands), and may be used to gather comprehensive data on genes specific to the cancer genome. Whereas tissue microarrays (Figure 10.2) enable examination of protein expression and most often use formalin-fixed, paraffin-embedded cells or tissue samples, cDNA microarrays are carried out using RNA extracted from unfixed material. The technique, shown in Figure 10.12, is based upon the preparation of cDNA (complementary DNA) mixtures from RNA extracts by reverse transcription. These are then hybridized to a microarray 'chip', a slide that carries thousands of 'spots' or probes made from cDNA or oligonucleotide sequences. Microarray chips are prepared using ink-jet or photolithography technology, where a geometrical grid of spots are immobilized onto a substrate made of glass, nylon

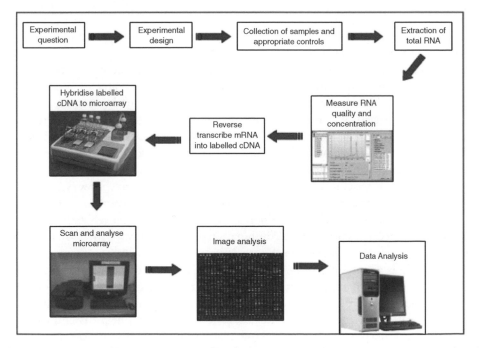

Figure 10.12 Revealing the cancer genome through cDNA microarray technology. Reproduced from Manning A.T. *et al.*, *EJSO* (2006), doi:10.1016/j.ejso.2006.09.002, Elsevier.

or silicon. Hybridization of homologous cDNA from the prepared cell or tissue extract to the cDNA probes on the chip produces a signal, which depending upon the type of chip used, may be radioactive, chemiluminescent or fluorescent. The chip may be imaged and digitally analysed in order to observe and calculate the relative strength of the signals produced at each spot, which will in turn reflect the level of gene expression in the sample being investigated. In doing so, the level of expression and regulatory parameters of multiple classes of genes known to be or potentially involved in cancer biology pathways may be compared across multiple tumour types.

Obtaining meaningful data from DNA microarrays depends upon adequate data analysis tools in the form of highly specialized software. DNA microarrays also do not stand alone in the isolation and validation of candidate novel drug targets. However, they are useful exercises in hypothesis generation, that is, to obtain preliminary data on gene expression distributions in different tumour types which will themselves indicate the genes or clusters of genes that warrant further investigation. To do this, data obtained from microarrays should be optimized to rule out any spurious observations arising from the shifting effects of experimental protocol on the expression and detection of the many genes represented on one microarray chip. To do this, additional mRNA analysis, for example, Northern blotting, reverse transcriptase-PCR-based assays should be carried out following microarray analysis on individual genes showing interesting expression characteristics.

DNA microarray studies may be designed to look at (a) differential expression of previously characterized genes between tumour types (class comparison); (b) gene expression profiles in a cohort of tumour samples as a prediction of phenotypic behaviour, for example, adverse prognosis, chemotherapy response (class prediction); or (c) new genes or gene clusters that may be specific to a tumour type and lead to the discovery of new therapeutic targets (class discovery).

Research or academic institutions often have a dedicated microarray facility, for example, the Cancer Research UK microarray facility at the Paterson Institute for Cancer Research, Manchester, United Kingdom and in the United States, the National Cancer Institute central microarray facilities at their Gaithersburg and Frederick facilities (see http://arraytracker.nci.nih.gov/). There are a number of commercial DNA microarray systems available, including the Affymetrix GeneChip system, used alongside bioinformatics software such as ArrayAssist, developed by Stratagene. The SuperArray Bioscience Corporation's pathway focused microarrays allow synchronized investigation of genes expressed in disease-specific pathways relevant to cancer such as angiogenesis, apoptosis and cell cycle signalling, as well as the Cancer PathwayFinder, a microarray that carries probes for a combination of these pathways. Microarray studies carried out using tumour tissue samples are often large scale and rely on the recruitment of large numbers of patients, for example, a study of the gene expression characteristics determining treatment response in childhood acute leukaemias currently underway at the Cancer Research UK Children's Cancer Group, Manchester, United Kingdom (see http://www.medicine.manchester.ac.uk/cancerstudies). To help disseminate data obtained from microarray studies taking place internationally, cancer microarray databases such as ONCOMINE (set up at the University of Michigan, United States) caARRAY (National Cancer Institute) and MIAME VICE (MIAME-compliant

Variations In Cellular Expression, Paterson Institute of Cancer Research Genechip facility where MIAME (Minimum Information About a Microarray Experiment) is a standard for reporting microarray data which are available to the scientific community for the deposit of new data and retrieval of information for future studies.

10.2.4 Three-dimensional in vitro tumour models

To bridge the gap between *in vitro* and *in vivo* research, a number of three-dimensional tumour models may be generated *in vitro* from cell lines which show some of the characteristics of tumour tissue existing in an animal model or a patient. Cell lines ordinarily grow either as monolayers, adherent to a surface such as a tissue culture flask, or in a cell culture suspension, for example, as a spinner culture. Conventional two-dimensional cell cultures are useful to carry out preliminary drug screens or for the rapid analysis of molecular biology pathways because they proliferate quickly and are simple to maintain and process. Unlike homogeneous cell cultures, however, tissue mass does not contain only one type of cell, but consists of a number of cell types that adhere and communicate within a tissue microenvironment. Although it is possible to grow more than one cell line as a co-culture to experimentally model how they interact, for example, tumour and endothelial cell lines in studies of tumour angiogenesis, these are still two-dimensional and therefore lack the microenvironmental conditions, tissue morphology and cellular architecture that arise in a tissue mass.

The typical histology of a tumour, as described in Chapter 2, consists of a mass of tumour cells within a stromal cell matrix that sit on a basement membrane, through which a tumour may invade. The stromal cell matrix may contain fibroblasts, endothelial cells, from which tumour microvasculature is derived, immune cells such as macrophages, pericytes and interstitial fluid. There will be a continuous interaction between cells of the same type (autocrine) and of different types (paracrine), where the production of growth factors and other chemokines determine the biological behaviour of the tumour as a whole. The extracellular matrix additionally provides a scaffold for mechanical integrity of the tumour mass, and often carries the tumour-derived blood supply, which supplies the tumour with nutrients. Cells within the tumour are held together via adhesion molecules such as E-cadherin, which determines the ability of tumours to disseminate and eventually form metastases.

As discussed in Chapter 12, the formation of a three-dimensional tissue mass rather than a monolayer has microenvironmental consequences, where diffusion gradients running from the peripheral to the inner parts of the mass determine the availability of oxygen, glucose and other nutrients. Changes in oxygen and glucose concentration have knock-on metabolic effects that lead to altered pH and the upregulation of genes associated with increased glycolysis, such as the glucose transporters, glycolytic enzymes, hypoxia-regulated carbonic anhydrases and the monocarboxylate (lactate) transporters. The cellular morphology and architecture will also change, where peripheral layers will be adequately oxygenated and viable, whereas inner layers will be necrotic. The consequences for anti-cancer drug development, therefore, are that monolayers will have a limited capacity to realistically predict the drug diffusion, distribution and toxicity that will occur in a three-dimensional tumour. For instance, a small molecule inhibitor that relies on diffusion through the plasma membrane will have to go through several layers to get to the inner regions of a tumour mass, which will in turn affect its toxicity, whereas this will not be an issue when using cell culture monolayers. On the other hand, a novel agent, for example, a bioreductive drug may be highly potent against hypoxic cells in a three-dimensional system, but not in a monolayer where there is little variation in nutrient supply. The limitations of three-dimensional cell culture techniques are that, although they counter some of the problems of growing cells as two-dimensional monolayers, they still lack important features of *in vivo* models, such as a host and tumour-derived blood supply and tumour-host interaction.

Tumour cell spheroids

The simplest way of generating three-dimensional cell cultures is to make multicellular tumour cell spheroids (Figure 10.13a and b) where cell lines that naturally aggregate and have been allowed to form colonies in monolayer culture, for example, human hepatoma HepG2, Chinese hamster lung V-79, human colon HT29, human breast T47D and human bladder EJ138, are cultured in suspension in spinner flasks to an approximate volume of 1 mm^3. These are visible to the naked eye, but upon fixation and examination by light microscopy, share many of the microenvironmental features of tumours grown *in vivo*, such as central necrosis and a viable but highly glycolytic hypoxic layer.

Microcarrier beads

These may be used to generate three-dimensional tumour masses where cell lines are attachment-dependent and therefore do not naturally aggregate when in monolayer culture. This technique is also suitable for sensitive cell lines that are difficult to culture such as endothelial cells, as well as for the co-culture of different cell types. Microcarrier beads are commercially available in a range of sizes, materials and coatings, which determine their properties and applications for example, Cytodex dextran beads (Sigma-Aldrich). The beads are seeded when cells adhere to and proliferate on their surface, in effect forming mini-spheroids (Figure 10.13d and e). The mini-spheroids will then grow larger and adhere with each other, eventually forming large spheroid-like bead and mini-spheroid clusters. This process is determined by the extent of cell adhesion and attachment, which are heavily influenced by microenvironmental factors such as pH, the net charge of the bead and its coating, and the expression and activity of cell surface receptors.

Scaffolds

Prefabricated three-dimensional scaffolds are intertwined fibres that are biodegradable and can be made from collagen or synthetic polymers. Following inoculation of the scaffold with cells, these will proliferate in the interstitial spaces formed by the fibres, eventually forming a three-dimensional tissue-like culture (Figure 10.13f). Scaffolds can be used to simulate the supportive structure of the extracellular matrix and its role in cell signalling, which are thought to promote migration, proliferation and differentiation of cells.

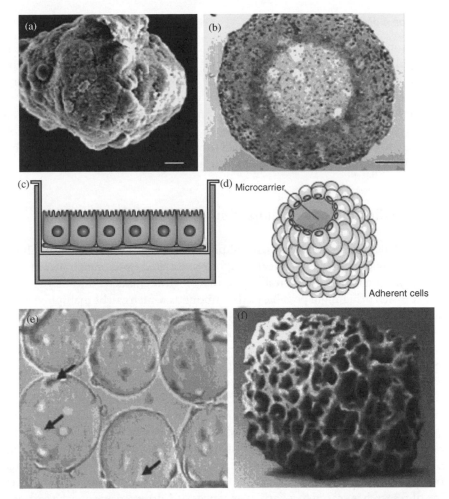

Figure 10.13 Scanning electron micrograph of a multicellular spheroid derived from the human hepatoma cell line HepG2 (a) along with a cross-section of a spheroid derived from the V-79 Chinese hamster lung cell line (b), clearly showing the necrotic inner core that has arisen due to diffusion gradients that limit the supply of oxygen and nutrients to the core. Reconstituted basement membranes, for example, Matrigel, simulate the basement membrane matrix on which epithelial tissue grows and through which epithelial-derived tumours may invade (c). Microcarrier beads (d) may be used where cell lines are sensitive and do not form aggregates easily. Cells growing on the surface will form micro-spheroids (shown by arrows, (e)), which adhere to those on adjacent microbeads, eventually forming large spheroid-like clusters of microbeads and cells. Prefabricated scaffolds (f) are intertwined fibres, often made of collagen, along which cells may be cultured. Interstitial spaces between the fibres provide room for cellular proliferation and the formation of three-dimensional cell cultures. (a), (b), (c) and (d) reproduced from Pampaloni *et al.* (2007) *Nat. Rev. Mol. Cell Biol.* AOP, published online 8 August 2007; doi:10.1038/nrm2236, Nature Publishing Group.(e) and (f) Reproduced from Kim (2005) *Semin. Cancer Biol.* 15: 365–377, Elsevier.

Extracellular matrix gels

These are sometimes referred to as reconstituted basement membrane, for example, Matrigel (BD Biosciences) (Figure 10.13c) and are designed to mimic the basement membrane on which epithelial-derived tumour cells can grow and form a tumour-like mass. Such three-dimensional cultures can be used to investigate tumour cell polarization, extent of adhesion and migration. Reconstituted basement membranes are also used in studies of tumour angiogenesis where endothelial cell lines seeded onto the membrane surface differentiate into luminal tubes and migrate through the membrane leaving detectable holes in the membrane surface.

10.3 Identification and optimization of lead drugs

Novel drugs may be derived from natural products, either directly or through semi-synthetic approaches, where chemical compounds isolated from plant material may be altered to bring about more desirable pharmacological characteristics. Drug screens may also be used to highlight possible lead compounds, which can be manipulated using medicinal chemistry. The National Cancer Institute has a range of drug repositories that may be screened for activity against a novel target. These repositories have been compiled from submissions of novel chemical compounds isolated or synthesized by cancer research groups within and external to the NCI, and include a natural products repository, containing approximately 50 000 plant samples and a pure chemicals repository, containing around 140 000 non-proprietary compounds that may be screened for antitumour activity. These are sometimes referred to as a diversity set, as the compounds available tend to be of widely varying chemical structure in order to increase the likelihood of finding a lead drug that best fits a biological target. Screening chemical compounds for antitumour activity is usually carried out initially using tumour cell lines, such as the NCI panel of 60 tumour cell lines (Figure 10.1). However, if a line of research is geared to a particular cancer site, drug screens may be carried out using a panel of tumour cell lines corresponding to that tumour type. The large number of chemical compounds involved means that this approach may be extremely labour intensive. Therefore, rational drug design approaches are used, which involve computational methods such as molecular modelling, that are used to map the tertiary or quaternary structure of a prospective drug target and to design candidate lead drug compounds. For a comprehensive account of the role of medicinal chemistry in anticancer drug discovery, see recommended texts below

- *Cancer Drug Design and Discovery:* Stephen Neidle (Editor) Academic Press; 1st Edition (24 Oct 2007)

- *Essential of Organic Chemistry:* Paul M. Dewick, Wiley-Blackwell; 1st Edition (13 April 2006)

- *Molecular Modelling: Principles and Applications*, Andrew Leach, Prentice–Hall; 2nd Edition (30 Jan 2001).

10.3.1 Screening for anticancer activity in vitro

The initial stages of drug screening often involve the evaluation of the toxicity of a large number of drug classes, and chemical variants of lead drugs isolated through rational drug design techniques. Desirable qualities of a drug screening assay include simplicity of design; they should enable reproducible analysis of a large number of compounds to provide a reasonably accurate assessment of chemosensitivity. The assay should also be inexpensive and quick to perform.

The MTT (3-(4,5-dimethylthiazol-2-yl)-2,5-diphenyltetrazolium bromide) proliferation assay, described by Mosmann (1983), is used routinely as a means of rapidly identifying new drug candidates with antitumour activity. Because the screen enables simultaneous measurement of drug toxicity in several tumour cell lines, the assay is also useful as a means of recognizing which cancer subtypes might be particularly susceptible to treatment with the novel drug or class of similar drug compounds. The MTT assay is based on the colorimetric measurement of mitochondrial dehydrogenase enzymes. These enzymes, which catalyse the reduction of the yellow tetrazolium salt MTT to a dark blue formazan dye, are only present in living cells, which are then stained blue (Figure 10.14). Therefore, after solubilization of stained cells with dimethyl sulfoxide (DMSO), the colorimetric absorbance of the resulting solution is proportional to the surviving fraction of cells remaining after exposure to the drug being screened.

The clonogenic assay is based upon the survival of colony-forming cells after drug exposure. Following treatment of plates of cells with drug compound, the remaining viable cells are allowed to recover and proliferate for some days, each forming a colony of healthy cells. The relative number of countable colonies in drug-treated and untreated controls provides a measure of drug activity. Although the clonogenic assay is time consuming, it is often believed to be more accurate, and as a consequence may be used to confirm data on promising drug compounds obtained using the MTT assay.

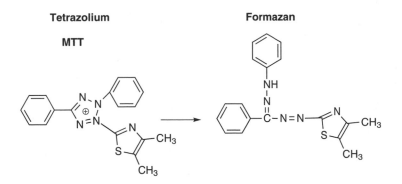

Figure 10.14 Structure of MTT and the reduced compound formazan. Mitochondrial dehydrogenases active in living cells catalyse the reduction of the tetrazolium salt MTT (yellow) to formazan (blue), where the resulting staining intensity corresponds to the number of viable cells. The assay offers a rapid means of measuring the surviving fraction of cells after exposure to a novel drug compound, and therefore the chemosensitivity of cell lines representing certain types of cancer. Reproduced with permission from American Association for Cancer Research, Scudiero et al. (1988) Cancer Res. 48:4827–33.

10.4 Preclinical pharmacology

A candidate drug must undergo toxicological testing *in vivo* before it is given to human subjects. This is a regulatory requirement, where data is submitted to the Medicines and Healthcare products Regulatory Agency (MHRA, the successor to the Medicines Control Agency), when seeking a clinical trials authorization. This will allow clinical trials to be initiated if ethical approval has been granted by the relevant ethics committee (ethical approval is usually obtained from the ethics committee that sits at the NHS trust where the trial is being conducted.

10.4.1 In vivo tumour models

In vivo tumour models are used in drug development to provide data on the pharmacology and toxicology of a new agent, and when used at basic science level, to highlight novel drug targets and pathways that may give rise to new drug strategies. In the United Kingdom, the use of animals in research is tightly regulated by the Home Office, which aims to enforce the animal experimentation legislation as laid down by the Animals and Scientific Procedures Act 1986. The Home Office is responsible for the issue of the *project licence*, which covers a programme of work carried out by a laboratory, and the *personal licence*, which must be obtained by individual personnel carrying out the experimentation after an acceptable level of training. In addition, the dedicated biological services unit within an institution, where housing and breeding of research animals takes place, is subject to stringent regulation and inspection by Home Office inspectors. To obtain a project licence, the type of procedure and the number of animals used must be justified, and are expected to conform to the philosophy of *reduction, refinement and replacement*, where the aim is to reduce the number of animals to the minimum that will provide a statistically significant set of data, to refine the technique so that the procedure causes the minimum pain and distress, and to replace the use of an animal with an alternative model where possible. The controversy surrounding the use of animals in research has led to the founding of various societies with a range of viewpoints, for example FRAME (Fund for the Replacement of Animals in Medical Experiments) found at www.frame.org.uk and the Research Defence Society at www.rds-online.org.uk. The *UKCCCR Guidelines for the Welfare of Animals in Experimental Neoplasia*, compiled by the United Kingdom Co-ordinating Committee on Cancer Research, also makes certain recommendations regarding the use of animals in cancer research. These guidelines are in two parts. The General Recommendations are applicable to all regulated procedures, whereas the Specific Recommendations are more directly targeted to the particular problems of experimental neoplasia, such as cancer-specific complications like cachexia (weight loss) and ulceration. These guidelines are available at the National Cancer Research Network (NCRN) web site www.ncrn.org.uk. Consequently, it is conventional practice for animal experimentation to take place following *in vitro* studies using tumour cell lines, which serves to predict the most promising drug target or agents in a drug screen, and to provide the focus for *in vivo* research. Animal models in cancer research provide a means of evaluating *in vitro* observations that may have been made in cell culture, but in the presence of a host response. For instance, the interaction between tumour cells and stroma, blood supply, and paracrine effects, as well as the occurrence of invasion/ metastasis to adjacent or distant tissues may be studied *in vivo*. Such models are also a regulatory requirement, in order to highlight possible adverse drug reactions and to gain approval for clinical trials in humans.

Tumour xenografts

Tumour xenografts are generated by the transplantation of tumour cells into immuno- deficient mice that will not 'reject' the tumour cells. Such mice strains include athymic mice (genotype *nu/nu* or nude mice) or severe combined immunodeficiency (SCID) mice. The procedure involves taking cells from either a human tumour (tumour explant), or established cell lines grown *in vitro*, and then injecting them into the mouse subcutaneously (Figure 10.15). If the tumour 'takes' a palpable tumour is detectable within 2–4 weeks. Tumour xenografts may be used to answer basic questions in cancer biology by studying the effects of host response on the growth of a tumour derived from a genetically manipulated cell line. Their use carries with it the advantages of a wide

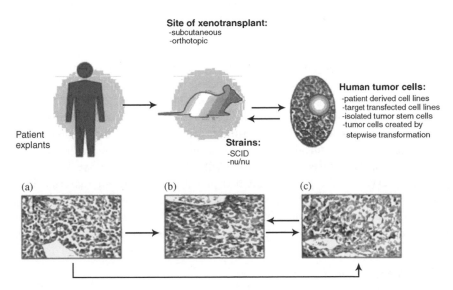

Figure 10.15 Xenograft models involve implantation of tumour cells into immunodeficient mice. Tumour cells may either be explants (cells taken directly from human tumours), or derived from established or genetically manipulated cell lines growing in culture. The xenografts above were all taken from a human non-small cell lung tumour designated LXFL 529. Although, (a) is the original tumour, (b) is a xenograft grown from an explant, and (c) is a xenograft derived from a able LXFL 529 cell line, the histological features appear similar. The close correlation between both the histological features and their sensitivity to chemotherapy (xenografts derived from patient explants predicted chemotherapy response in 90% (19/21) tumours and chemotherapy resistance in 97% (57/59) tumours) helped validate the use of xenografts as *in vivo* tumour models. Reproduced with permission from American Association for Cancer Research, Sausville and Burger. *Cancer Res.* 2006;66:3351–4.

range of available tumour types, which may originate from a number of sources, with the capacity to model certain tumour histologies or gene expression profiles. However, the disadvantage is that the host response to the xenografted tumour is different to that of human tumours in several ways. For instance, the blood supply and angiogenesis taking place in response to a xenograft of human tumour cells in a mouse will be host-rather than tumour-derived, and the stroma will be murine in origin. It is also practically very difficult to implant tumour cells orthotopically, for example, breast tumour cells into a mouse mammary gland; therefore tumours are generated subcutaneously, which is in an artificial tissue compartment.

A genetically manipulated xenograft may then be used to screen for agents that target a particular pathway that are activated or repressed in specific cancers. For example, in breast cancer, the preclinical evaluation of the HER2 inhibitor trastuzumab (Herceptin) was carried out using xenograft models of breast lines genetically manipulated to overexpress HER2, whilst the *in vivo* evaluation of the EGFR tyrosine kinase inhibitor erlotinib (Tarceva) has been carried out using a range of xenografts derived from, for example, lung and brain tumour cells. Xenograft models may also be used to gather preclinical data on the use of a novel anticancer agent in combination with more established therapies, for example, standard agent chemotherapy and/or radiation. The Developmental Therapeutics Program at the NCI routinely carries out evaluation of anticancer drug candidates using xenograft models of the NCI-60 panel of tumour cell lines.

It is desirable for a xenograft model to closely resemble a human tumour both in its natural history, that is, the way the morphological and histological features of the tumour changes with malignant progression, and in their treatment sensitivity. Accordingly, a study was carried out by the Freiburg group to determine whether xenograft models derived from human tumour explants may be used to predict chemo-response. This study specifically attempted to relate the response of the xenograft to chemotherapy administered to the mice with the chemoresponse that had been originally observed in the patient that had provided the tumour material. In doing so, a strong correlation was found, where sensitivity to chemotherapy in the xenografts predicted chemotherapy response in the patient in 90% (19/21) tumours and chemotherapy resistance in 97% (57/59) tumours, as well as showing similar histology.

Transgenic/gene targeted mice

Transgenic and gene targeted organisms are generated by the addition of an exogenous DNA vector construct into its genome. This is carried out either at the zygote level, where DNA is injected directly into an egg immediately following fertilization (Figure 10.16), or by *in vitro* genetic manipulation of embryonic stem (ES) cells (Figure 10.17), which are then injected into host blastocysts to produce a chimera (Figure 10.18). Transfer of DNA into a blastocyst involves either the injection of ES cells into the blastocoel cavity, or by morula aggregation. Morula are extracted from the oviducts of 2.5-day pregnant mice, where at this stage of embryogenesis cells are still capable of mixing undifferentiated ES cells before going on to form a blastocyst. Genetically manipulated ES cells may then be sandwiched between two morulae.

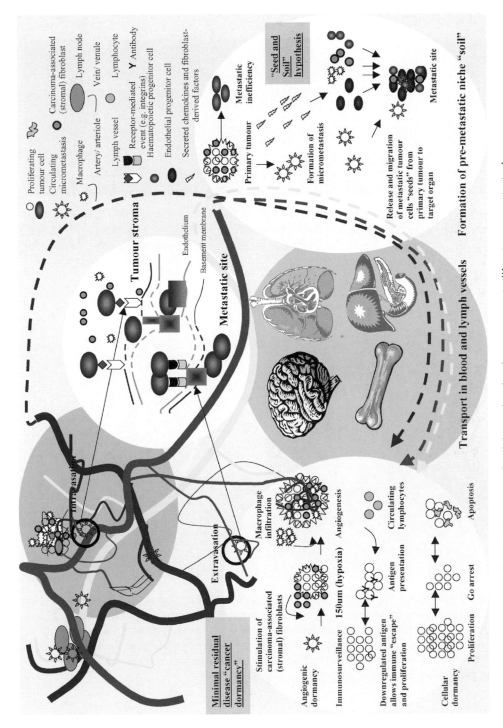

Map 1 Summary of cellular and molecular events controlling tumour metastasis.

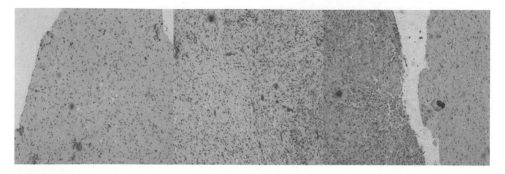

Figure 6.1 Pathology of glioblastoma: typical pathology shows a gradation between normal tissue, infiltrating border zones of hyperplasia and tumour tissue. These samples have been immunohistochemically stained for facilitative glucose transporter Glut-1 (brown). Reproduced with permission from an original photograph by Natalie Charnley, Academic Department of Radiation Oncology, University of Manchester.

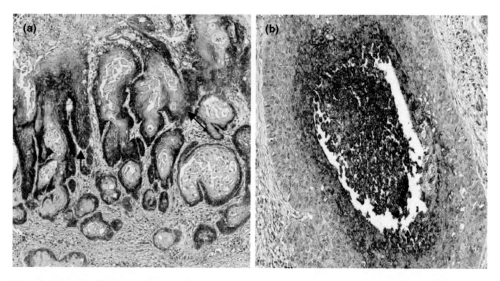

Figure 7.1 Facilitative glucose transporter Glut-1 expression (brown staining) detected by immunohistochemistry in samples of oral squamous cell carcinoma surgically removed from a patient. The highest level of expression was found in (a) invading tumour tissue (arrows) or (b) around necrosis, indicating a biological link with malignancy and hypoxia. Accordingly, Glut-1 may be used as a marker of malignancy, hypoxia and prognosis in a range of solid tumour types. Reproduced from Oliver *et al.* (2004) *Eur. J. Cancer*, 40, 503–7.

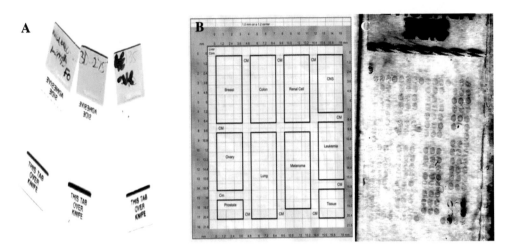

Figure 10.4 Tissue microarrays obtained from the National Cancer Institute TARP laboratory (a), consisting of cores of tumour samples taken from human patients, covering a range of tumour types including breast, colon, renal, central nervous system, ovarian, lung, skin, prostate and leukaemia (b). (c) basic immunohistochemistry was carried out to determine the variation of facilitative glucose transporter Glut-1 expression between normal tissue and across the different tumour types. The circular structures are tissue cores highlighted here by the blue haematoxylin counterstain, which stains cellular components such as nuclei and plasma membranes and provides structural context for immunohistochemical staining when observed by light microscopy.

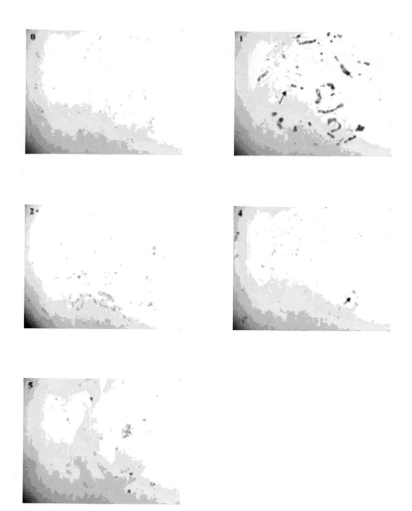

Figure 10.5 Microarrays may also be prepared using cores of agarose embedded pellets of formalin-fixed cell cultures. Pictured here are microarrays obtained from the National Cancer Institute TARP laboratory carrying the NCI-60 panel of tumour cell lines. These were stained for Glut-1 using immunohistochemistry and placed under ×400 magnification. The extent of Glut-1 expression was graded according to the area and intensity of staining (BT549 = 0; MCF7 = 1, OVCAR = 2; HCC2998 = 3, IGROV1 = 4; SNB19 = 5). Reproduced from Evans *et al.* (2007) *Cancer Chemother. Pharmacol.*, Springer.

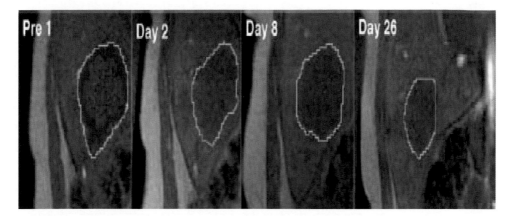

Figure 11.4 DCE-MRI images in a patient with liver metastasis from cholangiocarcinoma taking part in a phase I trial of BMS-582 664, a novel VEGFR/FGFR tyrosine kinase inhibitor. Post-treatment images demonstrate complete absence of contrast agent uptake into this tumor. The subject subsequently had a confirmed partial response by CT scan. Reproduced from Galbraith (2006) *NMR Biomed*. 19: 681–689, John Wiley & Sons Inc.

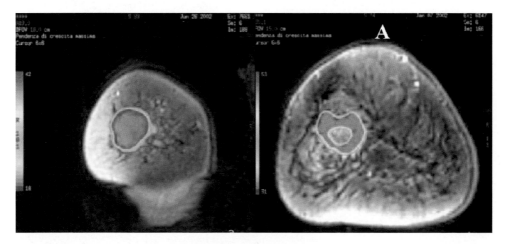

Figure 11.5 DCE-MRI image of a breast tumour in a patient taking part in a study aimed at evaluating MRI as a means of predicting histological response to primary chemotherapy (PCT). These images, showing two characteristic patterns, homogeneous (a) and ring like (b), were taken to provide baseline contrast enhancement values as a measure of tumour volume before treatment. Reproduced from Martincich et al. (2004) *Br. Cancer Res. Treat*. 83: 67–76, Springer.

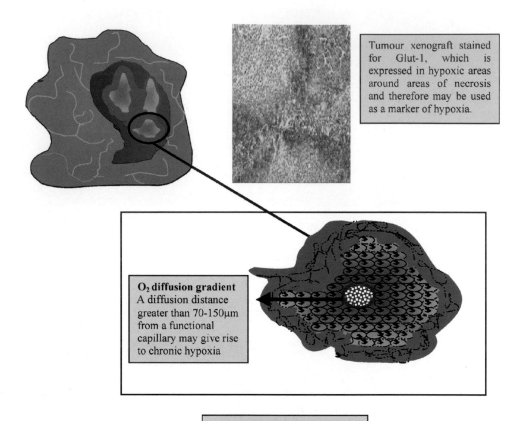

Tumour xenograft stained for Glut-1, which is expressed in hypoxic areas around areas of necrosis and therefore may be used as a marker of hypoxia.

O₂ diffusion gradient
A diffusion distance greater than 70-150μm from a functional capillary may give rise to chronic hypoxia

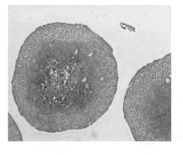

"Artificial tumours"
Tumour cell spheroids are grown *in vitro*, and behave like inside-out tumours. Oxygen and nutrients from the surrounding growth medium diffuse from the outside of the spheroid to the central core, which becomes necrotic. Cells surrounding this necrotic core are hypoxic, and express Glut-1 (Photograph courtesy of Dr Roger Phillips).

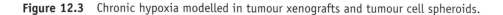

Figure 12.3   Chronic hypoxia modelled in tumour xenografts and tumour cell spheroids.

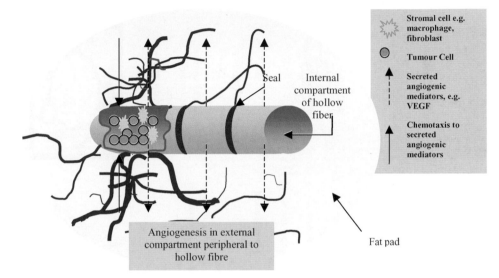

Figure 13.12 The hollow fibre assay for preclinical evaluation of anti-angiogenic agents.

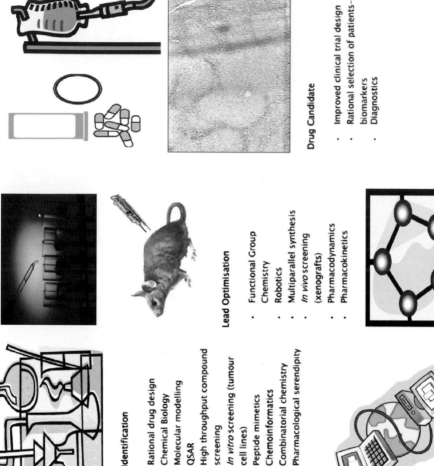

Target Identification and Validation

- Cancer genome sequencing
- Expression profiling of malignant versus non-malignant cell lines
- Gene cloning
- Functional Genomics and Proteomics

Lead Identification

- Rational drug design
- Chemical Biology
- Molecular modelling
- QSAR
- High throughput compound screening
- *In vitro* screening (tumour cell lines)
- Peptide mimetics
- Chemoinformatics
- Combinatorial chemistry
- Pharmacological serendipity

Lead Optimisation

- Functional Group Chemistry
- Robotics
- Multiparallel synthesis
- *In vivo* screening (xenografts)
- Pharmacodynamics
- Pharmacokinetics

Drug Candidate

- Improved clinical trial design
- Rational selection of patients – biomarkers
- Diagnostics

Map 2 The discovery, optimisation and clinical development of novel anticancer agents.

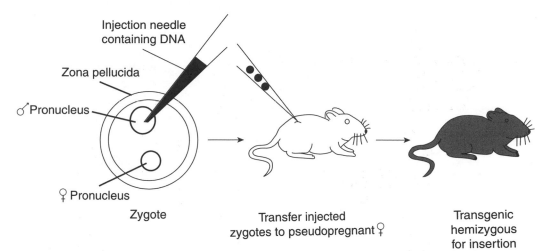

Figure 10.16 Transgenic mice may be made by zygote injection. Zygotes are extracted from the oviducts of female mice that have been mated the previous day and placed under a microscope fitted by two micromanipulator setups. One will carry a blunt micropipette that is used to hold the zygote in place, while the other will carry the injection needle which is filled with solution containing the DNA construct which will integrate into the mouse genome. After injecting the DNA into one of the zygote pronuclei, they are transferred to into the oviduct of a pseudopregnant female. Usually, 20 to 30 embryos are transferred at a time to ensure an adequate number of full-term births. Of these, 10–30% will be transgenic (hemizygous) and contain one site of DNA integration. Reprinted with permission from Sedivy and Joyner (1992).

The blastocyst or the morula aggregate is then injected into a pseudopregnant mouse (a female mouse in oestrus and mated with a vasectomized male) using a pair of micromanipulators. The resulting animals, or *founder* animals, are used to establish breeding colonies of genetically manipulated mice.

Transgenic organisms are usually generated to determine the biological effects of gain of function (knock-in) events such as overexpression or misexpression of a gene. Gene targeting experiments, however, involve targeted knock-out of the gene (Figure 10.19). As with tumour xenografts, virtually all cancer research involving transgenic organisms is carried out in mice.

A range of transgenic or gene targeted tumour mice (sometimes referred to as genetically engineered mouse models (GEMMs)), are in use corresponding to different tumour types. These typically involve the insertion of vectors containing an oncogene (*knock-in mice*). Often, this gene is placed under the control of a tissue-specific promoter that targets expression to the relevant tissue. For example, there are transgenic breast tumour models available that overexpress oncogenes such as *HER2* and *PyMT*, which when placed under the control of the mammalian mammary tumour virus (MMTV) in a transgenic plasmid vector, are specifically expressed in mammary gland tissue. This strategy overcomes the problem of embryonic lethality, which may occur if the genomic change is generalized. Figure 10.20 shows a plasmid vector used to generate

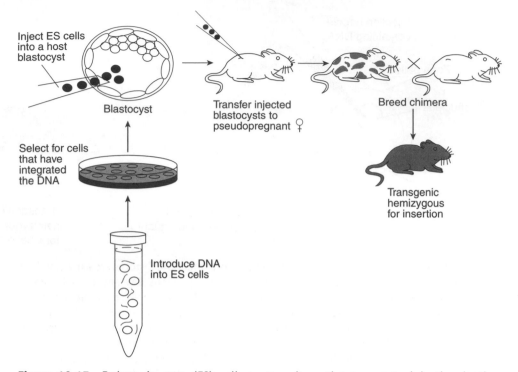

Figure 10.17 Embryonic stem (ES) cells are an alternative to zygote injection in the generation of transgenic mice. DNA is introduced into ES cells *in vitro* by electroporation, where a suspension of cells is given an electric shock to deliver DNA into the nucleus. The DNA construct will have a selection marker for example, *neo* (Figure 10.21) which will allow preferential growth of successfully transfected ES cells in selection medium. Cells from one clonal population (i.e. from a colony derived from a single transfected cell) will be used to produce a chimera, which when born and bred, will in turn produce ES cell-derived offspring. Of these, around 50% will be hemizygous for the newly integrated DNA. Reprinted with permission from Sedivy and Joyner (1992).

HER2-overexpressing mice. These models display many of the pathological features of human breast cancer. Alternatively, a cancer may result from a mutation or decreased activity of a tumour suppressor gene. A GEMM showing *knock-out* or *targeted mutation* of this gene loses its protective function and undergoes the malignant changes necessary to develop a tumour. There are a number of different strategies in the preparation of vectors, which are described very effectively in a recent review by Olive and Tuveson (2006). A mouse showing gene knock-out may be generated by the integration of a construct to create a null allele at the locus of the gene of interest. An idealized targeting construct (Figure 10.21) is built from four components. These are:

1. The targeting construct: this consists of a positive selection marker, for example, *neo*, which enables selection of cells that have incorporated the DNA into the genome. This is driven by a promoter which is active in ES, such as phosphoglycerate kinase.

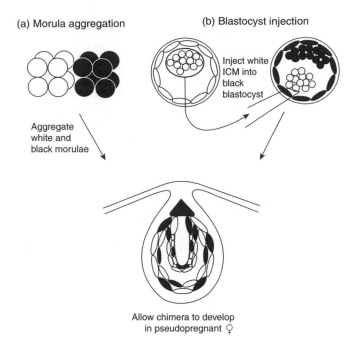

Figure 10.18 Making a chimera. Two procedures for making a chimeric embryo include morula aggregation (a), where genetically manipulated ES cells are sandwiched between two morulae that have been extracted from 2.5-day pregnant females. Alternatively, blastocysts may be directly injected with ES cells (b). The blastocyst or the morula aggregate is then injected into a pseudopregnant mouse (a female mouse in oestrus and mated with a vasectomized male) using a pair of micromanipulators. The resulting chimera is then allowed to develop in a pseudopregnant female. Reprinted with permission from Sedivy and Joyner (1992).

The sequence is surrounded by *lox P* sites, which will enable its eventual removal from the targeted allele. *Lox P* (locus of X-over P1) is a sequence of DNA which enables binding of the site-specific DNA-recombinase Cre (cyclization recombination). Cre catalyses a process known as *reciprocal recombination*, which occurs by cutting and pasting of double-stranded DNA between the two *lox P* sites, and will lead to removal of the selection cassette and eventual generation of the null allele.

2. A homologous, isogenic (coming from the same inbred strain of mouse) portion of DNA of approximate length 5–8 kb which is evenly split so as to flank the targeting construct both up and downstream. This is important so that the targeting construct integrates with the genomic DNA at the locus corresponding to the targeted gene. Therefore, in the genome of certain mouse cells, the genomic region that includes the gene of interest is now paired to DNA sequence that is complementary except for the gene of interest, which has been 'replaced' by an alternative *floxed* (flanked by *lox P* sites) DNA sequence, which typically codes for the selection marker that enables the screening and isolation of cells showing this mutation.

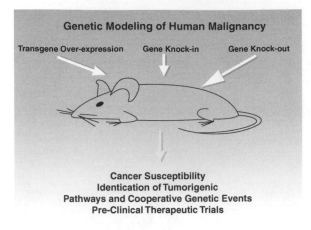

Figure 10.19 Strategies used in the design of genetically engineered mouse models (GEMMs) for the study of human malignancy.

3. A negative selection marker, such as DT-A, will be placed downstream of the 3′ homologous sequence to screen against random integration events.

4. A linearization site will be placed at some distance 3′ downstream of the negative selection marker to protect it from degradation of the ends after linearization of the plasmid, which may be carried out as part of the characterization, analysis and recycling of the gene targeting vector.

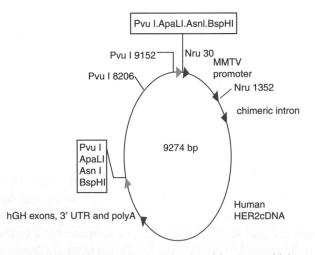

Figure 10.20 Map of the 9274 bp HER2 transgenic plasmid vector, which consists of a MMTV promoter that specifically targets expression of the *HER2* gene to mammary gland tissue. The Nru sites that flank the MMTV promoter are there to enhance *in vivo* expression of the gene. Reproduced with permission from American Association for Cancer Research, Carver and Pandolfi. *Clin. Cancer Res*. 2006;12:5305–11.

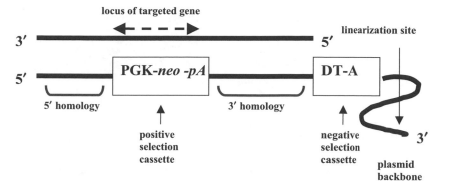

Figure 10.21 A generalized gene targeting construct (adapted from Papaioannou and Behringer (2005)).

The advantage of GEMM tumour models is that their development within the host more accurately reflects the natural history and stages of malignant progression in spontaneously occurring tumours, displaying features of malignant progression from hyperplasia to advanced carcinoma and the development of metastasis (Figure 10.22). The *PyMT* breast tumour model, for example, possesses morphological features and biomarker expression similar to that of human breast tumours (Figure 10.23). In this way, GEMMs may be used to model pathological criteria used in the staging of human tumours according to the tumour/node/metastasis (TNM) system (Section 6.2). GEMMs also provide a means of revealing important novel pathways in cancer. This may be approached either through observation of spontaneous tumours that may arise in genotypically novel tumour models, that is, showing knock-in or knock-out of a gene of interest (gene X), with as yet unknown phenotype, or by carrying out breeding crosses between such mice and another transgenic mouse model with an

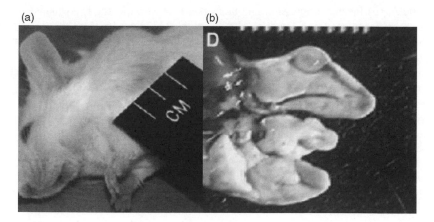

Figure 10.22 Transgenic breast cancer model with a palpable breast tumour appearing after weeks (a) and lung metastases (b). Reproduced with permission from American Association for Cancer Research, Finkle *et al.* (2004) *Clin. Cancer Res.* 10:2499–2511.

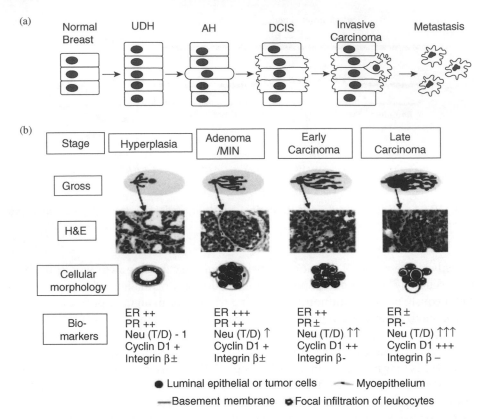

Figure 10.23   The natural history of human breast cancer as compared to the PyMT transgenic mouse model. (a) Normal breast epithelium will form premalignant lesions that may undergo transformation steps from usual ductal hyperplasia (UDH), through to atypical hyperplasia (AH) and then ductal carcinoma *in situ* (DCIS). Such premalignant lesions may go on to form invasive breast carcinoma and metastasis to other sites such as the brain or lung. Adapted from Tannock *et al.* (2005). (b) Tumour progression and biomarker expression in the PyMT mouse model of breast cancer (Reproduced from Lin *et al.*, *Am. J. Pathol.* 2003 Nov; 163(5):2113–26, High Wire Press Stanford University Libraries – US.), where four stages of malignant progression– hyperplasia, adenoma, early carcinoma and late carcinoma – emerge as the mouse ages, designated according to the extent of cellular proliferation and invasion from the ducts into the surrounding normal mammary tissue. Gross and microhistology are illustrated, as well as changes in cellular morphology and biomarker expression. In this model, analogous to human tumours, two markers of breast malignancy, HER-2 and cyclin D1, become more pronounced as the tumours progress. MIN - mammary intraepithelial neoplasia.

established tumour-generating phenotype (mouse Y). After several generations, offspring showing the genetic characteristics of both models will be produced, and their capacity to develop tumours evaluated. Any increase or decrease in the incidence and rate of malignant progression relative to the parental mouse Y will relate to the tumour-promoting or inhibiting role of gene X in the pathology of this type of cancer. The generation of such models may also be used as tailor made models in the preclinical evaluation of novel anticancer agents directed against these genes as targets. The mouse overexpressing the tyrosine kinase receptor HER2/erbB2 was developed by Genetech Inc (California, United States) and used in preclinical studies to gather data on the use of the monoclonal HER2-targeted antibody Herceptin in early stage HER2-positive tumours. Examples of GEMMs used to model a range of cancers are shown in Table 10.2.

10.4.2 Comparative oncology

The use of non-human animal tumour models is subject to the species differences which may influence the structure and function of tumours at cellular, molecular and tissue level. For instance, tumour cells may show species-dependent differences in the rate and degree of differentiation, the expression and activity of genes and cell signalling pathways. At the tissue level, there may be species-specific differences in the natural history and clinical course of certain cancers, such as aggressiveness, invasion and the pattern of metastasis. The aim of comparative oncology is to gather clinical and scientific data on inter-species differences that may be applied to the development of novel anticancer therapies, as well as to the optimization of current cancer treatment for human and veterinary use. As is the case for clinical trials in human patients, this depends on collaboration between experimental and clinical oncologists, but also makes use of the input of veterinary oncologists, who are responsible for animal patients and contribute to the collection of data on cancer occurring in companion animals. The potential input of comparative oncology in the development of anticancer agents for human cancers is illustrated by Figure 10.24. A study carried out by Dobson *et al.* (2002) between 1997 and 1998, which analysed data from pet insurance claims, aimed to analyse cancer incidence in dogs in the UK. In this cohort of 3242 claims, 2546 were identified as being related to canine neoplasia, which translated into a crude overall incidence estimate of 1948 cases per 100 000 dogs per year. Younger dogs were less likely to be affected, where the risk increased sharply after age 6 years and peaked at 10 years, where the incidence rate was 81 cases per 100 000 dogs. To exclude bias due to the higher proportion of younger dogs covered by pet insurance plans, epidemiological data was adjusted to an age-standardized incidence rate of 2671 cases per 100 000 dogs. Age-standardized incidence rates by tumour site are shown in Figure 10.25, the most prolific canine cancers affecting skin and soft tissue (1437 per 100 000) followed by the alimentary tract (210 per 100 000) and the mammary glands (205 per 100 000). Also of note was the incidence of bone cancers, including osteosarcoma, at 83 cases per 100 000, and nasal/respiratory cancers, which included lung tumours, at 32 cases per 100 000. Organizations such as the Veterinary Cancer Registry (www.vetcancerregistry.com), which collates clinical data submitted by veterinary oncologists, are providing a means of studying the epidemiology of companion animal cancers. Large scale sequencing projects such as the *Canine Genome Project*, a collaboration between the University of California, Berkeley, the University of Oregon, and the Fred Hutchinson Cancer Research Center; and the *Cat Genome Project*, based at the Laboratory of Genomic Diversity at the NCI, have also provided comprehensive data on the expression of genes

Table 10.2 Examples of GEMM tumour models

Tumour type	Genotypic alteration	Allele type	Promoter	Phenotype
Lung non-small cell lung carcinoma	K-rasG12D-LA2, K-rasLSLG12D, Or K-rasLSLG12V	Conditional knock-ins or transgenic	Endogenous or h-actin; Adeno-Cre	Multistage disease progression from AAH to Ad to Ad C.
Small cell lung carcinoma	RBFl + p53Fl	Conditional knock-outs	Endogenous; Adeno-Cre	Bronchiole hyperplasia; SCLC; metastases to bone, brain, adrenal gland, ovary and liver.
Breast	c-met ± c-myc	Transgenic	Tet-inducible MMTV or MSCV-LTR Syngeneic transplant	c-myc alone results in increased branching and hyperplasia c-met alone results in non-progressing MIN Combination results in multistage disease from high-grade neoplasia to Ad C.
Breast	HER2/ErbB2 +	Transgenic	MMTV	See Figure 10.20
Breast	PyMT	Transgenic	MMTV	See Figure 10.23
Prostate	NKX3.1-KO + PTEN-KO + p27-knock-out	Conventional knock-outs	Endogenous	NKX3.1; PTEN compound mutants display multistage disease progression from HYP to LG-PIN to HG-PIN/early carcinoma, including metastases to LNs p27 loss enhances progression and is sensitive to gene dosage. Androgen independence following androgen ablation.
Colon	APC$^{Fl-580S}$	Conditional knock-in	Endogenous; Adeno-Cre	Colorectal Ad, with half demonstrating submucosal invasion (Ad C).
Ovarian	SV40 T and t antigens	Transgenic	MISIIR	Poorly differentiated epithelial carcinomas; differentiated parts resemble serous Ad C. Testicular tumours in male mice.

(*continued*)

Table 10.2 (*Continued*)

Tumour type	Genotypic alteration	Allele type	Promoter	Phenotype
Pancreas	K-rasLSLG12D, p53LSLR172H ascites, pleural surfaces, and diaphragm	Conditional knock-ins	Endogenous; Pdx1-Cre or p48-Cre	Multistage disease progression from PanIN to ductal Ad C, including desmoplastic response. P53R172H mutation conferred decreased latency and genomic instability. Extensive metastases to lung, regional lymph nodes, liver, adrenal gland, ascites, pleural surfaces and diaphragm.

AAH, atypical adenomatous hyperplasia; Ad, adenoma; Ad C, adenocarcinoma; HG, high grade; HYP, hyperplasia; LG, low grade; MIN, mammary intraepithelial neoplasia; MMTV, mouse mammary tumour virus; PanIN, pancreatic intraepithelial neoplasia; PIN, prostatic intraepithelial neoplasia; SCLS, small cell lung carcinoma. Adapted from Singh and Johnson, 2006.

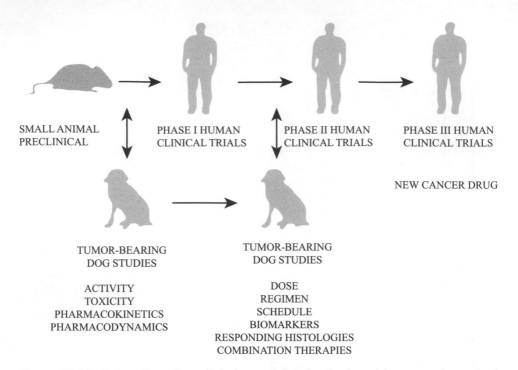

SMALL ANIMAL
PRECLINICAL

PHASE I HUMAN
CLINICAL TRIALS

PHASE II HUMAN
CLINICAL TRIALS

PHASE III HUMAN
CLINICAL TRIALS

NEW CANCER DRUG

TUMOR-BEARING
DOG STUDIES

ACTIVITY
TOXICITY
PHARMACOKINETICS
PHARMACODYNAMICS

TUMOR-BEARING
DOG STUDIES

DOSE
REGIMEN
SCHEDULE
BIOMARKERS
RESPONDING HISTOLOGIES
COMBINATION THERAPIES

Figure 10.24 Integration of preclinical experimental animal models, companion animal studies and clinical trials in humans. From the COTC brochure courtesy of www.cancer.gov. Dog studies may be integrated into a generalized preclinical and clinical research protocol following xenograft or GEMM mouse studies to gather pharmacological and toxicological data, or prior to phase II human studies, in order to provide comparative dose escalation studies, histological data, and supplementary data on treatment response. The advantage of using a larger species such as the dog is that the anatomy and physiology, as well as the natural history of the tumour, may more closely resemble that of humans.

	Malignant (%)	Benign (%)	Not specified (%)	Incidence rate (/100,000 dogs/year)
Skin and soft tissue	21	69	10	1437
Alimentary	44	6	50	210
Mammary	26	13	61	205
Urogenital	21	5	74	139
Lymphoid	97	2	1	134
Endocrine	8	1	90	113
Oral/pharyngeal	29	54	17	112
Bone	73	0	27	83
Nasal/respiratory	53	0	47	32
Central nervous system	38	6	56	26
All tumour sites	28	41	30	2671

Figure 10.25 Epidemiology of canine cancers by site. A study carried out between 1997 and 1998, which analysed data from pet health insurance claims, estimated the total age-standardized incidence rate of canine cancer to be 2671 per 100 000 cases. Reproduced from Dobson *et al.* (2002) *Journal of Small Animal Practice* 43, 240–246, Blackwell Publishing Ltd.

and therefore drug targets influential in tumorigenesis, which validate further study and use of companion animal cancers to develop novel therapies.

The core comparative oncology programme at the NCI, the Canine Comparative Oncology and Genomics Consortium (CCOGC), has been setup to promote and carry out preclinical and clinical studies involving canine tumours. The growing interest in comparative oncology is due to a number of factors. The ethical argument is that the study of spontaneously occurring companion animal cancers is commensurate with *reduction, refinement and replacement* as the animals involved are already being treated for cancer in a clinical setting. The scientific argument is that companion animals like dogs may present with certain features of cancer, such as tumour volume, heterogeneity, recurrence and metastasis that more closely resemble those of humans than the more widely used xenograft and GEMM models. The similarity in anatomy and size may also produce a more predictive model. Limitations of using companion animals, however, may include cost; the animal is larger therefore the dose of drug used is higher. Furthermore, although the average lifespan of the dog allows these 'clinical trials' to take place more rapidly than in humans, at a timescale of around 1–3 years, studies will still take longer to complete than those involving mouse models. Table 10.3 illustrates examples of spontaneous tumours arising in companion animals that are the subject of comparative oncology studies and preclinical evaluation of novel therapies.

Much of the work carried out in the field of comparative oncology seems to be in two fundamental areas. First, studies are carried out to determine the correlation between the biological and pathological features, the clinical course and epidemiology of human and companion animal tumours. As the species similarities and differences emerge, this knowledge may be applied to subsequent studies where companion animals with these cancers are recruited to preclinical studies where novel therapies may be evaluated. Canine osteosarcoma (Figure 10.26), for instance, is an aggressive, often metastatic bone cancer that shows many of the biological and epidemiological features of its human counterpart, with an incidence rate (according to the study carried out by Dobson *et al.*, 2002) of 70 cases per 100 000 dogs in the United Kingdom. Currently, the standard treatment in both humans and dogs is surgery, which, because it is most likely to affect the appendicular skeleton, involves amputation of the limb. This is usually followed by a chemotherapy regimen consisting of doxorubicin, methotrexate and cisplatin and/or radiotherapy, which in humans, leads to a 70% survival rate after 5 years, and in dogs, a 60% survival rate after 1 year. This disease has been the subject of a range of comparative oncology studies and, following on from these, preclinical studies to evaluate strategies such as the delivery of cisplatin in a STEALTH liposome formulation. This particular study was carried out in 2002 at the University of Wisconsin-Madison, allowing preclinical evaluation of a formulation with the potential to reduce the severity of cisplatin toxicity when used in man- this formulation proved to be tolerated at five times the dose than that of free cisplatin in the dogs involved in this study. Targeted inhibitors of proteins highly expressed in tumours such as insulin-like growth factor-1 and the receptor tyrosine kinases have also been the subject of canine osteosarcoma studies. The inhalation technology apparatus shown in Figure 10.27 is similar to the nebulizer system used for the delivery of bronchodilators for the treatment

Table 10.3 Examples of companion animal cancers that have been used or are amenable for use in the preclinical development of drugs

Species	Histology	Biology	Preclinical application
Breast			
Human	Ductal carcinoma *in situ*	• Risk related to lifetime oestrogen exposure	
	Lobular carcinoma	• Localized and regional at diagnosis	
		• 60% of are oestrogen receptor positive	
		• c-erbB-overexpression	
		• 86% 5 year survival	
Canine	50% mammary tumours are benign	• Early reduction in oestrogen exposure is protective	
	Malignant carcinoma most common; probably lobular in origin	• Canine sex-hormone cycle is distinct from humans	
		• 45% Oestrogen-receptor positive	
Lung			
Human	Non-small cell lung cancer most common (carcinoma, adenocarcinoma, large cell carcinoma)	• Common metastasis sites: pleura, lung, bone, brain,	• BCG (Bacillus Calmette-Guerin vaccine) combined with surgery
	Small cell lung cancer account for 18% of diagnoses	• pericardium, liver	• Immunotherapy (L–MTP-PEh (Liposomal muranyl tripeptide phosphatidylethanolamine))
		• 15% 5-year survival overall	• Leuteinizing hormone releasing hormone analogue

(continued)

Table 10.3 (*Continued*)

Species	Histology	Biology	Preclinical application
Canine	Adenocarcinoma most common	• Advanced disease at diagnosis • Mutations in *K-ras* identified • Survival <2 months following surgery if lesion >5 cm or metastatic • Survival >1 year if lesion <5 cm and not metastatic	• Interleukin-2 inhalation • Inhalational chemotherapy
Osteosarcoma Human	High grade Complex karyotype primary tumour with no consistent translocation	• Primary bone tumour most commonly appendicular • Aggressive metastatic phenotype, metastases to lungs • 70% survival at 5 years with chemotherapy	
Canine	High grade Complex karyotype with no consistent translocation	• Primary bone tumour most commonly appendicular • Aggressive metastatic phenotype, metastases to lungs common • 60% survival at 1 year with chemotherapy • Occurs in older dogs • More rapid disease course than in humans	• L-MTP-PEh (Liposomal muramyl tripeptide phosphatidylethanolamine • IL-2 and chemotherapy inhalation • STEALTH liposome encapsulated cisplatin • IGF-I blockage (OncoLAR) • Split tyrosine kinase inhibitor

Adapted from Hansen and Khanna (2004).

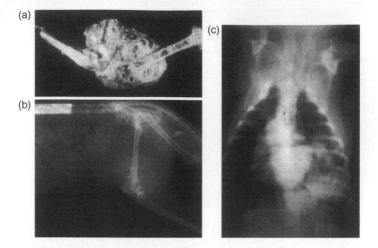

Figure 10.26 Spontaneous tumours occurring in companion dogs are being used to model human tumours for the development of novel drug strategies. The panel (from LAWHEAD/BAKER. *Introduction to Veterinary Science*, 1st ed. © 2005 Delmar Learning, a part of Cengage Learning, Inc. Reproduced by permission. www.cengage.com/permissions) shows (a) a case of the malignant bone tumour osteosarcoma (b) a radiographic image of the osteosarcoma; and (c) a radiograph of a dog with a metastasis in the chest resulting from a primary tumour elsewhere.

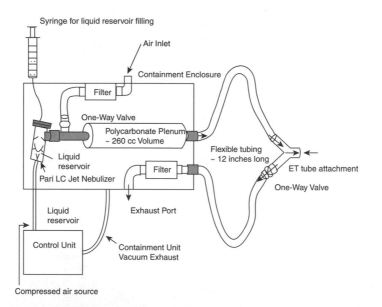

Figure 10.27 Device used for inhalational chemotherapy in clinical trials involving dogs with lung carcinoma. The study, carried out at the University of Wisconsin-Madison in 1999, was aimed at determining the safety and efficacy of inhaled chemotherapy in spontaneously arising primary and metastatic lung cancers. The dogs received new formulations of either paclitaxel or doxorubicin by the inhalation route every 2 weeks using the specially designed aerosol device, followed by radiographic assessment of response. In carrying out this study, it was possible to evaluate a novel means of delivering chemotherapy locally to lung tumours, with the objective of achieving adequate concentrations of drug in the tumour in the absence of serious systemic effects. Reproduced with permission from American Association of Cancer Research, from Hershey *et al.* (1999) 5: 2653–2659 *Clin. Cancer Res.*

of chronic obstructive airways disease, and has been used to deliver standard agent chemotherapy and experimental agents in canine cancer. When evaluating inhaled doxorubicin and cisplatin in dogs with lung cancer, results were again favourable in terms of reducing the toxicity of chemotherapy, where there was no observable systemic toxicity and only very limited clinical signs of local pulmonary toxicity. Other experimental agents used in canine studies include the immunotherapy LMTP-PE (liposomal muramyl tripeptide phosphatidylethanolamine), a liposome-encapsulated, synthetic macrophage activator, which has been evaluated in dogs with osteosarcoma and mammary cancer.

11
Clinical trials

11.1 Introduction

Clinical trials in cancer differ from those in other therapeutic areas particularly in phase I. In other therapeutic areas phase I trials are carried out in healthy volunteers whereas the risk of adverse effects from anticancer agents would render this unethical when evaluating anticancer agents. Phase I clinical trials are carried out to characterize the pharmacodynamics, pharmacokinetics, maximum tolerated dose (MTD), and dose limiting toxicity (DLT) of the new agent. These studies are carried out in patients with advanced cancer refractory to other treatment and with normal organ function, where the usual starting dose is one tenth the lethal dose (LD_{10}) in mice or the most sensitive animal model. The primary purpose of phase I studies is to carry out a dose escalation study, or to titrate the MTD that can be used in humans. The dose is typically escalated on a Fibonacci scale, for example, 1, 2, 3, 5, 8, 13, 21 mg/m^2, so that doses plateau out, that is, increase by decreasing multiples of the previous dose. Phase II and phase III trials have a similar design and objectives as for other disease groups. In phase II, a small cohort of patients diagnosed with the cancer for which the new agent is intended is recruited, in order to gather data on drug safety and efficacy. For phase II trials, larger numbers of patients are involved, where they are randomized to receive the new treatment or the 'gold standard', that is, the established treatment regimen. Rather than being placebo controlled trials, as is often the case for other therapeutic areas, phase II and III trials in cancer patients often involve comparison of drug combinations. Therefore, these studies may compare a standard treatment combination with the same combination plus the new treatment as an add-on therapy, or alternatively, the trial may be a comparison between a standard treatment combination of two or three anticancer agents and an alternative treatment combination where one of these agents has been 'swapped' for the novel agent. Clinical trials currently taking place for the treatment of cancer can be found at www.clinicaltrials.gov.

Clinical trials have defined endpoints relating to clinical outcome. Therefore the new anticancer agent is evaluated in terms of treatment response and the effect on survival

Cancer Chemotherapy   Rachel Airley
© 2009 John Wiley & Sons, Ltd.

rate. Treatment response is defined as:

- complete response (100% response, the tumour disappears)
- partial response (tumour volume reduced by 50%) -stable disease (no change)
- progressive disease (tumour has increased in size, metastasis).

The length of time for patient follow-up is typically 5 years, so that 5-year survival rates may be measured. These may be expressed as disease-free, metastasis-free, local-recurrence (relapse at the same site as the original tumour)-free or overall survival. The drug is also evaluated in terms of changes of prolongation of life, and the time to recurrence and/or metastasis. Survival rates are assessed statistically using Kaplan–Meier analysis, which estimates survival probabilities by comparing the 'events', that is, metastasis, recurrence or death taking place at a point in time during patient follow-up. Figure 11.1 shows Kaplan–Meier plots from a phase III trial of the HER2 targeted monoclonal antibody trastuzumab (Herceptin) in breast cancer post surgery, where there is a clear disease-specific survival advantage in the patients receiving Herceptin,

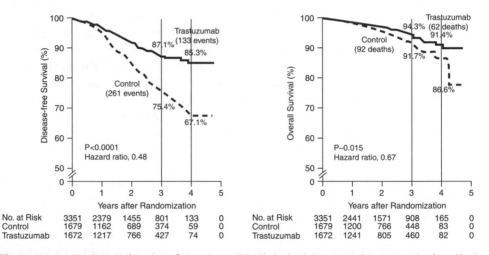

Figure 11.1 Kaplan–Meier plots from phase III clinical trials comparing a standard cyclical regimen of doxorubicin and cyclophosphamide followed by paclitaxel (control group) with the same regimen plus the HER2-targeted monoclonal antibody trastuzumab (Herceptin), in patients with surgically removed HER2-positive breast cancer (Reproduced with permission from Romond *et al.* (2005) *N. Engl. J. Med.* 353:1673–84, Copyright © 2005 Massachusetts Medical Society. All rights reserved.) Disease-free survival (left) is distinct from overall survival (right) as causes of death unrelated to the cancer are excluded from the data. After 5 years follow-up, it is clearly apparent that the patients who received Herceptin had a higher probability of surviving the cancer. However, the difference in overall survival rate between Herceptin and control groups is not as distinct, suggesting that in the patient group receiving Herceptin, mortality rate may in some measure be determined by factors other than the disease. For instance, Herceptin was found to increase the number of deaths due to congestive cardiac failure.

but a less significant difference in overall survival rates, perhaps as a result of factors unrelated to the cancer, such as the cardiac effects observed in the patients receiving Herceptin. In this way, Kaplan–Meier analysis can reveal changes in survival rate afforded by the addition of a new anticancer agent and make distinctions between the specific tumour response and the overall response of the patient.

11.2 Evaluation of treatment response

Evaluating treatment response involves a range of imaging techniques, such as Doppler ultrasonography (Figure 11.2), positron emission tomography (PET) (Figure 11.3) and magnetic resonance imaging (MRI) (Figures 11.4 and 11.5). PET is based on the use of proton-rich isotopes as tracers. These imaging techniques allow assessment of treatment response by calculating changes in tumour volume as well as metabolic changes such as glucose metabolism and blood perfusion, which provide a surrogate measure of tumour function but may also be necessary to evaluate the pharmacological activity of chemotherapy targeted against tumour vasculature or the tumour microenvironment. Imaging technology may also be used at an earlier stage in the drug discovery process, for instance, where microPET systems are used to image tumours in mice. The application of an imaging technology depends upon the tracer used, of which there are several (Table 11.1). The use of isotopes of fluorinated glucose [18F] fluorodeoxyglucose (FDG) is based upon the Warburg effect, which describes the increased uptake of glucose in malignant relative to normal tissue. FDG, like glucose, is phosphorylated to form FDG-6-phosphate upon entry into the cell by hexokinases, in order to maintain the concentration gradient required for facilitated uptake by membrane-bound glucose transporter proteins (Figure 11.6). During glycolysis, glucose-6-phosphate undergoes a series of metabolic steps to form pyruvate, which is then used to manufacture acetyl

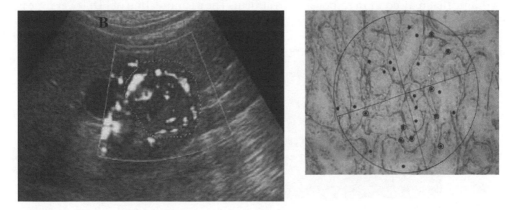

Figure 11.2 Echo contrast-enhanced power Doppler ultrasonography in renal cell carcinoma. This study was carried out to relate contrast parameters with angiogenesis, where the bright areas showing a high ratio of pixels to background corresponded to areas with high microvessel density measured using a graticule. Reproduced with permission from Kabakci, N. *et al.* (2005) *Journal of Ultrasound in Medicine*, 24, 747–753, American Institute of Ultrasound in Medicine.

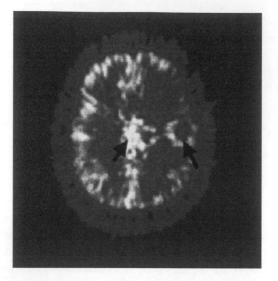

Figure 11.3   18F-FDG PET image from a patient with high grade glioma. Medial and lateral (see arrows) and normal grey matter show high tracer uptake, reflecting the high level of Glut-1 glucose transporter in tumour tissue as well as the blood-brain barrier. Reproduced from Aboagye and Price (2003) *New Drugs* 21:169–81, Springer.

CoA, for use in the Krebs' cycle or the synthesis of fatty acids. FDG, however, does not undergo isomerization, and therefore becomes trapped in the cell. The rate of FDG accumulation is proportional to the rate of glucose utilization by the cell, which, due to the Warburg effect, is higher in tumour cells. Thus, a radioactive isotope of FDG is detectable in larger quantities during a PET scan in tumours than the surrounding normal tissue, allowing an estimate of tumour volume, and any changes in tumour volume that may occur in response to treatment. The accumulation of FDG over time is

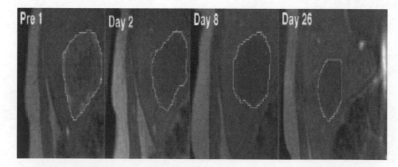

Figure 11.4   DCE-MRI images in a patient with liver metastasis from cholangiocarcinoma taking part in a phase I trial of BMS-582 664, a novel VEGFR/FGFR tyrosine kinase inhibitor. Post-treatment images demonstrate complete absence of contrast agent uptake into this tumor. The subject subsequently had a confirmed partial response by CT scan. Reproduced from Galbraith (2006) *NMR Biomed.* 19: 681–689, John Wiley & Sons Inc.

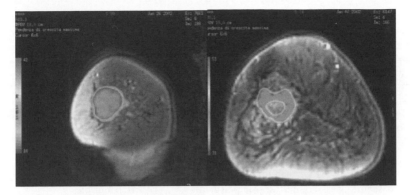

Figure 11.5 DCE-MRI image of a breast tumour in a patient taking part in a study aimed at evaluating MRI as a means of predicting histological response to primary chemotherapy (PCT). These images, showing two characteristic patterns, homogeneous (a) and ring like (b), were taken to provide baseline contrast enhancement values as a measure of tumour volume before treatment. Reproduced from Martincich et al. (2004) *Br. Cancer Res. Treat.* 83: 67–76, Springer.

measured using tracer kinetics, where parameters such as MR_{glc}, the metabolic rate of glucose; C_{glc}, circulating glucose, and the rate of glucose transport and phosphorylation are all interrelated. Alternatively, the standard uptake value (SUV) is a semiquantitative measure of FDG accumulation which assumes complete glucose uptake and negligible dephosphorylation, but takes into account the dose of tracer injected and the patient's volume of distribution. In the drug discovery process, FDG-PET may be used to measure generalized features of tumour response, such as a reduction in tumour volume, or as a surrogate measure of the activity of novel agents that block drug targets that interfere with glycolytic metabolism, for example hypoxia inducible factor-1 or

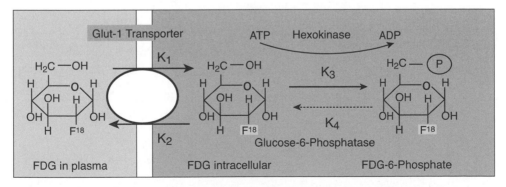

Figure 11.6 Transport and metabolism of the PET tracer fluorodeoxyglucose (FDG). This analogue of glucose is taken up by the facilitative glucose transporter, which is overexpressed in a wide range of tumours. The concentration gradient is maintained by rapid phosphorylation of FDG catalysed by the glycolytic enzyme hexokinase to form FDG-6-phosphate. This metabolite can undergo no further metabolism so accumulates in the cytoplasm of malignant cells. Reproduced with permission from American Association for Cancer Research, Kelloff et al. (2005) *Clin. Cancer Res.* (2005) 11: 2785–2808.

Table 11.1 Functional and molecular imaging techniques potentially useful in drug discovery programmes such as MRI and PET rely on the use of tracers that act as markers of tumour growth and/or functionality, or detect the expression and activity of the drug target

Imaging technology	Use	Marker/contrast agent
MRI	Tumour vascular function	Gadolinium DTPA
	Measurement of blood volume	Iron oxide particles
Diffusion weighted MRI	Rates and diffusion of water molecules through tissue/tumour	
BOLD MRI	Permeability and perfusion	Deoxyhaemoglobin
Ultrasound scanning (Doppler)	Tissue/tumour perfusion	Microbubbles
CT	Tumour size and function (tumour perfusion, blood–brain barrier breakdown)	Iodine-based contrast agents
MRS	Endogenous reporter molecules (metabolites) to evaluate tumour microenvironment	$[^{31}P]$ adenosine triphosphate, phosphomonoester, inorganic phosphate, intracellular pH $[^{1}H]$ lactate, choline, glutamine
	Exogenous reporter molecules to evaluate tumour microenvironment:	
	• Oxygenation	$[^{19}F]$ Perfluorocarbons
	• Hypoxia	$[^{19}F]$ SR-4554
	• Glucose utilization	$[^{18}F]$FDG
	Drug pharmacokinetics in tumour and normal tissues	$[^{18}F]$ 5FU, gemcitabine $[^{31}P]$ cyclophosphamide, ifosfamide
PET	Drug pharmacokinetics in tumour and normal tissues by labelling drug of interest with PET isotope	$[^{18}F]$ 5FU, $[^{11}C]$ temazolamide, $[^{13}N]$ cisplatin, $[^{11}C]$ BCNU, $[^{18}F]$ tamoxifen
	General antitumour effects	
	• Cellular proliferation	$[^{11}C]$ thymidine, $[^{18}F]$ fluorothymidine
	• Glucose utilization	$[^{18}F]$ FDG
	• Tissue perfusion	$[^{15}O]$ H_2O
	• Blood volume	$[^{15}O]$ CO
	• Amino acid metabolism	$[^{11}C]$ methionine,
	• Detection of thymidylate synthase inhibition	$[^{11}C]$ thymidine

Table 11.1 *(Continued)*

Imaging technology	Use	Marker/contrast agent
	Specific antitumour effects	
	• VEGF/VEGF receptor inhibition	^{124}I-labelled antibodies/peptides
	• Overexpression of erbB2	[^{124}I] anti-erbB2 antibody

Diagnostic imaging may be carried out on human patients in translational target validation or tumour biology studies, or in clinical trials to evaluate chemoresponse. The specialist equipment required is expensive but the technique is relatively non-invasive. The technology can also be used in preclinical studies involving mouse tumour models.

BOLD, blood oxygenation level dependent; CT, computerized tomography; MRS, magnetic resonance spectroscopy.

Adapted from Seddon and Workman (2003).

mTOR (discussed in Section 12.3 and Chapter 19, respectively). The European Organization for Research and Treatment of Cancer (EORTC), a translational research organization based in Brussels, have a set of criteria for the use of FDG-PET in clinical trials. These are based upon the use of SUVs as a surrogate measure of the clinical endpoints of complete/partial response, stable and progressive disease (Figure 11.7).

11.3 Assessment of vascularity and angiogenesis by nuclear medicine technology

A large group of novel drug therapies aim to block tumour blood supply by either targeting tumour capillaries directly (antivascular agents) or the synthesis of new blood vessels (anti-angiogenic agents, see Chapter 13). These may be evaluated using nuclear medicine techniques that measure vascular physiological function, that is, *flow*, or more specifically in a physiological system, *blood flow*, given as unit of blood per time per mass of tissue. This is distinct from *perfusion*, which is expressed in terms of the same dimensional units but refers to nutritive flow, or the exchange of nutrients (oxygen, glucose, etc.) and waste. The analysis of nutritive flow may be more appropriate for preclinical studies of angiogenesis, as changes in perfusion may lead to tumour micro-environmental phenomena such as hypoxia, which partially contribute to the increased production of angiogenic mediators in tumours. However, measurements of perfusion should be offset by consideration of any arteriovenous *shunting*, where blood flow takes place in the absence of nutrient and waste exchange, which may come about where there is a direct anatomical conduit that provides a flow path that bypasses the capillary bed. Any nuclear imaging technique ideally distinguishes between true perfusion and shunts, which may be particularly important if investigating therapies that target highly angiogenic tumours where vascular function is poor and the structure and morphology of blood vessels is disrupted. Tracers validated for perfusion imaging include ^{62}Cu-PTSM (^{62}Cu-pyruvaldehyde-bis-N4-methylthiosemicarbazonato)-copper (II), ^{13}N-labelled

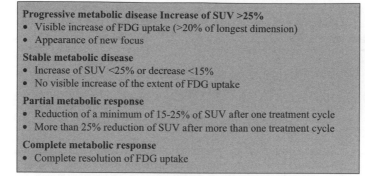

Progressive metabolic disease Increase of SUV >25%
- Visible increase of FDG uptake (>20% of longest dimension)
- Appearance of new focus

Stable metabolic disease
- Increase of SUV <25% or decrease <15%
- No visible increase of the extent of FDG uptake

Partial metabolic response
- Reduction of a minimum of 15-25% of SUV after one treatment cycle
- More than 25% reduction of SUV after more than one treatment cycle

Complete metabolic response
- Complete resolution of FDG uptake

Figure 11.7 Proposed European Organization for Research and Treatment of Cancer criteria for assessment of response by FDG-PET using the standard uptake value (SUV), a semi-quantitative measure of FDG accumulation used to image and estimate changes in tumour volume (Reproduced with permission American Association for Cancer Research, from Kelloff *et al.* (2005) *Clin. Cancer Res.* (2005) 11: 2785–2808.)

ammonia and ^{82}Rb-rubidium. The impetus for developing tracers for imaging perfusion characteristics stems from their application to cardiac disease, and is based on the Fick equation, which relates blood flow to the rate of clearance of the tracer from the tissue. Clearance of the tracer and therefore the quality of the data is influenced by parameters such as the half life of the isotope, albumin binding and metabolism of the compound. For instance, whereas the 9.3 minute half life of ^{13}NH$_3$ facilitates accurate signal counting, its tendency to bind serum albumin limits its use in non-cardiac studies. The tracer H$_2$^{15}O, an isotope of water, has the advantage of being metabolically and biologically inert, and the free diffusion of water in and out of tissues means that clearance rates represent perfusion rates more closely. However, the accuracy of data gathered using this tracer may be subject to the vascular heterogeneity prevalent in tumours, which affects the equilibrium between arterial and tissue water content. For this reason, techniques that image perfusion alongside hypoxia and/or total vascular volume have been suggested, where these may reflect the presence of vascular heterogeneity and dysfunction in tumour capillary structure and integrity. Hypoxia tracers that have undergone validation in human and animal tumor models include the 2-nitro-imidazoles, such as [18F] fluoromisonidazole and [18F] EF5, which are isotopes of hypoxia-activated bioreductive drugs (described in Section 12.2) but are pharmacologically inert. Hypoxia has also been imaged using isotopically labelled thiosemicarbazones, such as ^{99m}Tc or $^{62/}$^{64}Cu-labelled dithiosemicarbazone. Imaging vascular blood volume may provide a means of assessing vascular integrity, and therefore may be used to evaluate response to novel antivascular agents. Tracers such as ^{15}C-carbon monoxide bind irreversibly with haemoglobin to form ^{15}CO-Hb carboxyhaemoglobin. As long as blood vessels are intact the tracer metabolites remain exclusively within the vasculature providing an indication of total blood volume. However, where blood vessels are damaged, such as following administration of vascular targeting agents such as combretastatin, the tracer will leak into surrounding tissue causing a measurable reduction in blood volume.

Tracers used to measure specific pharmacodynamic effects of a novel agent include molecular probes that measure the production and biological activity of angiogenic mediators. For example, the new antitumour agents Vitaxin (see Section 13.2) and cilengitide, both currently in phase II clinical trials, target the integrin $\alpha v\beta 3$. To facilitate their pre-clinical and clinical validation, RGD (Arg-Gly-Asp) peptide-based probes, which themselves target integrins, have been used successfully to image integrin-positive tumours. Angiogenic growth factors such as vascular endothelial growth factor (VEGF) and fibroblast growth factor, or the monoclonal antibodies to their target tyrosine kinase receptor may also be labelled, for example, with ^{124}I to image the presence of growth factor or growth factor receptor expression. For instance, the immunoglobulin G1 monoclonal antibody VG76e, which binds to human VEGF may be labelled with the positron-emitting radionuclide, iodine-124 ($[^{124}I]$-SHPP-VG76e) to investigate levels of circulating VEGF *in vivo*. To measure receptor binding, $[^{125}I]$-VEGF is also undergoing validation. The tracers may assist in the rational selection of patients with tumours highly expressing these angiogenic factors for recruitment into clinical trials of novel agents that block these pathways and therefore specifically target the tumour, and clinical response may be directly related to the blockade of the targeted angiogenic pathway.

12

Tumour hypoxia

12.1 Introduction

Tumour hypoxia, or low oxygen tension, is frequently observed in solid tumours. Whereas the average level of oxygenation in normal tissues is around 40 mmHg, in malignant tissue, the level of oxygenation falls to below 20 mmHg, and levels of oxygenation of 0–1% frequently exist in some areas of a solid tumour. Hypoxia arises where oxygen demand surpasses oxygen extraction from the adjacent blood supply. In normal tissue, changes in oxygen demand are met by adjusting blood flow. However, in tumour tissue, vascularization is poorly organized: capillaries are often twisted, elongated or blind-ended, and are less able to make the vasomotor changes necessary to support fluctuating demands for oxygen. Coupled with the increased rate of proliferation seen in an aggressively growing tumour, which may coincide with the appearance of avascular areas, the tumour oxygen demand soon outgrows oxygen availability and patches of necrosis, or dead tissue, develop. The position of this necrotic tissue is determined by oxygen gradients relative to a patent blood capillary. Close to the capillary, there is sufficient oxygen available to support oxidative phosphorylation and therefore a comfortable rate of energy production and ATP synthesis to support the tumour cell. However, as these cells consume oxygen, cells at an increasing distance from the blood capillary have gradually less oxygen available to them. At a critical distance, cells are subjected to anoxia, or a complete lack of oxygenation, and as cells can survive only for a limited time in the complete absence of oxygen, cell death will occur. The distance between a patent blood vessel and necrosis is determined by the oxygenation of the blood it delivers – at the arterial end of a capillary, necrosis occurs at a distance of around 70 μm, whereas necrosis will develop at approximately 150 μm (Figure 12.1). Tumour hypoxia arising as a result of a diffusion gradient tends to be chronic, this type of hypoxia often being described as diffusion-limited hypoxia. Acute hypoxia, or perfusion-limited hypoxia, is a result of transient interruptions in blood supply, which may be caused by morphological changes in tumour vasculature, or spontaneous vasomotion in contiguous host arterioles that affect blood flow in downstream tumour capillaries. This in turn leads to micro regional fluctuations in tumour oxygenation.

Cancer Chemotherapy   Rachel Airley
© 2009 John Wiley & Sons, Ltd.

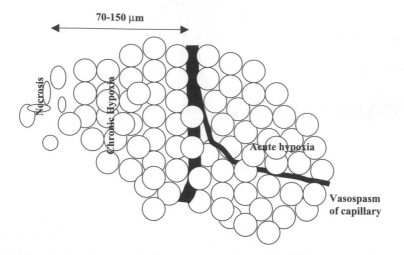

Figure 12.1 Chronic (diffusion-limited) hypoxia occurs where distance from a functional capillary exceeds the diffusion distance of oxygen. This usually occurs at a distance of around 70 µm from the venous end of a blood vessel (blood is deoxygenated) and 150 µm from the arterial end. Acute (perfusion-limited) hypoxia is a consequence of poor vasomotor function, where temporary shut-down of blood vessels causes intermittent episodes of local hypoxia.

Tumour hypoxia is a well-established therapeutic problem, causing changes in biology that lead to increased malignancy and likelihood of metastasis, as well as increasing resistance to radiotherapy and conventional chemotherapy. Hypoxia-linked chemoresistance occurs in 3 ways. Firstly, many conventional anticancer agents are larger molecules, for example, antitumour antibiotics. In the absence of a structurally and functionally normal blood supply, effective penetration of the drug into hypoxic regions of the tumour is prevented. Secondly, hypoxia causes cells to leave the cell cycle, that is, to enter G0 phase. Cells in G0 are not actively dividing, and many anticancer agents target DNA synthesis, replication or function, these cells will be refractory to treatment. Thirdly, some anticancer agents depend upon the presence of oxygen for activation. For example, the activation of bleomycin depends upon the formation of a DNA–bleomycin–ferrous ion–dioxygen complex that is oxidized in the presence of oxygen. Further, hypoxia may reduce levels of target molecules, for example, hypoxia-induced drug resistance of adriamycin and etoposide may be caused via the induction of glucose-regulated proteins which ultimately reduce the level of DNA topoisomerases, which are themselves important cellular targets of these anticancer agents. Hypoxia also causes induction of the multi-drug resistance efflux transporter p-glycoprotein, which prevents intracellular accumulation of substrate drugs to cytotoxic levels. Therefore, patients with tumours showing areas of hypoxia have poorer prognosis, and are more likely to be affected by local recurrence or metastasis after treatment.

The tumour microenvironment is hostile. Aside from oxygen deprivation, tumour cells may also suffer a restricted nutrient supply. Further, as there is little oxygen available for oxidative phosphorylation, ATP stores are maintained through an increased rate of anaerobic glycolysis, leading to raised lactate levels and low intratumoral pH. To survive this environment, tumour cells undergo a range of adaptive changes regulated via the transcription factor hypoxia-inducible factor-1 (HIF-1). The discovery of HIF-1 in the 1990s has led to a significantly increased understanding of how tumours not only withstand hypoxic conditions, but also undergo physiological changes that give rise to poor prognosis and aggressive behaviour, such as metastasis. HIF-1 is a complex of two subunits; HIF-1α and HIF-1B. HIF-1α is rapidly degraded in normoxic conditions via the E3 ubiquitin ligase von Hippel–Lindau complex (see Section 18.3), so that accumulation and subsequent complexation with HIF-1B, a binding partner constitutively expressed independently of local levels of tissue oxygenation, only occurs in hypoxic conditions. HIF-1B is also capable of forming complexes with HIF-2α or HIF-3α, which were discovered relatively recently, although their precise function is still poorly understood; as well as with the aryl hydrocarbon receptor (AHR), which mediates the xenobiotic response, that is, activation of enzymes that metabolize drugs and exogenous toxins such as the cytochrome P450 system. The formation of the HIF-1 heterodimer induces a conformational change that allows binding of the transcription factor to the hypoxia-response element (HRE), an enhancer sequence of DNA found in the promoter region of hypoxia-inducible genes. This effects activation of hypoxia-regulated genes coding for proteins that promote three major changes: a switch to anaerobic glycolysis, supported by increased expression of the facilitative glucose transporters Glut-1 and Glut-3; adaptation to low pH, via increased expression of the tumour-specific carbonic anhydrases CAIX and CAXII; and angiogenesis, or the growth of new blood vessels with which to support a rapidly growing tumour. Angiogenesis is stimulated by a number of hypoxia-inducible growth factors such as vascular endothelial growth factor (VEGF), epidermal growth factor and its receptor (EGF/EGFR) and basic fibroblast growth factor (bFGF). Hypoxia also decreases the expression of pro-apoptotic proteins such as Bid and Bax, allowing tumour cells to survive and proliferate. When treating a tumour, therefore, hypoxic cells enjoy a survival advantage, leading to the persistence of residual cells that are biologically aggressive and chemo- and radioresistant. The rapid proliferation of these cells will once again lead to pockets of hypoxia, exerting a positive selection pressure on genotypically similar cells and promoting the formation of a local recurrence or metastasis, for example, by allowing tumour-cell derived angiogenesis (described in depth in Section 5.5. The interaction between tumour growth and metastasis, hypoxia and angiogenesis is summarized in Figure 12.2. The characterization of the molecular mechanisms allowing adaptation to hypoxia has involved the modelling of tumour hypoxia *in vitro*, in three-dimensional tumour cell spheroids; *in vivo*, in xenografted tumours derived from tumour cell lines, and *ex vivo*, in clinical biopsy samples (Figure 12.3). The data obtained from the study of hypoxia-regulated events in clinical biopsies has been key to the validation of hypoxia-regulated genes and proteins as therapeutic targets, as these translational studies have shown their ability to predict poor survival. These studies are prolific in number, where HIF-1α, Glut-1 and CAIX predict poor survival in a wide range of cancer types, including breast, cervix, lung and bladder cancers.

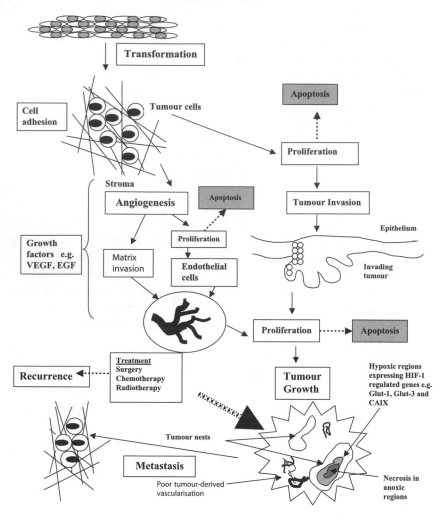

Figure 12.2 The influence of tumour hypoxia at different stages of malignant progression. Malignantly transformed tumour cells gain the potential to invade, metastasize and recur after treatment with chemotherapy, radiotherapy or surgery. This is deeply influenced by the hypoxic tumour microenvironment, where hypoxia confers a survival advantage that allows tumour cells to proliferate and evade cell death (apoptosis). The hallmarks of tumour hypoxia are angiogenesis, an increased rate of glycolytic metabolism; and the increased expression of pH regulating enzymes and transporter proteins, themselves mediated by changes in the expression of hypoxia-regulated genes induced via the HIF-1 transcription factor. Hypoxia-regulated genes include vascular endothelial growth factor (VEGF) and epidermal growth factor (EGF), which signal for angiogenesis; the facilitative glucose transporter Glut-1; glycolytic enzymes such as the hexokinases, pyruvate kinase and lactate dehydrogenase; the carbonic anhydrases CAIX and CAXII and the monocarboxylate transporters MCT 1 and MCT4. Reproduced from Airley, R.E. and Mobasheri, A. (2007) *Chemotherapy* 53:233–56, Karger, Basel.

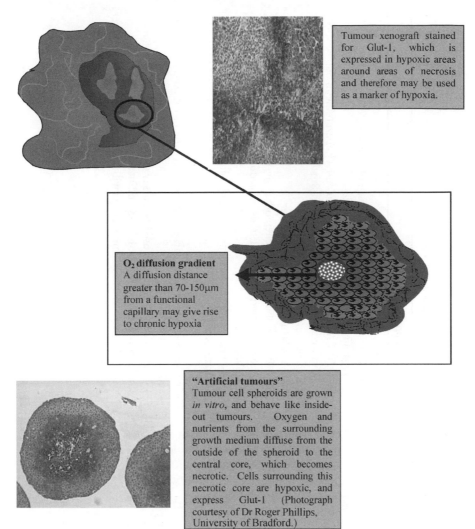

Tumour xenograft stained for Glut-1, which is expressed in hypoxic areas around areas of necrosis and therefore may be used as a marker of hypoxia.

O₂ diffusion gradient
A diffusion distance greater than 70-150μm from a functional capillary may give rise to chronic hypoxia

"Artificial tumours"
Tumour cell spheroids are grown *in vitro*, and behave like inside-out tumours. Oxygen and nutrients from the surrounding growth medium diffuse from the outside of the spheroid to the central core, which becomes necrotic. Cells surrounding this necrotic core are hypoxic, and express Glut-1 (Photograph courtesy of Dr Roger Phillips, University of Bradford.)

Figure 12.3 Chronic hypoxia modelled in tumour xenografts and tumour cell spheroids.

12.2 Bioreductive drugs

Efforts to overcome and exploit tumour hypoxia include several strategies, described in Table 12.1. Bioreductive drugs may act as radiosensitizers, to overcome radioresistance, or hypoxia-activated prodrugs which are selectively activated to cytotoxic metabolites in hypoxic conditions within a tumour. Initially developed as radiosensitizing agents such as the 2-nitroimidazoles metronidazole and misonidazole (Figure 12.4), these agents behaved as 'oxygen mimetics' which were able to stabilize or 'fix' the reversible DNA damage caused by radiation. Although there were several clinical studies carried

Table 12.1 Novel agents in preclinical and clinical development that target hypoxia or hypoxia-regulated genes

Strategy	Drug	Clinical development
Bioreductive Drugs	*N-oxides*	Tirapazamine
	Tirapazamine, AQ4N	Phase II: Small cell lung cancer, thoracic radiotherapy followed by tirapazamine, cisplatin and etoposide.
	Nitroaromatics/heterocyclics	Phase III CATAPULT studies (Cisplatin and Tirapazamine in Subjects with
	CI-1010	Advanced Previously Untreated Non-Small-Cell Lung Tumors).
		AQ4N (*banoxantrone*)
	Quinones	Phase I: advanced oesophageal cancer
	Mitomycin C	Phase I: in combination with chemotherapy/radiotherapy.
	RH1	EO9 – 'Eoquin' entering phase II trials in bladder cancer.
	Porfiromycin	RH1 – phase I trials
	EO9	PR-104 – phase I clinical trials in advanced solid tumours, phase II trial will
	PR-104	evaluate its use in small cell lung cancer.
	2-nitroimidazoles	*Pimonidazole*: evaluation as a marker of hypoxia in patients with cervix and head
	Bioreductive markers: pimonidazole,	and neck tumours.
	misonidazole, EF5	*(18)F-Misonidazole*: PET tracer used as marker of hypoxia and prognosis, most
	Radiosensitizing agent: misonidazole	studies involving patients with head and neck cancer.
		Misonidazole: phase III trial in combination with radiotherapy in cervical cancer
		showed little benefit.

Hypoxia-regulated genes

HIF-1	
7-hydroxystaurosporine (UCN-01) PX-478 YC-1	Phase 1: UCN-01 plus prednisolone in refractory solid tumours and lymphomas. Phase I trial initiated 2007 in advanced solid tumours and leukaemias. Evaluated as an inhibitor of hypoxia-induced angiogenesis in xenografts.
Glut-1	
Glucose analogue radiosensitizers e.g. 2-deoxyglucose	Clinical trials initiated including phase I/II trials of 2-deoxyglucose in combination with radiotherapy in glioma; and in combination with chemotherapy, e.g. a phase I/II trial to evaluate its use as a single agent in advanced cancer and hormone refractory prostate cancer; and in combination with docetaxel in a phase I trial involving patients with advanced solid malignancies.
2-glu-SNAP- conjugate of glucose and nitric oxide donor	*In vitro* testing in ovarian, breast and glioblastoma cell lines.
Glufosfamide – conjugate of glucose and isophosphoramide mustard, an alkylating agent.	Phase I trial in combination with gemcitabine for the treatment of solid tumours. Phase III trial for the treatment of metastatic pancreatic adenocarcinoma previously treated with gemcitabine in progress. Phase II trials evaluating its use in platinum-resistant ovarian cancer, recurrent sensitive small cell lung cancer and soft-tissue sarcoma in progress.
CAIX	
Fluorinated sulfonamide derivatives	Phase II trial of E7070 (indisulam) in advanced non-small cell lung cancer; and separate phase I studies in combination with carboplatin and capecitabine in refractory solid tumours have been reported. Clinical trials in progress evaluating use in melanoma, colorectal and renal cancers.
G250 (Rencarex) anti-CAIX chimerized monoclonal antibody	Phase I/II clinical trials investigating G250 as monotherapy and in combination therapy with cytokines (IL-2 and IFN) in metastatic renal cell carcinoma showed improved long term survival and a good safety profile. Phase III trial evaluating its use as monotherapy in patients that have undergone surgery for non-metastatic kidney cancer is currently in progress.

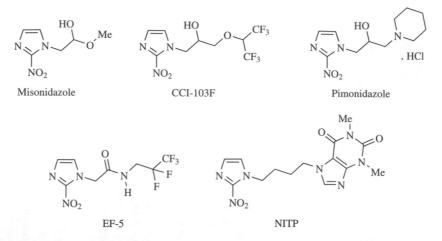

Misonidazole   CCI-103F   Pimonidazole

EF-5   NITP

Figure 12.4 2-nitroimidazoles are similar in structure to the antimicrobial agent metronidazole, and in a similar fashion, target hypoxic cells. These have been evaluated as hypoxia markers in clinical studies involving patients with cervix and head and neck tumours, to assess their ability to predict prognosis and their suitability for allowing the rational administration of hypoxia-targeted agents or radiotherapy according to hypoxic status. Misonidazole was also evaluated as a radiosensitizing agent in a number of clinical studies, although there has been no evidence of any additional benefit.

out to evaluate the radiosensitizing effect of misonidazole, mostly carried out in the 1980s and 1990s, but the most recent being a phase III study reported in 2004 involving patients with cervical cancer, there has been no observable benefit. Instead, the 2-nitroimidazoles are now used as bioreductive hypoxia markers, which have been modified in various ways to produce an inert compound capable of detecting hypoxia. This may be carried out immunohistochemically, for example, pimonidazole (Hypoxyprobe), where mouse monoclonal antibodies are used to detect intracellular pimonidazole adducts that become linked to cellular components in hypoxic tissue; or via a radioactive isotope for example, [18F]-fluoromisonidazole, which may be used as a tracer. In the search for biomarkers that can reliably, non-invasively and inexpensively measure tumour hypoxia, these have been evaluated along side the HIF-1-regulated genes Glut-1 and CAIX in xenografts and in patients.

Bioreductive cytotoxic agents are reduced under certain conditions in their target tissue by means of a one or two electron reduction process. Although the degree of hypoxia-selectivity varies in bioreductive agents developed so far, the aim is to find agents that have a large *hypoxic differential*, that is, are ineffective in normoxic normal tissue but highly effective in hypoxic tumour tissue. There are currently 4 classes of bioreductive drug in development, examples of which are shown in Figures 12.5 and 12.6: the quinones, which encompass the lead bioreductive drug mitomycin C and its analogue porfiromycin, together with the more recent indolequinones such as EO9 (apaziquone) and the diaziridinylbenzoquinone RH-1; the nitroaromatics,

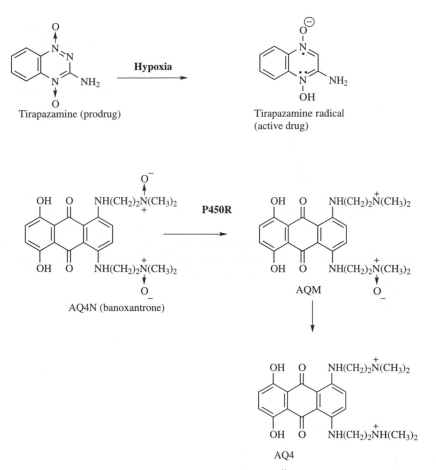

Figure 12.5 Hypoxia-dependent activation of the bioreductive agents tirapazamine and AQ4N (banoxantrone), both undergoing evaluation in clinical trials.

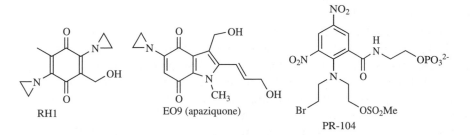

Figure 12.6 Other classes of bioreductive drugs in clinical development include the quinone bioreductive drugs, such as the diaziridinylbenzoquinone RH1 and the indolequinone EO9 (apaziquone); and the dinitrobenzamide mustard PR-104.

which include the dinitrobenzamide mustards such as PR-104; the aliphatic N-oxides, such as AQ4N (banoxantrone); and the heteroaromatic N-oxides, which include the most clinically advanced hypoxia-targeted bioreductive drug tirapazamine.

The bioreduction process of mitomycin C and related quinone bioreductive agents is discussed in Section 8.3.1. In a similar fashion, the activation of tirapazamine and banoxantrone is catalysed by reducing enzymes such as NADPH: cytochrome P450 reductase (P450R), the cytochrome P450 group enzymes, NQO1 (DT-Diaphorase) and nitric oxide synthase (NOS), which in hypoxic conditions reduce the prodrug to a cytotoxic radical (Figure 12.5), where the tirapazamine radical acts as a strand-breaking agent by abstracting hydrogen from DNA, whilst the active intermediate of banoxantrone, AQ4, is an inhibitor of topoisomerase I. Whereas tirapazamine and AQ4N have a large hypoxic differential, the bioreductive drugs mitomycin C and EO9 show less oxygen-dependence; activation being mediated chiefly by the action of the reducing enzyme DT-Diaphorase in normoxic or hypoxic conditions. Tirapazamine was originally licensed to Sanofi-Aventis, where two phase III clinical trials, CATAPULT I and CATAPULT II, evaluated its use in non-small cell lung cancer. In CATAPULT I, patients were given cisplatin, the standard treatment for this type of cancer, or cisplatin plus tirapazamine; a concept that had been informed by *in vitro* observations of synergy between the two drugs. When data from CATAPULT I showed the improved clinical response to this combination, CATAPULT II was initiated, which compared treatment with cisplatin plus tirapazamine with cisplatin plus etoposide. Although tumour response was better in the cisplatin plus tirapazamine arm, there was a reduced survival benefit compared to that of cisplatin plus etoposide. At this point, it was suggested that tirpazamine might be useful in triple agent combination chemotherapy. Since then, another phase III trial has been reported, carried out by the Southwest Oncology Group, also in patients with non-small cell lung cancer, in combination with carboplatin and paclitaxel. The results of this trial were somewhat disappointing, however, as the addition of tirapazamine to the two-drug regimen increased toxicity in the absence of any survival benefit. There have been a number of phase I and II clinical studies evaluating tirapazamine in several cancer types, including phase II trials in patients with cancer of the uterine cervix in combination with paclitaxel, in gastric cancer in combination with docetaxel and cisplatin and in ovarian cancer in combination with cisplatin. Another tactic, where hypoxia markers are used to predict which patients may gain most clinical benefit from the use of bioreductive drugs, is also being pursued. In a substudy involving patients with squamous cell carcinoma of the head and neck enrolled in a phase II trial comparing treatment with radiotherapy plus tirapazamine and cisplatin versus fluorouracil plus cisplatin, positron emission tomography (PET) was carried out using the bioreductive tracer [^{18}F]-fluoromisonidazole as a means of scanning for hypoxia prior to and during treatment. Retrospective analysis showed that, as expected, patients with hypoxic tumours were more likely to develop local recurrences. However, patients with hypoxic tumours as diagnosed using the bioreductive marker, that had received tirapazamine, showed significantly fewer local recurrences. This indicated both that tirapazamine was specifically targeting hypoxic cells and that hypoxia markers might be incorporated into clinical studies of hypoxia-targeted chemotherapy in order to gain a more representative picture of their efficacy. Following on from this, and the reacquisition of the tirapazamine licence by SRI International, there is now a study in planning which will attempt to correlate the response of patients with cervical cancer to tirapazamine with the level of tumour hypoxia measured before and after treatment using Glut-1 and other HIF-1-regulated genes detected immuno-histochemically in biopsy samples. An alternative mode of action has also been postulated, where there is evidence that tirapazamine acts as a vascular disrupting agent, an effect brought about by the inhibition of the enzyme NOS, the consequent reduction in nitric oxide production leading to tumour blood vessel constriction. Banoxantrone is currently being evaluated in a number of phase II trials, including haematological malignancies and glioblastoma. These have followed completed phase I studies such as an initial dose escalation study carried out in patients with oesophageal tumours and a further phase I study carried out in patients with bladder cancer, both in combination with radiotherapy. Banoxantrone is also being evaluated in combination with cisplatin in a phase I trial involving patients with advanced solid tumours. A phase I study was recently reported (2008) which evaluated the use of banoxantrone in patients with advanced solid tumours, where retrospective analysis of tumour samples showed a significant correlation between hypoxia, measured using the endogenous hypoxia marker Glut-1, and the hypoxia-selective conversion of the prodrug to active AQ4. The quinone bioreductive drug apaziquone (EO9), following on from phase I trials evaluating its pharmacokinetics in the 1990s, showed little activity in phase II trials looking at its use in non-small cell lung, foregut and colorectal cancers. However, like the earlier quinone mitomycin C, indications are that apaziquone is a potential novel treatment for superficial bladder cancer, where around a decade later, a phase II trial in this cancer type yielded promising results, the drug being well tolerated and inducing an ablative tumour response. A placebo-controlled phase III trial in a larger group of patients with superficial bladder cancer is now recruiting. So far, the preclinical evaluation of the dinitrobenzamide mustard PR-104 has concentrated on the characterization of its bioreduction process and its mechanism of action, revealing an interesting activation pathway that involves hydrolysation of PR-104 to the alcohol PR-104A. This metabolite behaves as the hypoxia-selective prodrug, which is converted to the active hydroxylamine metabolite PR-104H and eventually to the amine PR-104M. The cytotoxicity of the active metabolite is attributed to its ability to cross-link DNA. PR-104 has now entered phase I clinical trials for dose escalation and safety profiling in advanced solid tumours, and a phase II trial is currently recruiting, which will evaluate its use in small cell lung cancer.

12.3 Inhibitors of HIF-1 and HIF-1-regulated genes

There are currently a number of therapeutic strategies targeting HIF-1 and hypoxia-regulated genes in preclinical and clinical development, summarized in Table 12.1. The validation of HIF-1 as a therapeutic target has involved the use of HIF-1α and HIF-1B-deficient tumour xenografts in order to model the effect of an incomplete HIF-1-response in tumour formation, growth and treatment response. This has been beset with a degree of controversy, where separate studies have on one hand shown that although the rate of tumour growth is not inhibited by an incomplete HIF response, there is a significant delay in the initiation of tumour formation in the HIF-1 deficient tumours. On the other hand, other groups have found that increased HIF-1 signalling is pro-apoptotic and therefore inhibits tumorigenesis. To complicate matters further, another study suggested that a complete HIF-1 response in just a small proportion of cells within a tumour is sufficient to rescue the entire tumour from the effects of HIF-1-deficient growth, an effect that may be mediated by the production of secretion of hypoxia- regulated angiogenic growth factors such as VEGF.

In spite of this, there has been a considerable interest in the development of HIF-1 blocking agents (Figure 12.7), which have varying degrees of HIF-1 specificity. For instance, one agent in development, 7-hydroxystaurosporine (UCN-01), is a protein kinase C (PKC) inhibitor that also has the ability to block HIF-1-mediated gene transcription. UCN-01 has been evaluated or are currently recruiting for separate phase I trials for treatment of advanced solid tumours and haematological malignancies, such as pancreatic, ovarian, renal and skin cancers. Trial regimens include combination of UCN-01 with a range of agents, such as irinotecan and topotecan, fluorouracil, cisplatin and the novel Akt inhibitor perifosine (see Chapter 16). The first phase II trial to be reported has been a study by the Princess Margaret Hospital Phase II consortium, which evaluated UCN-01 in combination with topotecan in recurrent ovarian cancer. However, in this group of patients there was no significant clinical activity. Further phase II trials planned include a study involving patients with large cell and mature T-cell lymphomas and small cell lung cancer in combination with topotecan. YC-1 (3-(5′-hydroxymethyl-2′-furyl)-1-benzylindazole) is a novel agent initially developed for its antiplatelet activity for the treatment of circulatory disorders. However, observations using Hep3B hepatoma cells showed an apparent effect on the expression of HIF-1-regulated genes such as erythropoietin (EPO) and VEGF. YC-1 has therefore become a lead compound in the search for HIF-1 inhibitors. The anti-platelet activity of YC-1 is brought about by the activation of platelet soluble guanylate cyclase (sGC) and the increased expression of cyclic guanosine monophosphate (cGMP). Activation of these enzymes also induces vasodilatation and therefore changes in local tissue perfusion. For this reason it was initially thought that YC-1 inhibited the HIF-1 pathway via a reflexive suppression of the hypoxia response. This hypothesis was abandoned, though, when the presence of other sGC inhibitors failed to block this response. Since then, experiments carried out in tumour xenografts have shown that YC-1 has HIF-1-dependent anti-angiogenic activity, where areas of YC-1 treated tumour showing a morphologically abnormal and poorly developed blood supply coincide with immunohistochemical detection of HIF-1α protein. Other studies have offered alternative explanations, one showing that YC-1 decreases the expression of hypoxia-regulated genes via a direct effect on HIF-1 transactivation, by inducing degradation of the C-terminal transactivation domain (Figure 12.8) and consequently blocking proteasomal inhibition. Another study, however, failed to detect either a decreased HIF-1α half life or an increased level of HIF-1 transcription (mRNA); instead proposing that HIF-1 inhibition occurred via suppression of the PI3K/Akt/mTOR/4E-BP pathway, which regulates HIF-1α translation. Another mechanism by which YC-1 inhibits HIF-1 activity may be via an effect on the nuclear factor-κB (NFκB) transcription factor. NFκB

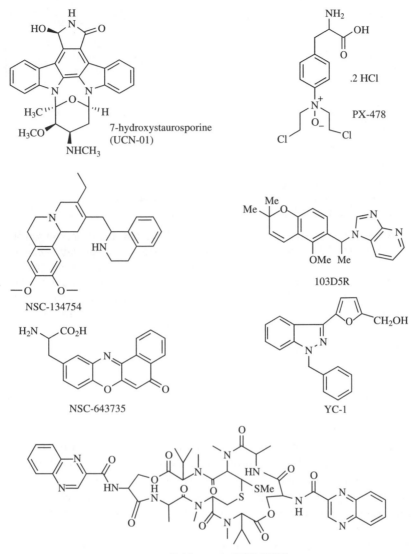

Figure 12.7 Examples of novel compounds identified as having HIF-1 inhibiting activity. Efforts by various research groups to find lead small molecule inhibitors of HIF-1 have identified a number of compounds from diversity screens such as the natural products echinomycin (NSC-13 502) and the 2,2-dimethylbenzopyran 103D5R; the actinomycin D aglycone analogue NSC-643 735 and NSC-134 754, a semisynthetic analogue of the plant alkaloid emetine; other novel agents shown to inhibit HIF-1 include PX-478 (S-2-amino-3-[4V-N,N,-bis(2-chloroethyl) amino]phenyl propionic acid N-oxide dihydrochloride), believed to inhibit HIF-1 by a number of mechanisms, inhibiting HIF-1 mRNA synthesis and translation and decreasing the stability of HIF-1α; YC-1 (3-(5′-hydroxymethyl-2′-furyl)-1-benzylindazole), a novel agent initially developed for its anti-platelet activity for the treatment of circulatory disorders but observed to have anti-angiogenic activity by virtue of its ability to inhibit HIF-1; and the protein kinase C (PKC) inhibitor UCN-01 but also blocks HIF-1-mediated transactivation of hypoxia-inducible genes.

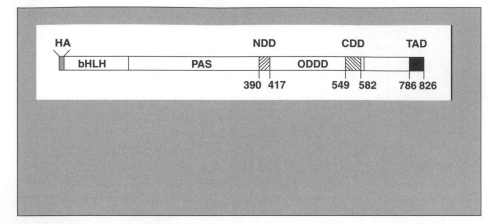

Figure 12.8 Structure of HIF-1α, a basic helix loop helix (bHLH) type transcription factor that includes the N-terminal degradation domain (NDD); the C-terminal degradation domain (CDD), believed to be targeted by the lead HIF-1 inhibiting agent YC-1; the oxygen-dependent degradation domain (ODDD), which gives HIF-1α its oxygen sensitivity; and the transactivation domain (TAD), which binds DNA sequences in the promotor region of hypoxia-inducible genes (HA, haemagglutinin; PAS, per-ant-sim domain, which promotes heterodimerization with binding partners such as HIF-1β). Reproduced with permission from Kim, H.L., Yeo, E.J., Chun, Y.S., Park, J.W. *Int. J. Oncol.* 2006;29:255–60, Spandidos.

is now known to mediate the induction of HIF-1α via cytokines such as interleukin (IL)-1β and tumour necrosis factor (TNF-α). NFκB also acts as a downstream signal for Akt-induced HIF-1α expression, where overexpression of NFκB successfully reverses the downregulation of HIF-1-inducible reporter gene expression by Akt inhibitors such as wortmannin. Pre-clinical studies continue to show promise, more recent data revealing that YC-1 inhibits hypoxia-induced tumour cell migration and metastasis using Matrigel invasion assays and tumour xenografts in mice; where tumour cells were implanted into the spleen to generate liver metastases and into the pleural cavity to induce invasion into the lung.

The heterodimerization of HIF-1α and HIF-1β depends upon the presence of PAS (per-ant-sim) domains, where both proteins have two PAS domains, PAS-A and PAS-B. The PAS domain also has a role in the complexation of complete HIF-1 with the HRE of hypoxia-regulated genes. Therefore targeting a PAS domain may provide an alternative approach to the design of HIF-1 inhibitors.

A number of potential HIF-1 inhibitors have been identified by screening libraries of compounds, such as the National Cancer Institute diversity sets, for HIF-1α inhibiting activity. Typical methodology is to use genetically manipulated cell lines containing HIF-1–reporter gene constructs, where a gene such as luciferase, which is readily detectable by measurement of its chemiluminescence, is put under the control of a HRE enhancer sequence. The extent of HIF-1 inhibition upon exposure to a range of novel drug compounds can then be easily measured by integrating this method into high throughput screening technology. One such compound identified in this way is PX-478 (S-2-amino-3-[4V-N, N,-bis (2-chloroethyl) amino] phenyl propionic acid N-oxide dihydrochloride), a small molecule HIF-1 inhibitor that decreases both constitutively amplified and hypoxia-induced HIF-1α. Whilst PX-478 is believed to modulate HIF-1α stability by inhibiting its deubiquitination, which in turn leads to increased levels of polyubiquitinated HIF-1α, this effect is not blocked by a proteasomal inhibitor, so that increased proteasomal degradation is not likely to be the primary effect of exposure to this agent. Instead, the more significant mechanism of action is now thought to be via the inhibition of HIF-1α mRNA synthesis and translation, where decreased levels of nuclear HIF-1α protein are detected in tumour cell lines treated with of PX-478. In a study which evaluated its antitumour effects in a range of xenografts derived from a panel of tumour cell lines, there was a significant correlation between tumour response and HIF-1α levels, together with a reduction in HIF-1-regulated genes such as Glut-1. The antitumour activity, represented by reduction in tumour volume and growth delay, was also highly promising, particularly in lung xenografts, where there was 100% regression (treatment was curative). At the time of writing, a phase I trial sponsored by Biomira Inc. (Oncothyreon) to evaluate PX-478 in advanced solid tumours or leukaemias is in the recruitment stages.

Efforts by various research groups to find lead small molecule inhibitors of HIF-1 have yielded a number of lead compounds from diversity screens such as the natural products echinomycin (NSC-13 502), the 2,2-dimethylbenzopyran 103D5R, the actinomycin D aglycone analogue NSC-643 735 and NSC-134 754, which is a semisynthetic analogue of the plant alkaloid emetine. Also undergoing preclinical investigation is the flavonoid Vitexin (apigenin-8-C-β-D-glucopyranoside) and deguelin, a naturally occurring rotenoid. Topoisomerase-1 (TOPO I) inhibitors such as topotecan inhibit HIF-1α translation. However, this is believed to occur via an effect on transcriptionally mediated events rather than by a mechanism associated with its cytotoxic activity (described in Section 8.4.3). One explanation is that TOPO I–DNA cleavage complexes form at the loci of active genes, leading to the arrest of RNA transcription machinery and downstream inhibition of HIF-1α protein accumulation.

Since the characterization of the HIF oxygen-sensing pathway and the discovery of facilitative glucose transporters in the 1980s and 1990s, the increased rate of glycolysis observed in malignant tissue is now more often associated with tumour hypoxia, despite the observation that the rate of glycolysis in malignant tissue is increased in both aerobic and anaerobic conditions. This phenomenon, known as the Warburg effect, was first observed as early as the 1930s. In fact, although ubiquitously expressed and linked with poor prognosis in virtually all cancer types, there are differences in constitutive Glut-1 expression between tumours and tumour cell lines which are likely to be dependent upon other factors, such as the expression of transforming oncogenes, for example, H-Ras and c-myc. However, the dual control of Glut-1 in hypoxic conditions via the HIF-1 pathway and on a number of levels through a reduction in oxidative phosphorylation (Figure 12.9) lends to its validity as a means of targeting hypoxic tissue in tumours. Initial efforts taking place in the late 1970s to exploit this effect predated the characterization of the molecular pathways controlling glucose transport and metabolism, and chiefly concentrated on the use of glucose analogues as antimetabolites that

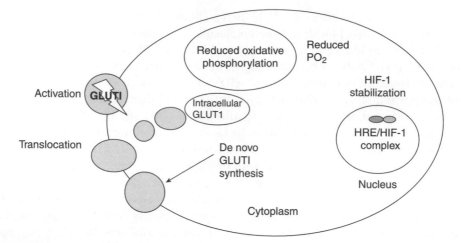

Figure 12.9 Regulation of glucose transport by hypoxia is triphasic. Initially, the decreased rate of oxidative phosphorylation taking place in acutely hypoxic cells necessitates an increase in the rate of anaerobic glycolysis to make up for the shortfall in ATP production. This stimulates the activation of facilitative glucose transporter Glut-1 preexisting on the plasma membrane, and if hypoxia persists, translocation of additional Glut-1 molecules to the plasma membrane from intracellular vesicles. In chronically hypoxic cells, HIF-1 signals for the *de novo* synthesis of Glut-1, and in a small range of tumour types such as those occuring in the CNS, Glut-3. Reproduced from Airley, R.E. and Mobasheri, A. (2007) *Chemotherapy* 53:233–56, Karger, Basel.

would block glycolysis, such as 5-thio-D-glucose (5TG) and 2-deoxy-D-glucose (2DG), where selective toxicity would be achieved through the increased uptake of glucose analogues into cancer cells. At the time, it was also observed that these compounds were more toxic to hypoxic cells *in vitro*, although this approach was eventually shelved due to the dose-limiting effects of normal tissue toxicity in mice, presumably due to non-specific inhibition of glycolysis. Another approach that has been used more successfully is to use 2DG alongside radiotherapy as a radiosensitizing agent, where the glucose analogue is believed to reduce the ability of tumour cells to undergo DNA repair and to inhibit the survival of resistant hypoxic cells dependent upon an increased rate of anaerobic glycolysis. A phase I/II clinical trial involving patients with gliomas has shown treatment with 2DG in combination with a radiotherapy (5 Gy/fraction/week) to be well tolerated with no significant signs of acute toxicity or late radiation-induced damage to normal brain tissue. It has also been suggested that 2DG inhibits the neutralization of reactive oxygen species such as superoxide and peroxide radicals by glucose, rendering radiation more cytotoxic. At the time of writing, another phase I dose-escalation study is ongoing which will test this hypothesis by evaluating the use of 2DG in combination with stereotactic radiosurgery in patients with intercranial metastases. This involves treatment with a high intensity beam of radiation focused at the point of the tumour. In line with the increased understanding of how hypoxia induces an upregulation of Glut-1 and the glycolytic enzymes, there has now been a re-emergence of research activity concentrating on the use of glucose analogues as

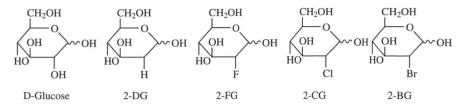

Figure 12.10 Analogues of d-glucose, such as 2-deoxy- (2-DG), 2-fluoro- (2-FG), 2-chloro- (2-CG), and 2-bromo-D-glucose (2-BG) are undergoing evaluation as glycolytic inhibitors which will selectively target hypoxic cells. Reproduced from Lampidis *et al.* (2006) *Cancer Chemother. Pharmacol.* 58: 725–734, Springer.

a means of achieving differential toxicity towards hypoxic tumour cells by selective uptake of drug via Glut-1. Crucially, preclinical and clinical studies are showing that, rather than applying glucose analogues non-specifically to tumours, they should be rationally applied on the basis of Glut-1 expression. Preclinical studies have looked at the use of 2DG and more recently the 2-halogen substituted D-glucose analogues such as 2-fluoro-2-deoxy-D-glucose (2-FG), 2-chloro-2-deoxy-D-glucose (2-CG) and 2-bromo-2-deoxy-D-glucose (2-BG) (Figure 12.10) to induce cell kill by binding to the HIF-1-regulated glucose-phosphorylating enzyme hexokinase. Commensurate with this data, another study shows that HIF-1 expression, mediating overexpression of hexokinase, results in 2DG resistance, highlighting the potential for a future application in combination with HIF-1 inhibitors. They have also been evaluated *in vivo* as an adjunct to adriamycin and paclitaxel in osteosarcoma and non-small cell lung cancer, resulting in significantly increased tumour response. Two further phase I/II clinical studies are currently in the recruitment stage: one evaluating the use of 2DG in patients with advanced cancer and hormone-refractory prostate cancer, and the other to evaluate its use in combination with docetaxel in advanced solid tumours. An alternative strategy has been the design of glucose conjugates consisting of a cytotoxic species linked to a glucose molecule, which is preferentially transported into the tumour cell by Glut-1. Such agents include 2-glu-SNAP (Figure 12.11), the glyco conjugate of the nitric oxide donor *S*-nitroso-*N*-acetyl-penicillamine (SNAP). Here, nitric oxide is toxic to tumour cells, where it is known to cause a range of adverse effects including disruption of the mitochondrial respiratory chain and DNA synthesis. One of several

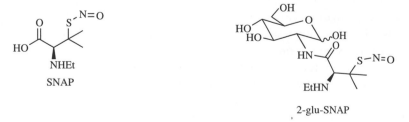

Figure 12.11 2-glu-SNAP, consisting of glucose conjugated to a nitric oxide donor. This is preferentially taken up into tumour cells via Glut-1.

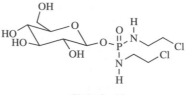

Glufosfamide

Figure 12.12 Glucose conjugates are designed to achieve preferential uptake into tumour cells overexpressing facilitative glucose transporters. Glufosfamide is a conjugate of glucose and the ifosfamide metabolite isophosphoramide mustard, which acts as an alkylating agent.

glyco-conjugates synthesized, 2-glu-SNAP has been tested *in vitro* using ovarian, breast and glioblastoma cell lines, producing increased activity relative to the unconjugated SNAP molecule that is also dependent upon the expression of Glut-1.

Another glucose conjugate in development is glufosfamide (Figure 12.12), a conjugate of glucose and the ifosfamide metabolite isophosphoramide mustard, which acts as an alkylating agent. Glufosfamide was initially evaluated in several phase I and II clinical trials under the auspices of the European Organization for Research and Treatment of Cancer, where an initial phase I dose escalation carried out in patients with refractory solid tumours yielded promising data, showing tumour response despite evidence of renal toxicity. This study therefore paved the way for progression to phase II trials. The first of these to be reported evaluated the use of glufosfamide in pancreatic cancer, followed by another in close succession in patients with glioblastoma, and a third carried out in patients with advanced non-small cell lung cancer who had previously been treated with platinum-based chemotherapy. In this group of clinical trials, however, activity was modest or insignificant. The development of glufosfamide is being sponsored by Threshold Pharmaceuticals, who have also sponsored clinical trials evaluating combination chemotherapy with 2DG and docetaxel. However, this ultimately suffered a set back when interim analysis highlighting the poor performance of glufosfamide in a phase II trial in small cell lung cancer led to discontinuation of the trial. Despite this, clinical development of glufosfamide has continued, where a recently published phase I trial (2008) has shown the potential for combination with gemcitabine for the treatment of solid tumours informed by pre-clinical studies showed that combination of these agents enhanced antitumour activity. A phase III trial evaluating glufosfamide for the treatment of metastatic pancreatic adenocarcinoma previously treated with gemcitabine is in progress, as well as further phase II trials evaluating its use in patients with platinum-resistant ovarian cancer, recurrent sensitive small cell lung cancer and soft-tissue sarcoma.

Overexpression of Glut-1 may confer a survival advantage to hypoxic tumour cells, a hypothesis born out by *in vivo* studies showing that Glut-1 antisense successfully inhibited the proliferation of HL60 leukaemia cells and MKN45-derived xenografts. This may be due to Glut-1-linked alterations in glucose metabolism, where a study analysing metabolite levels in Glut-1 overexpressing xenografts using magnetic resonance spectroscopy showed higher levels of the phospholipid metabolite PDE (phosphodiester), which relates to the degradation of phospholipids and suggests a mechanism by which Glut-1 increases tumour cell proliferation and turnover. The same study also showed that in the absence of intact HIF-1, Glut-1 overexpression increased the growth rate of hepatoma-derived xenografts, and a consistent link was found between Glut-1 expression and chemoresistance. A third approach, therefore, may be to specifically target Glut-1, and approach that might be less severe in terms of adverse toxicity than complete abrogation of glucose metabolism by glucose antimetabolites. The Glut-1 ATP-binding cassette, which determines the conformation of Glut-1 and therefore its ability to transport glucose into the tumour cell, may offer a means of pharmacological intervention, where it has been shown previously that flavone ATP-binding tyrosine kinase inhibitors such as genistein and quercetin bind to and inhibit transport of glucose through Glut-1.

The increased rate of anaerobic glycolysis in tumour cells takes place to counter the shortfall in ATP production occurring as a result of the decreased rate of oxidative phosphorylation taking place in hypoxic conditions. Under normoxic conditions, glycolysis produces pyruvate, which is converted to acetyl CoA, providing a carbon source for the tricarboxylic acid cycle and ultimately for oxidative phosphorylation via the electron transfer chain. However, in hypoxic conditions, pyruvate will be converted to lactate, the end product of anaerobic glycolysis. The production of lactate and pyruvate is in equilibrium, the position of which depends upon the catalytic activity of the terminal glycolytic enzyme lactate dehydrogenase (LDH). LDH exists in five isoforms, which differ in their constituent H (heart) or M (muscle) subunits, each containing a combination of four subunits. Whereas the H subunit has high catalytic activity, the M unit has low catalytic activity; therefore the level of catalytic activity and consequently the production of pyruvate from lactate depend upon the relative number of H and M subunits that constitute the LDH isoform. Where the predominantly expressed isoform is LDH1, which contains four H subunits, catalytic activity is high and there is little production of lactate, but where the predominant isoform is LDH5, which contains four M subunits, there is a high rate of lactic acid production. LDH5 is a HIF-1-inducible enzyme, therefore it is expressed in tandem with Glut-1 and glycolytic enzymes such as hexokinase in hypoxic tumours. Therefore, increased glucose uptake and metabolism in hypoxic tumours is accompanied by the production of excess lactic acid, which is at least partially responsible for the low pH existing in the tumour microenvironment. To compensate for this, a microenvironmental buffering system exists to ensure homeostatic regulation of pH (Figure 12.13). This is dependent upon, firstly, the activity of the H^+-linked monocarboxylate transporters (MCTs), two important MCT isoforms in tumour biology being MCT1 and MCT4. MCT1 is a high affinity transporter that is ubiquitously expressed, and like Glut-1, was characterized initially as an erythrocyte-type transporter. This isoform is capable of transporting a wide range of short chain monocarboxylates, such as lactate and butyrate, into cells for energy production, whilst exporting excess lactate from the cell in hypoxic conditions. MCT4, however, is a low affinity transporter specifically geared for excess lactate efflux from highly glycolytic cells, which may be of particular consequence in tumour pH regulation due to its induction in hypoxic conditions by HIF-1. The regulation of pH in tumours also

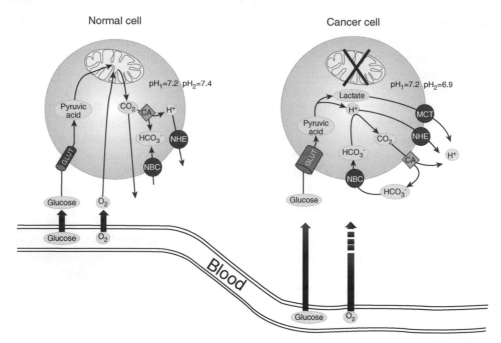

Figure 12.13   Hypoxia determines the interplay between glucose metabolism and microenvironmental pH in normal and malignant cells, revealing the potential for novel therapeutic targets. In normal cells, ATP is liberated from oxidative phosphorylation, which uses pyruvate generated from glycolysis. In tumour cells, however, hypoxia induces a switch to anaerobic glycolysis as a source of ATP, fueled by glucose transported into the cell via hypoxia-induced facilitative glucose transporter Glut-1. The end products of anaerobic glycolysis are CO_2 and lactic acid. Excess CO_2 levels are countered by hypoxia-induced carbonic anhydrase, for example, CAIX, which catalyses the conversion of CO_2 to extracellular carbonate (HCO_3^-) ions, and mono-carboxylate transporters (MCTs), also induced by hypoxia, which transport lactic acid out of the cell. To stabilize pH, HCO_3^- and H^+ ions are cycled between extracellular and intracellular compartments by means of sodium dependent HCO_3^- cotransporters (NBCs) and a Na^+/H^+ exchange pump mechanism (NHE). Reproduced from Swietach *et al.* (2007) *Cancer Metastasis Rev.* 26: 299–310, Springer.

depends upon the conversion of tissue CO_2 to HCO_3^- and H^+ by the catalytic addition of water molecules, where HCO_3^- is then transported out of the cell. This process is facilitated by the enzyme carbonic anhydrase; the predominantly expressed isoform in tumours being the HIF-1-regulated tumour associated carbonic anhydrase CAIX. Ultimately, HCO_3^- and H^+ ions are cycled between extracellular and intracellular compartments by means of sodium dependent HCO_3^- transporters (NBCs) and a Na^+/H^+ exchange pump mechanism (NHE).

CAIX has gained interest as a novel therapeutic target due to its overexpression in a wide range of tumours, where it predicts poor prognosis and is implicated in metastatic pathways. Aside from helping to maintain tumour pH, CAIX is also thought to play a role in tumour cell invasiveness by interfering with E-cadherin-dependent cellular

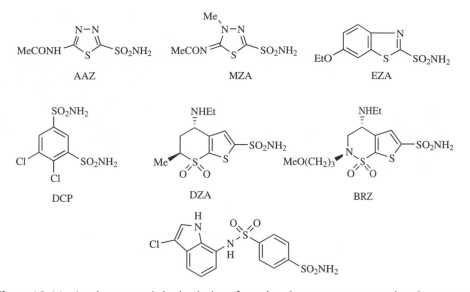

Figure 12.14   Lead compounds in the design of novel anticancer agents targeting the tumour-associated carbonic anhydrase CAIX. The carbonic anhydrase inhibitors acetazolamide (AZZ, Diamox), dorzolamide (DZA) and brinzolamide (BRZ) are sulphonamides used for the treatment of glaucoma, pictured here alongside further examples methazolamide (MZA), ethoxzolamide (EZA), dichlorphenamide (DCP) and E7070 (indisulam), in clinical trials as an antitumour agent. Reproduced from Vullo *et al.* (2004) *Bioorg. Med. Chem. Lett.* 14: 2351–2356, Elsevier.

adhesion. The design of CAIX inhibitors has achieved a head start due to the availability of lead inhibitor compounds such as the sulphonamides acetazolamide, dorzolamide and brinzolamide which are routinely prescribed for glaucoma as a means of reducing intraocular pressure. These compounds, however, show little selectivity towards CAIX relative to the isoforms CA1 and CAII which are highly expressed in normal tissue. Therefore, in an effort to maximize CAIX specificity, a series of fluorinated derivatives were synthesized and investigated (Figure 12.14), which included the novel drug candidate E7070 (indisulam). To date, indisulam has been evaluated in phase II clinical trials as single-agent second-line therapy for non-small cell lung cancer, although only minor tumour responses were seen. Following on from this, indisulam is now undergoing investigation in combination with other agents, where separate phase I studies have evaluated its use alongside carboplatin and capecitabine. At the time of writing, further trials are underway which will evaluate the activity of indisulam in combination with irinotecan in a phase II study involving patients with metastatic colorectal cancer. More phase I trials have also been initiated, looking at clinical response in melanoma and renal cancers.

Another CAIX inhibiting strategy is a chimeric mouse monoclonal antibody preparation raised against CAIX, alternatively described as the G250 antigen or MN. This antibody has been used in many experimental studies for the immunohistochemical detection of CAIX in human tumour samples, where the antigen is found in 85% of renal cell carcinomas. However, its application as an antitumour agent that induces antibody-dependent cellular cytotoxicity in cells displaying the antigen is currently undergoing clinical investigation. Phase I/II studies have evaluated its use in patients with renal cell carcinoma, both as monotherapy and in combination with cytokines such as IL-2 and interferons (IFN), in an effort to increase efficacy. The G250 formulation (Rencarex) is licensed to the pharmaceutical company Wilex and is currently undergoing evaluation in a phase III trial as monotherapy in patients that have undergone surgery for non-metastatic kidney cancer. It is proposed that Rencarex will fill a niche as a treatment for clear cell renal cancer, for which there is to date no approved treatment.

13

Antiangiogenic and antivascular agents

13.1 History of angiogenesis as a therapeutic target

Antiangiogenic anticancer agents target the processes that lead to new blood vessel formation in tumours, whereas vascular disrupting agents disrupt the structure or function of previously formed blood vessels.

If there were to be a cancer research 'hall of fame', angiogenesis would rightfully take its place for several reasons. First, angiogenesis research was a significant evolutionary leap, representing the first departure from the application of traditional anticancer pharmacology which at the time concentrated on cytotoxic agents that targeted DNA synthesis and replication, where the idea was to aim for maximum tumour cell kill. Second, it provided the impetus for a wealth of work aiming to characterize the tumour microenvironment, and helped shift the collective scientific consciousness towards thinking of the tumour as a collaboration of different cell types, its supportive matrix and vascular network, rather than as a ball of cells. Third, it demonstrates extremely effectively the time course along which an anticancer agent is developed, with the initial characterization of the tumour blood supply taking place in the 1960s but the first anti-angiogenic agents only entering clinical trial in the 1990s. Initial studies reported by Goodall *et al.* (1965) involved the observation of vascular patterns using window chamber devices containing tumour material that were implanted into the cheek pouches of Syrian golden hamsters (Figure 13.1). The window chambers offered clear visibility of the growing tumour as it developed its own blood supply, which showed a characteristic pattern according to tumour type. Significantly, these studies allowed the initial observations of the torturous, blind-ended vascular morphology, abnormal flow characteristics and intravascular clotting now firmly established as the cause of the adverse physiological conditions existing in the tumour microenvironment. Characteristic tumour-specific patterns included leashes, or arboreal arrangements with infrequent anastomoses, found in melanoma xenografts; or nets, that described reticular arrangements that were either irregular, as found in mammary carcinoma xenografts, or regular, found in haemangiopericytoma xenografts. The characterization of a distinctive

Cancer Chemotherapy   Rachel Airley
© 2009 John Wiley & Sons, Ltd.

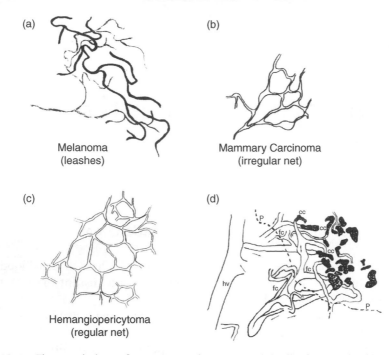

Figure 13.1 The morphology of tumour vasculature was originally characterized in an early but influential study carried out by Goodall *et al.* (1965), using window chamber devices containing tumour material that were implanted into the cheek pouches of Syrian golden hamsters. As the tumour material grafted and increased in volume, distinctive patterns of angiogenic growth typical of tumour type could be observed through the 'window', including (a) leashes, or arboreal arrangements with infrequent anastomoses found in melanoma xenografts; and nets, or reticular arrangements that were either irregular, as found in mammary carcinoma xenografts (b), or regular, found in haemangiopericytoma xenografts (c). The contribution of host versus tumour-derived vasculature was also described in relation to tumour blood flow (d), highlighting the pattern of intermittent and regurgitant flow, together with the intravascular clotting now known to be typical of tumours (p, periphery of xenograft; hv, host vessel; cc, cylindrical clot; fc, functional capillaries; arrows show direction of blood flow, with the double headed arrows representing regurgitant flow. Adapted from Goodall *et al.* (1965).

tumour blood supply provided the springboard for a paradigm shift introduced by Folkman in a seminal paper (Folkman, 1971), which put forward the hypothesis now known as *angiogenic dormancy*, where the growth of a new, tumour-derived blood supply allowed microscopic solid tumours that pre-existed as small populations of cells and dependent upon the diffusion of oxygen and nutrients from the host blood supply to gain the potential to expand to a volume beyond the diffusion distance and to become metastatically able. Folkman proposed that angiogenesis was induced by means of a 100 kDa tumour-derived mediator given the term 'tumour angiogenesis factor' (TAF) and for the first time proposed anti-angiogenesis as a new therapeutic strategy, citing TAF immunization as a possible approach (Figure 13.2). He also defined the term anti-angiogenesis as the prevention of new vessel sprouts rather than as the vasoconstriction

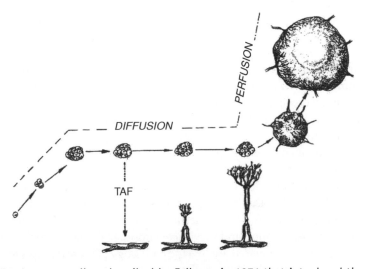

Figure 13.2   A new paradigm described by Folkman in 1971 that introduced the concept of angiogenic dormancy (see Section 5.6.1) and the novel therapeutic strategy anti-angiogenesis- arguably the first example of a departure from the traditional use of DNA or cell proliferation as an anticancer target. During angiogenesis, the growth of new capillaries allowed a rapid growth of the tumour beyond the diameter dictated by the diffusion gradiant of oxygen and nutrients from the host-derived blood supply. This switch from diffusion to perfusion, or nutritive blood flow, was attributed to the not yet fully characterized 'tumour angiogenesis factor' (TAF). Reproduced from *The Journal of Experimental Medicine*, 1971, 133: 275–288. Copyright 1971 The Rockefeller University Press.

or infarction of blood vessels already connected to the tumour. Interestingly, the original article incorporated a question and answer session with Folkman regarding the nature of TAF, which in this study was isolated from tumour implants. On being asked if TAF would be found in spontaneous tumours showing a normoxic periphery but anoxic or necrotic core, the response was as follows:

"When we attempt to isolate TAF from human tumours, we are careful to discard the necrotic portions, which are usually in the centre. To my mind, the necrotic centre of a large tumour was at an earlier time well vascularised. However, the enormous pressures that build up within a large tumour could diminish blood flow to the centre."

Thus, a tentative connection between the physiological tumour microenvironment and its typical manifestations of raised interstitial pressure, tumour hypoxia and the effects of changing vascularity was made more than two decades before the discovery of hypoxia- inducible factor-1 (HIF-1) and its ability to induce angiogenesis. Since then, the speculatively named TAF has given way to a more thorough understanding of the endogenous regulators of angiogenesis, as well as the molecular mechanisms that control their production. As discussed previously (Section 5.6.1), targeting angiogenesis offers a means of blocking the 'angiogenic switch' that provides a subclinical population of tumour cells the capability of malignant progression, that is, to proliferate, survive, invade into the surrounding tissue and produce metastases. There are only two known biological circumstances in which angiogenesis takes place. These are during development, for example, of new capillaries or during osteogenesis (bone development), where there is an ingress of capillaries into the medullary cavity of the forming bone. The other involves pathology, which includes malignant progression in cancer pathology; the formation of new tissue in wound healing, and several pathologies where there is an inflammatory component such as rheumatoid and osteoarthritis, reperfusion injury after myocardial or cerebral (stroke) infarction and inflammatory bowel diseases. All of these have the commonality of a hypoxic microenvironment, where hypoxia regulates many of the pathways that lead to angiogenesis, such as the production of vascular endothelial growth factor (VEGF), epidermal growth factor (EGF) and its receptor EGFR; as well as the proliferation and survival of endothelial cells themselves, through its regulation of apoptosis. The shared angiogenic pathology of these diseases has also led to cross talk between the drug development strategies adopted by research groups developing therapies to treat these diseases, a good example being the development of the matrix metalloproteinase and integrin inhibitors discussed in the following sections.

13.2 Anti-angiogenic drug targets

Since the discovery of TAF, a number of endogenous pro- and anti-angiogenic factors have been discovered, as described in Figure 13.3. Angiogenic activators such as VEGF, platelet-derived growth factor and basic fibroblast growth factor are themselves therapeutic targets, whilst inhibitors are under investigation either directly or as lead compounds in the search for novel anti-angiogenic agents. There are a number of possible sites of pharmacological intervention (Figure 13.4) which define the different

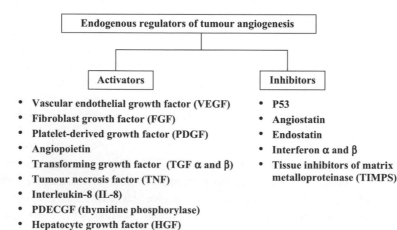

Figure 13.3   Endogenous angiogenic activators and inhibitors. Reproduced from Chen QR, Zhang L, Gasper W, Mixson AJ. *Mol. Genet. Metab.* 2001 Sep–Oct;74(1–2):120–7, Elsevier.

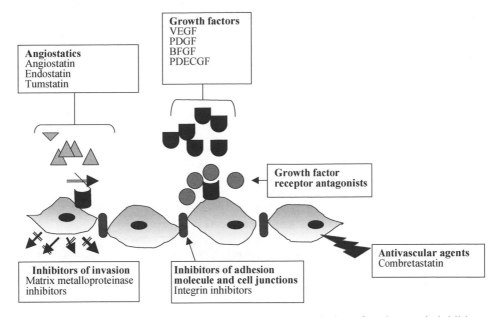

Figure 13.4 Sites of pharmacological intervention in the design of angiogenesis inhibitors.

classes of anti-angiogenic agent either approved or under investigation, as shown by Table 13.1. The first to be investigated were the angiostatic agent endostatin, a 20 kDa internal fragment of type XVIII collagen; closely followed by angiostatin, a cleavage product of plasminogen, which is the precursor of the thrombolytic serine protease plasmin. Work on these compounds lead to much excitement after an article was published in the *New York Times* in May 1998[1] that reported the 'cure' of tumours in mouse models. Observations that repeated doses of angiostatic agent maintained tumour dormancy also introduced the concept that cancer might become a chronic disease that was kept in check rather than eradicated by chemotherapy. However, it has proved more difficult to achieve the same effect in clinical trials in humans, where a phase I trial of endostatin initiated in 1999 involving patients with a broad range of solid tumours demonstrated its good safety profile, but did not show treatment response. The drug did progress to phase II trials, however, in patients with melanoma and neuroendocrine tumours. This time, with higher doses, the drug seemed to stabilize tumour progression, but the lack of tumour response failed to justify the high cost of production at that time. Now reintroduced as Endostar, where the original compound has been manipulated to increase solubility, it is in phase III trials in combination with other angiogenesis inhibitors in China. The pharmacodynamics of the angiostatics are yet to be fully understood, but it is believed that they directly target endothelial cell proliferation via a number of signal transduction pathways that include the MAPK pathway and the intrinsic and extrinsic apoptosis pathways (Figures 15.1 and 2.3). They also inhibit

---

[1]Kolata G, Hope in the lab: a special report; A Cautious Awe Greets Drugs that Eradicate Tumors in Mice. *New York Times*. May 3rd 1998.

Table 13.1 Summary of anti-angiogenic drug targets and associated therapies

Target	Therapy
Growth factors	
VEGF	Anti-VEGF mAb
bFGF	Interferon α
	Thalidomide (inhibitor of VEGF. bFGF and TNF-α)
	Lenalinomide
Growth factor receptor	
EGFR	Gefitinib (Iressa)
VEFGR	FTK787
	Bevacizumab (Avastin)
	Sunitinib (Sutent)
Matrix metalloproteinase	*Broad spectrum*
	Marimistat (BB2516)
	Batimastat
	Neovastat
	Selective-spectrum
	Metastat (COL-3)
	BMS-275 291
	Tanomastat (BAY-12-9566)
	Cipemastat (Trocade)
	Prinomastat
	S-3304
	Third generation MMPIs
	MMI-166
Integrins	Vitaxin (humanized monoclonal antibody to the integrin αvb3 vitronectin receptor CNTO 95 (mAb to alpha v family of integrins)
	Cilengitide (small cyclic RGD, peptide αvb3 and αvβ5 inhibitor)
	E7820 (Sulfonamide derivative, inhibits α2)
	Volociximab (M200) (α5β1 inhibitor)
	ATN-161 (5-amino acid peptide, inhibits α5β1, αvβ3)
Vascular targeting	Combretastatin A4
Endothelial cell proliferation	Endogenous inhibitors
	Endostatin
	Angiostatin
	Tumstatin

mAb, monoclonal antibody.

endothelial cell proliferation by inducing cell cycle arrest at the G1/S transition by downregulating the expression of proteins such as cyclin-D1 and cyclin-dependent kinase (CDK). Another angiostatic agent is tumstatin, which is composed of the 28 kDa fragment of type IV collagen.

Tumstatin may exert its anti-angiogenic effect by blocking αVβ3 integrin, which in a signalling cascade specific to endothelial cells activates mTOR-induced protein synthesis and therefore endothelial cell proliferation (see Section 19.1 for control of cellular proliferation by mTOR). Subsidiary effects of the angiostatics include interference with integrin signalling, necessary for endothelial cell communication and the formation of endothelial cell layers; and the matrix metalloproteinases, where matrix degradation is essential for the tunnelling of new vessels through tissue mass.

The subsequently developed anti-angiogenic therapies have a clearer cut mechanism of action, which has been cited as the reason why their development has surpassed that of the angiostatics. The design of the matrix metalloproteinase (MMP) inhibitors as a novel class of inhibitors is based upon the discovery of the exogenous tissue inhibitors of matrix metalloproteinase (TIMPS). These compounds specifically prevent invasion of newly formed vessels through the extracellular matrix by inhibiting a range of MMP isoforms depending upon their isoform selectivity.

The MMP isoforms are tissue specific and grouped according to their catalytic functionality (Figure 13.5), these properties indicating their role in cancer and their relevance as drug targets. Overall, the matrix metalloproteinase isoforms carry out isoform-specific catalytic breakdown of matrix components including the collagens,

Collagenases
- MMP1 (Collagenase 1-interstitial)
- MMP8 (Collagenase 2- neutrophil)
- MMP13 (Collagenase 3)

Stromelysins
- MMP3 (Stromelysin 1)
- MMP10 (Stromelysin 2)
- MMP11 (Stromelysin 3)

Gelatinases
- MMP2 (Gelatinase A)
- MMP9 (Gelatinase B)

Membrane-type (MT)
- MMP-14 (MT1-MMP)
- MMP-15 (MT2-MMP)
- MMP-16 (MT3-MMP)
- MMP-17 (MT4-MMP)

Others
- MMP12 (Metalloelastase)
- MMP7 (Matrilysin)

Figure 13.5 The MMP family of enzymes.

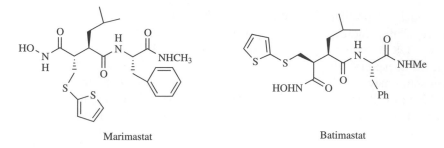

Marimastat   Batimastat

Figure 13.6 The broad spectrum peptidomimetic agents marimastat and batimastat, which target a range of MMP isoforms.

gelatins, fibronectin, fibrin and its precursor fibrinogen, laminin, vitronectin, elastins, tenascin, aggrecan, decorin and entactin. Certain MMPs are also able to activate MMP precursors. The MMPs are zinc-dependent enzymes that exist in active or latent form and share a common structure consisting of three domains – the catalytic, amino-terminal or propeptide domain, and the carboxy-terminal domain – where differences within the catalytic domain determine substrate specificity and the propeptide domain confers enzyme latency, by way of the PRCGxPD motif, where the C (cysteine) residue interacts with the zinc atom at the active site. Enzyme activation depends upon disruption of this interaction when the zinc atom interacts with water- the 'cysteine switch'. To date, there have been a number of attempts to target MMPs which, although they are still evolving, have been met with a limited degree of success. The first were the low molecular weight hydroxamates (Figure 13.6) batimastat and ilomastat, followed by the orally active marimastat, which were broad-spectrum zinc-binding peptidomimetic inhibitors based upon the structure of collagen. However, clinical trials proved disappointing, where patients suffered musculoskeletal toxicities such as severe joint pain and the consequent dose reduction abrogated any significant antitumour response. An explanation for this lies with the promiscuous nature of MMP functionality, where certain MMPs might be described as 'anti-targets', or enzymes that are essential for normal tissue function, so that their inhibition leads to collateral toxicity. Initially, this led to a change in rationale towards the design of more selective MMP inhibitors, including the small molecule non peptidomimetic inhibitors tanomastat (BAY-12-9566), which showed increased selectivity towards MMPs 2, 3 and 9 and no activity against MMP1, and prinomastat (AG 3340), which has selectivity to MMPs 2 and 3. However, both these agents were discontinued after phase III clinical trials: tanomastat after trials involving patients with pancreatic, ovarian and lung cancers; and prinomastat after trials in patients with prostate and non-small-cell lung cancers showed little efficacy. Therefore, it has become crucial to establish the function and so validate MMPs individually as anticancer targets. So far, efforts to establish which MMPs act as anti-targets have indicated MMP8, whose overexpression has been linked with cancer susceptibility and increased invasion and metastasis; MMP12, which is able to generate the production of angiostatin and inhibit angiogenesis; and MMP14, believed to be necessary for normal skeletal development. MMP 3 and MMP9, incidentally, have been shown to have both pro- and antitumorigenic activity, interesting in light of the

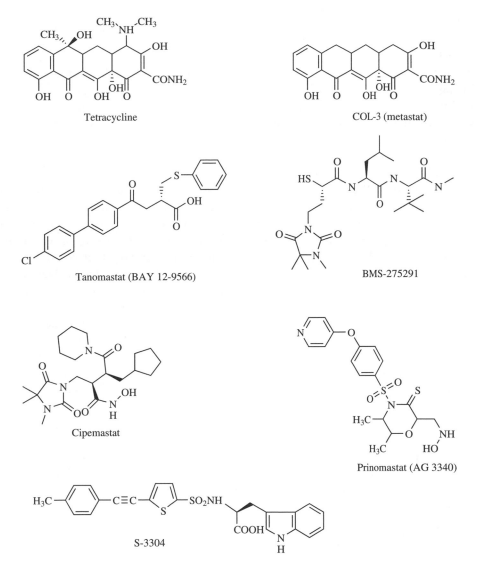

Figure 13.7 Selectivity of the newer, more specifically targeted MMP inhibitors. These include the small molecule MMP inhibitors, for example, tanomastat, which is lacking in activity against MMP1; and BMS-275291, which shows increased specificity towards MMP2 and MMP9 along with the tetracycline derivative MMP inhibitor COL-3.

increased selectivity towards these isoforms shown by the more selective spectrum MMP inhibitors. The development of second-generation MMP inhibitors continues (Figure 13.7), including another small molecule non peptidomimetic BMS-275291, selective for MMPs 2 and 9; the shark cartilage extract neovastat (AE-941); and the peptidomimetic agent cipemastat (Trocade), which are also, at the time of writing, in clinical trial.

Most recently, a new compound S-3304, a derivative of D-tryptophan, has been developed. This agent shows selectivity towards MMP2 and MMP9 but does not target MMP1, MMP3, or MMP7, which may protect against the musculoskeletal side effects seen with previous inhibitors- as demonstrated by the good tolerability profile observed during the trial. The tetracycline derivatives were investigated as potential MMP inhibitors by virtue of their ability to inhibit connective tissue breakdown by mechanisms unrelated to their antimicrobial activity (inhibition of amino acyl tRNA during protein synthesis). Following on from a series of interesting studies that demonstrated the antiproliferative activity of doxyxcycline *in vitro*, a series of chemically modified tetracyclines were synthesized. To date, one such derivative, metastat (COL-3) shows activity against MMP2 and 9, and their anti-angiogenic nature has been demonstrated with functional experiments that showed inhibition of tube formation by the human umbilical vein endothelial cell (HUVEC) cell line. Metastat is currently in phase I/II clinical trials in patients with progressive or recurring brain tumours. Ironically, at the time of writing, the only approved MMP inhibitor is periostat, licensed for the treatment of periodontal disease, which if nothing else demonstrates the significant overlap existing between the matrix pathologies of the malignant and inflammatory diseases. To this end, the design of third-generation MMP inhibitors will focus on achieving selectivity towards target MMPs, which will depend upon the precise modelling of the active sites of individual isoforms. So far, the rational design of MMP inhibitors has involved the synthesis of compounds that contain a zinc-binding group, a supporting scaffold that orientates the zinc-binding group and varying side chains that aid binding to the enzyme. The zinc-binding groups, which bind the catalytic domain of the MMPs, have included the hydroxamates, discussed above, as well as reversed hydroxamate, carboxylate, thiolate, phosphinate and phosphonate groups. Lately, novel compounds containing zinc binding groups such as pyrone, carboxylic ester and *N*-hydroxyurea have been investigated, as have compounds that do not contain a zinc-binding group, the example shown in Figure 13.8 being a compound discovered by

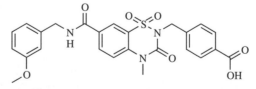

MMP-1 $IC_{50} > 10^5$ nM
MMP-3 $IC_{50} > 3 \cdot 10^4$ nM
MMP-7 $IC_{50} > 3 \cdot 10^4$ nM
MMP-9 $IC_{50} > 10^5$ nM
MMP-13 $IC_{50} = 4.85$ nM
MMP-14 $IC_{50} > 10^5$ nM

Figure 13.8 Novel MMP inhibitors are being developed from lead compounds that show increased isoform specificity during toxicity screening. The above compound is a selective MMP13 inhibitor (note the extremely low IC_{50} value) identified through high throuput drug screening at Pfizer. Reproduced from Pirard (2007) *Drug Discovery Today* 12: 640–646, Elsevier.

high throughput screening at Pfizer that shows a high degree of specificity towards MMP13.

The integrin inhibitors represent an anti-angiogenic strategy that target cell to cell and cell-matrix adhesion. Tumour-derived blood vessels constitute endothelial cells that overexpress certain integrins relative to normal blood vessels such as the αv integrin receptor family that include the integrins $\alpha5\beta1$, $\alpha v\beta3$ and $\alpha v\beta5$. These cell-surface glycoproteins are necessary for the formation of the endothelial cell layer within the new blood vessel that depends upon the existence of cell–cell junctions and promotes endothelial cell survival. Integrin receptors also mediate binding of endothelial cells to the extracellular matrix via arginine–glycine–aspartic acid (RGD) amino acid sequences found on matrix proteins, allowing migration of newly generated blood vessels through surrounding tissue.

There are several approaches being used in the design of integrin antagonists. These include RGD-containing peptide analogues such as cilengitide, which inhibits the $\alpha v\beta3$ and $\alpha v\beta5$ integrins. Cilengitide has been evaluated in a range of phase I/II trials, including a phase I trial involving patients with recurrent malignant glioma, where the treatment was well tolerated and complete or partial responses were observable in a small proportion of patients. However, in a phase II trial to evaluate the use of cilengitide in advanced pancreatic cancer, where it was given in combination with gemcitabine, although there was favourable tolerability, there was no significant improvement in clinical response relative to gemcitabine alone. Phase I and II trials evaluating the use of cilengitide in a range of cancers are still underway. Another strategy is the use of monoclonal antibodies that specifically target integrins, the most advanced in terms of clinical development being vitaxin, a humanized monoclonal antibody directed against the $\alpha v\beta3$ integrin, currently in phase II trials.

Vitaxin has been closely followed by the generation of the monoclonal antibody products CNTO 95, a monoclonal antibody targeting the αv family of integrins that is currently in phase I trials to evaluate its use in solid tumours; and volociximab, an inhibitor of $\alpha5\beta1$ in phase II clinical trials involving patients with renal cell carcinoma, melanoma, non-small cell lung and pancreatic cancer. Other integrin inhibitors in clinical development include ATN-161, a peptide antagonist of $\alpha v\beta3$ and $\alpha5\beta1$; and E7820, a sulfonamide derivative which inhibits $\alpha2$ integrins, both currently in phase I clinical trial.

13.3 The return of thalidomide

Thalidomide is an anticancer agent that was originally used as a sedative and to treat morning sickness, but was withdrawn in 1961 when it proved to be teratogenic, resulting in the birth of between 8000 and 12 000 'thalidomide babies' with characteristic severe limb deformities. The discovery that thalidomide had immunomodulatory and anti-angiogenic effects came out of important work carried out in the 1990s, culminating in its approval by the FDA in 1998 for the treatment of erythema nodosum leprosum (ENL), a dermatological proliferative disorder with characteristic skin lesions; and subsequently for the treatment of multiple myeloma in 2006. Thalidomide stood out as a potential new therapy for multiple myeloma because of the combined anti-angiogenic and immunomodulatory effects that could be used to target the complex signalling taking place within the bone marrow microenvironment in patients with this disease.

The investigation of thalidomide as an anti-angiogenic agent was inspired by the belief that the teratogenicity of thalidomide was a result of impaired vasculogenesis which led to limb bud malformations. Later work showed this to be mediated by the suppression of the angiogenic growth factors VEGF and basic fibroblast growth factor (bFGF), produced by tumour cells, associated immune cells such as macrophages and bone marrow stromal cells. Thalidomide also interferes with the release of important pro-inflammatory cytokines from monocytes and macrophages, primarily tumour necrosis factor-α (TNF-α), but also the transcriptional regulator NF-κB, the enzymes cyclooxygenase-2 (COX-2), the cytokines transforming growth factor-β (TGF-β) and other cytokines such as the interleukins IL-1β, IL-8, IL-6 and IL-12. This occurs alongside the stimulation of T-helper cells to produce IL-2 and interferon-γ (IFN-γ), these factors in turn activating cytotoxic natural killer (NK) cells. There is also evidence that thalidomide increases the activation of $CD4^+$ and $CD8^+$ T-cells. Another site of action is the bone marrow microenvironment, where paracrine signalling taking place between tumour and stromal cells is reduced via modulation of the adhesion proteins intercellular adhesion molecule 1 (ICAM-1) and vascular cell adhesion molecule 1 (VCAM-1) leading to suppression of processes such as cell migration. Thalidomide also induces apoptosis by interfering with the extrinsic apoptosis pathway (Figure 2.3), leading to G1 growth arrest. This is mediated in a number of ways, through increased activation of caspase-8 occurring in response to Fas induction; increased activity of the apoptotic inducer TNF-related apoptosis inducing ligand (TRAIL); and downregulation of the anti-apoptotic protein cellular inhibitor of apoptosis protein-2.

A synthetic glutamic acid derivative, thalidomide (α [N = phthalimido] glutarimide) has a single chiral centre, therefore exists as a racemic mixture of two enantiomers, $S(-)$ and $R(+)$ (Figure 13.9). At first, it was thought that the $S(-)$ enantiomer was teratogenic whilst the therapeutic, sedative properties were attributed to the $R(+)$ enantiomer, leading to attempts to manufacture formulations containing the latter. This approach was abandoned, however, when subsequent studies indicated that both enantiomers were teratogenic. Meanwhile, the $S(-)$ enantiomer 3-amino-thalidomide (ENMD-0995), granted orphan drug status in 2002 (see Section 8.4.2) shows increased anti-angiogenic activity *in vivo*, where it is a potent inhibitor of TNF-α release from peripheral monocytes. Accordingly, phase I trials have now been initiated to evaluate this agent as a therapy for multiple myeloma.

Whereas the isomerization of thalidomide presents a pharmaceutical problem to be overcome in order to establish its place in the clinic, clinical problems associated with its use include a range of adverse effects, the most severe being neutropenia and thrombocytopenia, deep vein thrombosis, neuropathy, sedation and constipation. Development of this class of anti-cancer agents therefore progressed down the route of designing analogues with improved anticancer activity as well as decreased toxicity. The most clinically advanced of these, lenalidomide (CC-5013, lenalinomide, revlomid, (α-(3-aminophthalimido) glutarimide), was approved by the FDA for the treatment of

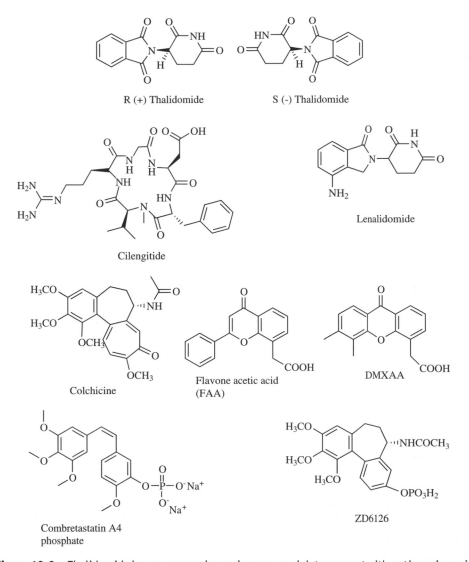

Figure 13.9 Thalidomide has re-emerged as an immunomodulatory agent with anti-angiogenic activity and has been approved for the treatment of multiple myeloma along with the thalidomide derivative lenalidomide; cilengitide is a small cyclic RGD peptide inhibitor of the integrin αvβ3 currently in phase I/II trials for the treatment of pancreatic, lung, skin, brain and haematological malignancies; the antivascular agents including those derived from colchicine, such as combretastatin A4 phosphate, a soluble prodrug of the natural product combretastatin A4 which was isolated from the African Bush Willow *Combresta caffrum*; flavone acetic acid (FAA) and the more potent derivative 5,6-dimethylxanthenone-4-acetic acid (DMXAA); and ZD6126, a phosphate prodrug of N-acetylcolchinol which causes blood stasis.

multiple myeloma shortly after thalidomide in 2006. This agent is significantly more potent at activating T-cell production and the release of the cytokines IL-2 and IFN-γ, and this occurs in the absence of the sedation and constipation experienced with thalidomide, with the neurotoxic reactions also being significantly reduced. Other analogues based on the thalidomide metabolite 5'-OH-thaliomide are currently in preclinical development, having been designed to optimize anti-angiogenic activity. Promising compounds include the N-substituted and tetrafluorinated analogues CPS45 and CPS49, where their anti-angiogenic activity has been evaluated *in vitro*. This is carried out using assays that measure the effect of candidate anti-angiogenic agents on proliferation and luminal tube formation by vascular endothelial cells, usually the HUVEC cell line. The thalidomide analogue CC-4047 (Actomid) has been evaluated in a phase I trial in patients with multiple myeloma, producing significant activation of T-cells, monocytes and macrophages. Phase II trials are now planned to evaluate its use in myelofibrosis and sickle cell anaemia.

13.4 Monoclonal antibodies as anti-angiogenic agents

Therapeutic monoclonal antibodies may be used to specifically inhibit proteins involved in malignant progression. The most clinically successful monoclonal antibodies developed as anti-angiogenic agents target angiogenic growth factors such as VEGF and its receptor VEGFR, the epidermal growth factor receptor EGFR and the related erbB receptor HER2. These tyrosine kinase type receptors are also the target of small molecule receptor tyrosine kinase inhibitors discussed in Chapter 14. The first of its class was trastuzumab (Herceptin), which targets the HER2 receptor, and was approved in 1998 for the treatment of HER2-positive breast cancer. The use of trastuzumab has been subject to its cardiotoxic effects, and there are also issues with chemoresistance believed to be due to *HER2* mutation and amplification of other members of the erbB family not targeted by trastuzumab. The agent is therefore the subject of ongoing clinical trials that aim to optimize its use with regard to predictive markers, scheduling and combination with other anticancer agents. A further EGFR targeted monoclonal antibody, cetuximab (Erbitux), was approved by the FDA in 2004 for the treatment of EGFR expressing colorectal cancer and then in 2006 for squamous cell carcinomas of the head and neck.

Bevacizumab (Avastin) was approved by the FDA in 2004 for the treatment of metastatic colorectal cancer in combination with fluorouracil containing regimens, and additionally in 2006 for the treatment of advanced, nonsquamous, non-small cell lung cancer in combination with carboplatin and paclitaxel. Two key phase III trials contributing to the approval process were the Eastern Cooperative Oncology Group 4599 trial, completed in 2006, which evaluated the use of bevacizumab in combination with carboplatin/paclitaxel in patients with lung cancer, and a phase III trial reported in 2004 evaluating a regimen consisting of bevacizumab plus irinotecan, fluorouracil and folinic acid for the treatment of metastatic colorectal cancer. Bevacizumab is the first monoclonal antibody preparation targeting VEGF. Like trastuzumab, it is a humanized monoclonal immunoglobulin G antibody (Figure 13.10) derived from a

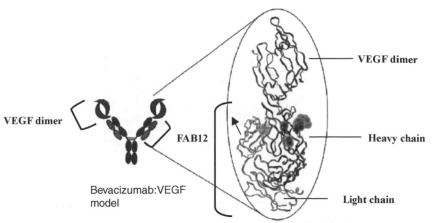

Figure 13.10   Structure of the bevacizumab : VEGF complex. The Fab fragment of the humanized antibody was prepared by manipulation of amino acid residues within the parent antibody A4.6.1 (the above version designated FAB12) and this is complexed to VEGF-A dimer. Adapted from Lien, S. and Lowman, H.B. (2008) Therapeutic anti-VEGF antibodies, in *Handbook of Experimental Pharmacology* (eds A Chernajovsky and A. Nissim), Springer-Verlag, Berlin Heidelberg, vol 181, pp 131–50.

parental murine monoclonal antibody, which itself would not be suitable for use in patients due to its immunogenicity. The parental antibody used to manufacture bevacizumab is the murine monoclonal antibody to VEGFA, A4.6.1, which blocks the binding of all active VEGF isoforms to the receptors VEGFR1 and VEGFR2. Manipulation of amino acid residues within the bevacizumab complex has produced an antibody with a human framework and a murine VEGF binding region. Another monoclonal antibody to VEGF, ranibizumab (Lucentis), was approved in 2006 for use in acute macular degeneration, an ophthalmic condition characterized by neovascularization of the choroid.

The first monoclonal antibody to target the EGFR, panitumumab, was approved by the FDA in late 2006 for the treatment of EGFR-expressing metastatic colorectal cancer. At the time of writing, a phase III trial is underway, aiming to evaluate the clinical efficacy of adding panitumumab to a combination chemotherapy regimen consisting of bevacizumab, irinotecan, fluorouracil and folinic acid as first line treatment for metastatic colorectal cancer.

13.5 The hollow fibre assay as a drug screen for anti-angiogenic drugs

The use of subcutaneously implanted hollow fibres as an *in vivo* angiogenesis assay (Figure 13.12) is a modification of the hollow fiber assay originally developed as a rapid *in vivo* drug screen by the National Cancer Institute, where fibres containing one of a panel of tumour cell lines were implanted into mice before dosing with drug. By removing the fibre and measuring the clonogenicity of the cells they contained, a rapid

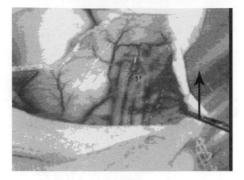

Figure 13.11   Morphology of blood vessels developing around implanted hollow fibers (arrow) (Reproduced with permission from Sadar *et al. Molecular and Cancer Therapeutics* 2002, American Association for Cancer Research.)

determination of *in vivo* drug response could be made without the necessity of developing transgenic tumour models or generating xenografts. The use of this technique as an angiogenesis assay arises from the observation that extension of implantation times beyond the stipulated 6 day period (Clear protocols for the technique are provided by the NCI on the following web site http://dtp.nci.nih.gov/branches/btb/hfa.html#HollowFiberAssay) results in extensive vascularization around the fibres in the subcutaneous site   (Figure 13.11). The vascularized tissue may be removed after dosing the animal and the extent of angiogenesis imaged in a number of ways, for instance by preparing whole mounts of the fixed tissue and analysing capillary number by semiquantitative histomorphometric analysis – there are a number of computer programs available with which to do this.

The technique also allows *in vivo* assessment of the effects of anti-angiogenic agents on vascular functionality, where imaging techniques such as positron emission

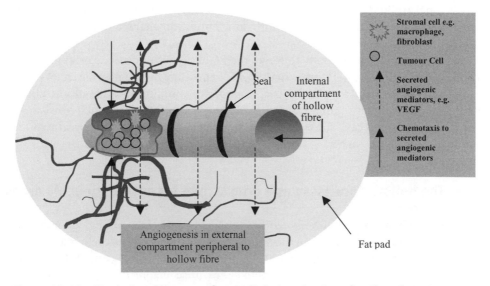

Figure 13.12   The hollow fibre assay for preclinical evaluation of anti-angiogenic agents.

tomography may be used alongside isotopes of CO and water to measure altered perfusion dynamics and blood vessel leakiness that may arise as a consequence of treating the animal with anti-angiogenic agents. Live intravital imaging, using lysine dextran labelling of blood vessels, allows detection of the developing neovascularization relative to any inhibition of the angiogenic process by the agent. Another advantage is that the fibres may be filled with co-cultures of cell lines that may more accurately reflect the make-up of a tumour, for example, using a combination of tumour and macrophage or fibroblast cell lines. By varying the nature of the cell lines used and other biological conditions, the assay may provide another means of identifying and validating novel targets for anti-angiogenic drug development.

13.6 Vascular disrupting agents

Vascular disrupting agents cause rapid collapse and shut down of established tumour blood vessels leading to regional tumour ischaemia and necrosis. These agents may be broadly categorized as tubulin-binding agents, such as combretastatin A4; and the flavonoids, which include the analogue of flavone acetic acid 5,6-dimethylxanthenone-4-acetic acid (DMXAA) (Figure 13.9). To date, most work carried out to characterize the pharmacodynamic effects of vascular disrupting agents has involved combretastatin A4, which is the most clinically advanced compound of this class. Several effects have been identified, which include changes in the actin cytoskeleton and certain signal transduction cascades that alter blood flow and cause endothelial cell death. Combretastatin A4 is a natural product of the African Bush willow tree *Combresta caffrum*, administered in the form of the more soluble prodrug combretastatin A4 phosphate. This agent, which is licensed to the pharmaceutical company OXiGENE, has been evaluated in phase I/II trials involving patients with advanced solid tumours, separate trials evaluating its use in combination with the anti-angiogenic monoclonal antibody bevacizumab (Avastin) and paclitaxel/carboplatin. Phase II trials have also been initiated to specifically evaluate its use in tumours of the lung and thyroid gland. Combretastatin A4 is classed as a tubulin-binding vascular disrupting agent, where its chemical structure is similar to the classical tubulin inhibitor colchicine, whose vascular disrupting properties are well established despite the agent being too toxic at doses necessary to achieve chemoresponse. These agents act directly upon endothelial cells, where, in a similar fashion to tubulin-binding agents acting on tumour cells such as the vinca alkaloids and the taxanes (Section 8.4.4), binding to tubulin subunits leads to depolymerization of the microtubules that make up the actin cytoskeleton and altered actinomyosin contractility. In the case of tubulin-binding vascular disrupting agents, however, selectivity to tumour rather than normal vascular endothelium is achieved by way of dissimilarities in morphology and physiology such as the rate of endothelial cell proliferation, lack of extravascular pericytes and the increased fragility afforded by the abnormal basement membrane, thin muscular wall and reduced vasomotor control characteristic of tumour blood vessels. These differences make endothelial cells more vulnerable to the effects of tubulin binding agents, whose primary effect of disturbing actinomyosin contractility is not just to inhibit mitotic spindle formation, but to initiate

cellular remodelling that compromises the shape, motility and the invasion characteristics of endothelial cells that are necessary to maintain the correct conformation,
attachment and permeability of the blood vessel within the tumour matrix. These effects
are mediated via the Rho-GTP pathway, where depolymerization of microtubules
activates the GTPase RhoA, in turn activating the downstream effector enzyme RhoA
kinase. RhoA kinase catalyses the phosphorylation of myosin light chains, increasing
cytoskeletal contractility, as well as inducing the formation of focal adhesion complexes
and the disassembly of the V- and E-cadherins necessary to maintain the integrity of cell
to cell junctions. Combretastatin also activates the stress protein SAPK2 (stress-
activated protein kinase 2), leading to the formation of stress fibres and F-actin
polymerization. Misalignment of focal adhesion complexes and the formation of thick
F-actin bands induce membrane blebbing at the endothelial cell surface, which further
compromises plasma membrane integrity and increases vascular permeability, eventually leading to endothelial cell necrosis. The increased cytoskeletal contractility is also
mechanically linked to the increase in vascular permeability, where increased contractility leads to a rise in the tensional forces acting towards the interior of the cell,
which oppose the adhesion forces holding cell junctions together. Increasing vascular
permeability has two effects, first to increase interstitial fluid pressure within the
tumour mass, which may restrict blood flow by restricting local microcirculation; and
second, to increase leakage of plasma, the resulting increase in blood viscosity further
reducing blood flow. This effect is exacerbated by erythrocyte stacking and the
activation of platelets. In addition, blebbing of endothelial cells, which precedes
apoptosis, may be observed where these structures also increase vascular resistance.

The flavonoid vascular disrupting agents are based upon flavone acetic acid, which is
believed to restrict blood flow by an NFκB-dependent pathway, leading to increased
production of TNF-α and other cytokines, which decreases tumour blood flow, whilst
at the same time stimulating the production of nitric oxide which increases vascular
permeability. DMXAA is a derivative of flavone acetic acid which is 16-fold more
potent, and is currently in phase II trials, including one currently underway which is
evaluating its use in combination with docetaxel in patients with hormone refractory
metastatic prostate cancer. Other vascular disrupting agents in clinical development
include another tubulin binding agent derived from colchicine, ZD6126, a phosphate
prodrug of N-acetylcholchinol which causes blood stasis and is currently being
evaluated in renal cancer.

14

Tyrosine kinase inhibitors

14.1 Introduction

A broad range of molecular pathways controlling malignant progression depend upon the expression of receptors or intermediate proteins with tyrosine kinase activity. When activated by binding of endogenous ligands, tyrosine kinases catalyse the transfer of phosphate groups from ATP to tyrosine residues on effector proteins. This transfers a signal that regulates the transcriptional control of genes influencing cell survival, proliferation, progression through the cell cycle, and critical events in invasion, metastasis and angiogenesis. Tyrosine kinases (Figure 14.1) may be classified as receptor tyrosine kinases, where the enzyme forms part of a plasma membrane bound receptor, or non receptor tyrosine kinases, which are in the majority of cases located within the cytoplasm or associated with the endofacial surface of the cell. Receptor tyrosine kinases, such as the vascular endothelial growth factor receptor (VEGFR), the epidermal growth factor receptor (EGFR) and platelet derived growth factor receptor (PDGFR are activated via ligand binding to the extracellular domain which triggers dimerization of the receptor. This induces transphosphorylation of the cytoplasmic intracellular domain, activating an ATP-binding region within the catalytic core of the tyrosine kinase, which to accept ATP, must be in an 'open' conformation. The ATP-binding site may also provide a docking site for cytoplasmic signalling proteins, for example, those homologous to Src, allowing their accumulation within the locality of the receptor and subsequently initiating a signal transduction cascade. There are a number of non-receptor tyrosine kinase families. These include Abl, found in the cytoplasm, where it is associated with the function of the actin cytoskeleton, and in the nucleus, where it may be involved in transcriptional regulation via an interaction with RNA polymerase II, the transcription factor E2F and the tumour suppressor protein Rb. Another group of enzymes, the Src kinases, are found in the cytoplasm associated with the inner face of the plasma membrane, where they are able to bind to intracellular tyrosine residues of ligand activated receptor tyrosine kinases such as PDGFR, CSF-1R, FGFR and EGFR, this in turn communicating a signal to pathways such as the Ras/Raf/Erk and Akt signal transduction cascades. Src kinases also mediate the activation of signal transduction cascades by receptors that themselves lack tyrosine kinase activity. Further functions

Cancer Chemotherapy   Rachel Airley
© 2009 John Wiley & Sons, Ltd.

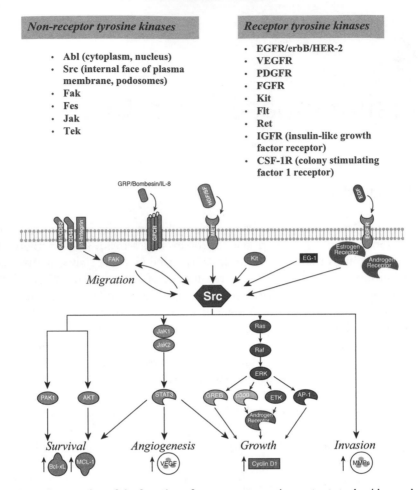

Figure 14.1 Integration of the function of non-receptor and receptor tyrosine kinases in signal transduction cascades. Endogenous ligand binding to the domain of plasma membrane bound receptor tyrosine kinases activates non-receptor tyrosine kinases such as Src, stimulating signal transduction cascades such as the Ras/RAF/ERK and Akt pathways that regulate tumour cell proliferation, survival and angiogenesis. Reproduced from Chang *et al.* (2007) *Neoplasia* 9: 90–100, Nature Publishing Group.

may arise from the coupling of Src kinases to antigen and cytokine receptors such as CD4 and CD8. Non receptor tyrosine kinases are also ATP-dependent, where structurally they possess a variable number of signalling domains and a kinase domain.

In general, the ATP-binding tyrosine kinase consists of two (N-terminal and C-terminal) lobes, between which lays a cleft where ATP binds (Figure 14.2). This ATP-binding cleft is the target for rationally designed small molecule tyrosine kinase inhibitors for novel therapeutics based on structural analogues of ATP, such as the bcr-abl inhibitor imitanib (Gleevec) and the EGFR inhibitors gefitinib (Iressa) and erlotinib (Tarceva). Early examples of ATP analogue tyrosine kinase inhibitors were flavonoids such as the naturally occurring soy bean isolate genistein, the cyclin-dependent kinase inhibitor flavopiridol and quercetin (Figure 14.3). The design of tyrosine kinase

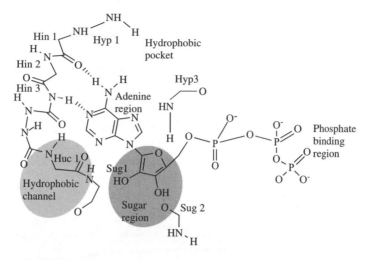

Figure 14.2 The ATP-binding site of tyrosine kinase is an important site for pharmacological intervention. The first ATP-binding tyrosine kinase inhibitors to be approved were the non-receptor tyrosine kinase bcr-abl inhibitor imatinib (Gleevec) and the receptor-binding EGFR tyrosine kinase inhibitor gefitinib (Iressa), an inhibitor of the receptor tyrosine kinase EGFR. Reproduced with permission from Paul and Mukhopadhyay (2004) *Int. J. Med. Sci.* 1: 101–115, Ivyspring International Publisher.

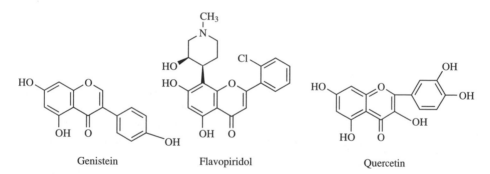

Genistein   Flavopiridol   Quercetin

Figure 14.3 Flavonoid ATP-binding tyrosine kinase inhibitors.

inhibitors based upon their analogy with ATP, however, also gives rise to the potential for non-specific interactions with ATP-binding cassette (ABC) type membrane-bound transporter proteins, such as the drug efflux transporters multidrug resistance protein (MRP), breast cancer resistance protein (BCRP) and p-glycoprotein (see Section 22.4.1) and facilitative glucose transporters such as Glut-1. The expression of these carrier proteins within tumours may therefore impact on response to these treatments and diagnostic imaging by FDG-PET (Chapter 11).

14.2 Tyrosine kinase inhibitors targeting angiogenesis

The tyrosine kinase activity of a large number of angiogenic growth factor receptors means that the design of novel receptor tyrosine kinase inhibitors has proved to be a

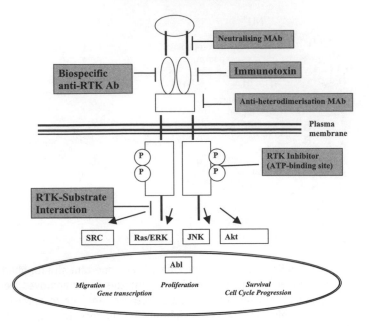

Figure 14.4 Structure of a generalized heterodimeric receptor tyrosine kinase showing potential sites of pharmacological intervention, including the ATP-binding site. Adapted from Gschwind *et al.* (2004).

successful therapeutic approach in angiogenesis research, with a number of agents approved and a still larger number currently undergoing preclinical and clinical development. The generalized structure of the receptor tyrosine kinase, shown in Figure 14.4, offers a number of sites for pharmacological intervention. The largest group so far interacts with the ATP-binding site of angiogenic growth factor receptors. These may be selective (Figure 14.5), where the first anti-angiogenic receptor tyrosine kinase inhibitor approved by the FDA was the EGFR inhibitor gefitinib in 2003 for the treatment of advanced non-small cell lung cancer. Second-generation EGFR inhibitors are now in clinical use, such as erlotinib, approved for non-small cell lung cancer (2004) and pancreatic cancer (2005) and lapatinib (Tykerb), approved in 2007 for use in combination with capecitabine in patients with HER2 expressing advanced metastatic breast cancer. Alternatively, multi-kinase inhibitors (Figure 14.6) bind the ATP-binding region of a number of tyrosine kinases. These include sunitinib (Sutent), which was approved by the FDA in early 2006 for the double indication of gastro-intestinal stromal tumours and renal cell carcinoma and targets a number of angiogenic growth factor receptors including the VEGFR, Flt-3, PDGFR, c-kit, stem-cell factor receptor and Fms-like tyrosine kinase receptor 3. This closely followed the FDA approval of sorafenib (Nexavar), an inhibitor of both the receptor tyrosine kinase VEGFR2 and the non receptor Raf serine/threonine kinases, for the treatment of renal cell carcinoma in late 2005, an indication for hepatocellular carcinoma being added in late 2007.

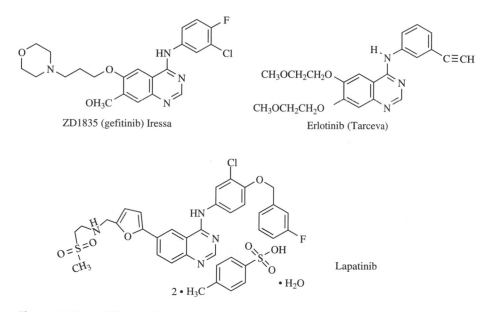

Figure 14.5 Inhibitors of the epidermal growth factor receptor (EGFR) tyrosine kinase.

Another site of interaction with the receptor tyrosine kinase that has yielded novel anti-angiogenic agents is at the extracellular ligand binding domain. So far, this has generated the monoclonal antibody preparations to the HER2 receptor, trastuzumab (Herceptin) and to the EGFR receptor, cetuximab (Erbitux) (Section 13.4).

14.3 Non-receptor tyrosine kinase inhibitors

The design of non receptor tyrosine kinase inhibitors (Figure 14.7) has focused mainly on bcr-abl and Src kinase. The bcr-abl tyrosine kinase is a feature of the Philadelphia chromosome found in patients with chronic myeloid leukaemia, whilst the Src kinase shows increased activity especially in colorectal and breast cancers and is coded for by the proto-oncogene *v-Src*, a transforming gene of the Rous sarcoma virus. Of those currently approved or in clinical development, the bcr-abl inhibitor imatinib (Gleevec) was the first small molecule tyrosine kinase inhibitor to enter clinical use, having been approved by the FDA in 2001 for the treatment of Philadelphia positive chronic myeloid leukaemia, and subsequently for paediatric use in 2003. A second-generation bcr-abl inhibitor, nilotinib (Tasigna), has now been approved by the FDA (late 2007) for patients with chronic myeloid leukaemia showing intolerance or resistance to imatinib. Although it was initially thought that imatinib was selective for bcr-abl, it is now known to have other targets, such as c-kit, which was the basis of its approval in 2002 for the treatment of gastrointestinal stromal tumours. Another recently approved non-receptor tyrosine kinase inhibitor is dasatinib (Sprycel), approved by the FDA in 2006 for the treatment of Philadelphia positive adult chronic myeloid and acute lymphoblastic leukaemias refractory or intolerant to prior therapy. Dasatinib is a dual

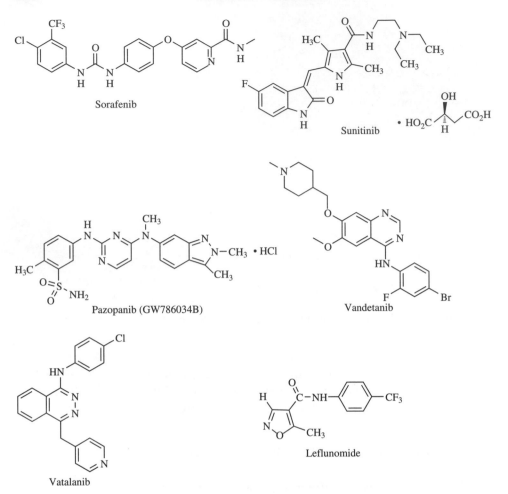

Figure 14.6 Multikinase receptor tyrosine kinase inhibitors, including sorafenib, an inhibitor of Raf serine/threonine kinases and the tyrosine kinase receptors vascular endothelial growth factor receptor-2 (VEGFR2), platelet-derived growth factor receptor (PDGFR), Flt-3, c-Kit, and p38; sunitinib, which inhibits VEGFR, PDGFR, stem-cell factor receptor and Fms-like tyrosine kinase receptor 3 receptor tyrosine-kinases; pazopanib, an inhibitor of VEGFR 1,2 and 3; vandetanib, which targets VEGFR2, EGFR and RET; vatalanib, an inhibitor of VEGFR1 (Flt-1) and VEGF2; and leflunomide, an inhibitor of PDGFR.

inhibitor of bcr-abl and Src kinase, which also targets c-kit and PDGFR-B. Efforts to develop inhibitors of Src have produced a number of compounds in preclinical and clinical development. Most, like dasatanib, despite showing potent Src inhibitory activity, also target bcr-abl and kit, as is the case with bosutinib, a Src/Abl inhibitor that has undergone phase I clinical evaluation in advanced solid tumours; along with AZD0530 and PP1. Novel approaches include the investigation of trisubstituted

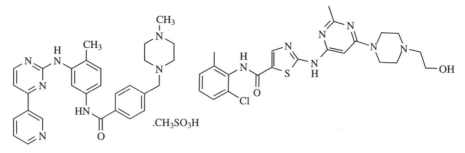

ST1571, imatinib (Gleevec)

Dasatinib

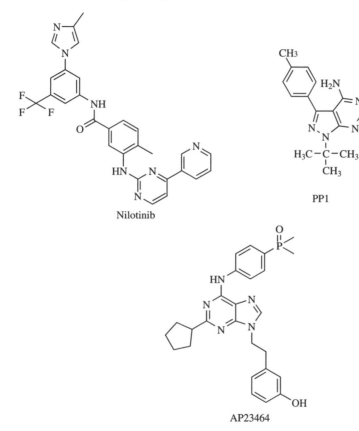

Nilotinib

PP1

AP23464

Figure 14.7 Non-receptor bcr-abl tyrosine kinase inhibitors imatinib and nilotinib; the Src inhibitors PP1 and AP23464; and the dual bcr-abl and Src inhibitor dasatinib.

purines such as the 2,6,9-trisubstituted purine derivative AP23464, a cyclin-dependent kinase (CDK) inhibitor that has shown Src inhibitory activity in structure-activity studies, making it a suitable lead compound for the future development of Src inhibitors.

15

Ras inhibitors

Ras is a proto-oncogene occurring in three forms, *H-Ras*, *N-Ras* and *K-Ras*, coding for a GTPase that localizes to the endofacial surface of the plasma membrane and activates growth factor-mediated signal transduction pathways regulating proliferation and survival of cells. The Ras GTPase is in its active state when bound to GTP but inactive when bound to GDP. In normal circumstances, cycling between the two states occurs, where this process is dependent on the relative activity of guanine nucleotide exchange factors (GEFs), which favour production of the active form by inducing dissociation of GDP and allowing GTP binding, and GTPase activating proteins (GAPs), which induce hydrolysis of bound GTP and allow a return to the inactive state. Oncogenic transformation occurs when single point mutations in codons 12, 13, 59 and 61 of *Ras* result in the loss of GAP functionality, leading to a prevalence of the constitutively active GTP-bound form. Consequently, in tumours expressing the *Ras* oncogene, there is an amplification of the signal transduction pathways mediating malignant transformation a progression.

To carry out its function, Ras must undergo post-translational modifications that allow anchorage to the inner surface of the plasma membrane. This is carried out by farnesyl transferase, a heterodimeric metalloenzyme that catalyses the transfer of a hydrophobic farnesyl isoprenoid group from farnesyl diphosphate, a biological intermediate in cholesterol synthesis, to the C terminal tetrapeptide CAAX motif (cysteine, aliphatic amino acid, any amino acid) of the Ras protein. Increasing the hydrophobicity of Ras allows association with the plasma membrane phospholipid bilayer, where it is activated in response to signalling by membrane bound receptor tyrosine kinases such as the EGFR and PDGFR (Figure 15.1). The Ras farnesyl transferase has therefore become an attractive target for novel anticancer agents (Figure 15.2). An earlier approach was to make structural analogues of the farnesyl transferase substrate farnesyl pyrophosphate, for example, (α-hydroxyfarnesyl) phosphonic acid, although these showed little antitumour activity *in vivo*. A more promising approach has been the development of the CAAX peptidomimetics, which initially showed poor cellular accumulation due to their large size, negative charge and vulnerability to proteolytic cleavage, but were then modified to create second generation membrane permeable FTIs by synthesizing prodrugs or integrating more rigid spacer groups into

Cancer Chemotherapy   Rachel Airley
© 2009 John Wiley & Sons, Ltd.

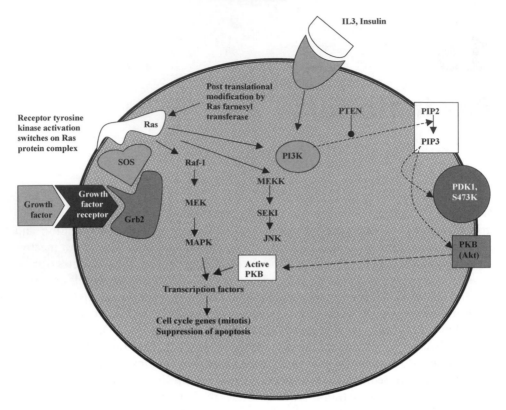

Figure 15.1 The Ras signal transduction pathway may be activated by binding of a growth factor ligand to its receptor tyrosine kinase, activating the Ras GTPase via post translational farnesylation catalysed by the enzyme Ras farnesyltransferase. Ras activation in turn stimulates the production of transcription factors regulating progression through the cell cycle and suppression of apoptosis by activating the signal transduction proteins MEK, MEKK and, via PI3 Kinase, Akt. Ras farnesyl transferase has therefore become a target for novel anticancer agents. Adapted from Buolamwini (1999).

their molecular structure. One example, L778 123, was evaluated in a number of phase I clinical trials until development was halted due to unacceptable toxicity. Non-peptidomimetic CAAX analogues are also in clinical development, the most advanced being tipifarnib (R1157 777, Zarnestra), a compound identified through high throughput screening which has undergone phase II evaluation in children with high grade glioma and neuroectodermal tumours such as medulloblastoma and in adults with myeloid leukaemias, colorectal and breast cancer. At the time of writing, tipifarnib is awaiting approval from the FDA after submission of trial data from a range of phase III trials which include a placebo-controlled trial in patients with refractory colorectal cancer and another trial evaluating the agent for the treatment of pancreatic cancer in combination with gemcitabine. Another non-peptidomimetic FTI, lonafarnib (SCH66 336, Sarasar), has been evaluated in phase I trials. In one study involving patients with advanced solid malignancies, lonafarnib was administered in combination with cisplatin and gemcitabine, although results proved disappointing, where there

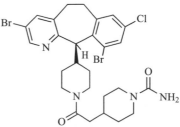

(α-hydroxyfarnesyl) phosponic acid

Lonafarnib (SCH66 336)

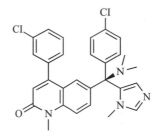

L778 123

Tipfarnib (R115 777, Zarnestra)

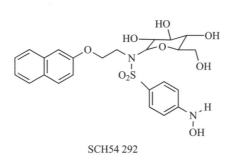

SCH54 292

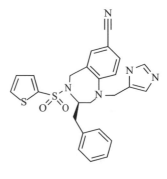

BMS214 662

Figure 15.2 Inhibitors of the *Ras* oncogene including the Ras farnesyl transferase inhibitors (FTIs), such as the farnesyl diphosphate analogue (α-hydroxyfarnesyl) phosphonic acid; the CAAX peptidomimetic agents, for example, L778123; and BMS214 662, tipifarnib and lonafarnib, three non-peptomimetic FTIs identified by high throughput compound screening. SCH54 292 inhibits Ras GTPase activity by binding to the Switch-II region involved in the interaction of nucleotide exchange factors.

was no evidence of farnesyl transferase inhibition and a significant level of toxicity. However, combination with paclitaxel in another phase I trial did not increase the level of toxicity above that of paclitaxel alone, justifying a phase II trial evaluating a similar combination in patients with taxane resistant non-small cell lung cancer. Although this trial was eventually discontinued due to interim reports of lack of efficacy, like tipifarnib, the use of lonafarnib is being explored in myelogenous leukaemias and paediatric brain tumours. A third non-peptidometic FTI, BMS214 662, has undergone a range of phase I trials in advanced solid tumours in combination with paclitaxel or platinum-based compounds.

Alternatively, it may be possible to target the Ras protein itself, for example by preventing conversion to the active Ras-GTPase. The compound SCH54 292 achieves this by forming a complex with the Switch-II region of the inactive Ras-GDP, which inhibits binding of GEFs.

16

Inhibitors of the Akt/PKB pathway

The *Akt* oncogene encodes a serine/threonine protein kinase that activates many tumorigenic processes, including mTOR driven protein synthesis (Chapter 19), growth factor mediated angiogenesis, tumour cell proliferation and survival via the enzyme phosphatidylinositol-3 kinase (PI3K). Akt is itself activated by another serine/threonine kinase (PDK1), which phosphorylates a site on threonine 308 of the protein. The enzyme is ubiquitously expressed in cancers as three isoforms designated Akt1, Akt2 and Akt3, individually expressed to varying degrees in different cancer types, particularly in glioma, lung and gastric cancers, as well as in the haematological malignancies. There are candidate inhibitor compounds currently under investigation which target Akt, PI3K and PDK1 (Figure 16.1). Among these are the PI3K inhibitors wortmannin and LY294002, most frequently used as experimental tools in the field of pharmacology to detect Akt-driven processes, but also providing lead compounds in the design of novel PI3K inhibitors. Prospective PDK1 inhibitors include BX-320, this compound showing promise *in vivo* in melanoma xenograft models, and the opioid antagonist naltrindole, which in one study inhibited growth and induced apoptosis in small cell lung cancer cell lines and may also prove to be a lead compound in the design of novel inhibitors of the Akt pathway. Small molecule inhibitors of Akt such as Akti-1, Akti-2 and Akti1, 2 are reversible, allosteric inhibitors that directly block the activity of Akt1, Akt2 or both isoforms respectively, as well as blocking phosphorylation and activation of the enzymes by PDK1. So far, *in vitro* studies carried out in tumour cell lines have revealed pro-apoptotic activity via the induction of caspases. Analogues of the Akt and PDK1 substrate phosphatidylinositol (3, 4, 5) triphosphate (PI), such as the alkyl phospholipid perifosine, inhibit the Akt pathway by decreasing the plasma membrane localization of Akt and consequently Akt phosphorylation. This has a pro-apoptotic effect, where *in vitro* studies using non-small cell lung cancer cell lines showed activation of both caspases 8 and 9, respective hallmarks of the extrinsic and intrinsic pathways in apoptosis (Figure 2.3), the major effect being upon the extrinsic apoptotic pathway via the tumour necrosis factor-related apoptosis-inducing ligand (TRAIL) death receptor (tumour necrosis factor is also a death receptor ligand). Aside from its pro-apoptotic effect, perifosine also induced morphological changes reminiscent of cell differentiation in prostate tumour cells *in vitro*, such as cellular

Cancer Chemotherapy   Rachel Airley
© 2009 John Wiley & Sons, Ltd.

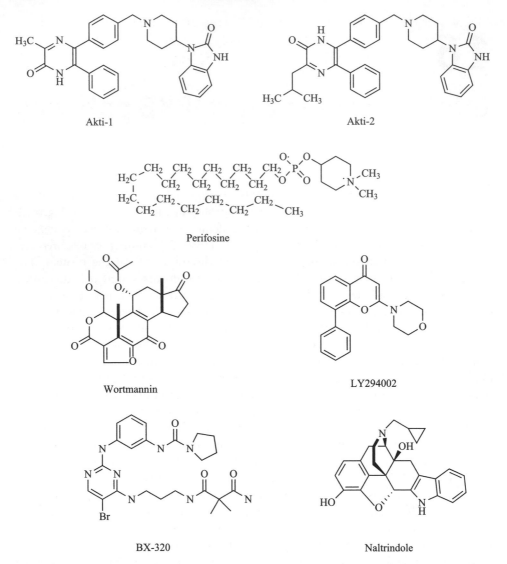

Figure 16.1 Structures of the Akt inhibitors Akti-1 and Akti-2; the lead inhibitors of PI3K, wortmannin and LY294002, used experimentally to define the role of PI3 kinase in cellular processes; and PDK1 inhibitors such as BX-320 and the opioid antagonist naltrindole, which prevent Akt activation. Akt activation is also prevented by the phospholipid analogue perifosine.

enlargement and granulation, where increased cellular differentiation is converse to malignancy. Perifosine is the most clinically advanced Akt inhibitor, where there have been a number of phase II clinical studies. Although there has been limited success with perifosine as single agent therapy in trials involving patients with prostate and head and neck cancers, there are a number of studies currently to be published or still in progress evaluating its use in renal, ovarian and non-small cell lung cancers, melanoma, glioma, sarcoma and haematological malignancies. There are also phase II trials in the pipeline that will evaluate its use in combination with anti-angiogenic agents such as the multikinase inhibitors sorafenib and sunitinib in advanced renal cancer and lenalidomide in multiple myeloma. Such an approach applies especially well to the use of EGFR inhibitors in prostate carcinoma, where a poor clinical response was observed in clinical trials, but *in vitro* studies show increased chemosensitivity when prostate tumour cell lines are treated with a combination of perifosine and the EGFR inhibitor erlotinib.

17

Targeting stress proteins: HSP90 inhibitors

Heat shock proteins (HSPs) are produced in response to heat stress in order to protect proteins vulnerable to damage and denaturation in these conditions. Several HSPs have been identified and characterized, such as HSP104, HSP70 and HSP90, which are cytoplasmic stress proteins, and the glucose-regulated proteins GRP94 and GRP78, found in the endoplasmic reticulum. Heat shock proteins form complexes with 'client' proteins, acting as molecular chaperones that maintain the protein in its folded state, mediate repair or degradation of partially denatured protein and initiate refolding of misfolded proteins. HSP90 has a wide range of client proteins, but has been the focus of anticancer drug design because of the involvement of a large proportion of these proteins in signal transduction in tumour proliferative and regulatory processes, such as the oncogenes *Src* and *HER2*; the signal transduction kinase MEK; the transcription factor HIF-1; cyclin-dependent kinases, mutant p53 and the oestrogen receptor. Inhibition of HSP-90 leads to defective client protein functionality and increased treatment sensitivity. HSP90 consists of 3 domains; the N-terminal, which binds ATP, the core domain, and the C-terminal, to enable homodimerization with another HSP90 molecule. The formation of a complex between the HSP90 homodimer and the client protein, via a 'molecular clamp' is an ATP-dependent process induced by the interaction between the two N-terminal domains. The HSP90 inhibitors such as the antitumour antibiotic geldanamycin bind the N-terminal ATP-binding site and therefore prevent the association of the N-terminals and complexation with the client protein (Figure 17.1). This may have several implications. Firstly, HSP90 binding assists the repair, or alternatively the ubiquitylation and proteasomal degradation of partially denatured client proteins, so that its inhibition leads to the accumulation of non-functioning forms of the protein. Conversely, HSP90 also protects undamaged client proteins, so that exposure to an inhibitor renders functional forms vulnerable to proteolytic degradation. Secondly, client proteins will not be in the correctly folded conformation for ligand binding and activation of signal transduction. HSP90 inhibitors therefore have multiple modes of action, such as the suppression of growth factor production, inhibition of kinases associated with progression through the cell

Cancer Chemotherapy Rachel Airley
© 2009 John Wiley & Sons, Ltd.

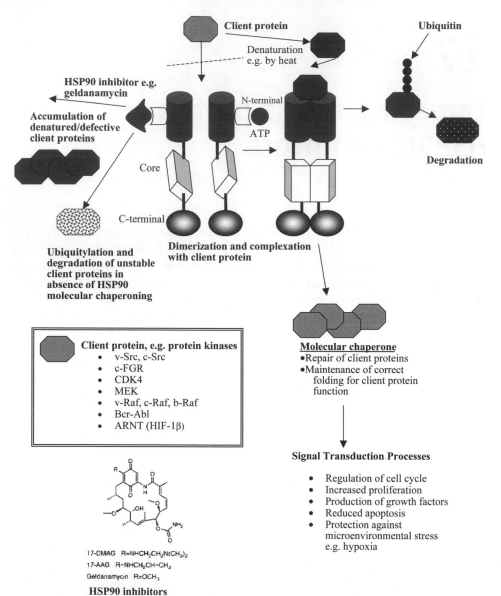

Figure 17.1 HSP90 functions as a homodimer that binds client proteins in an ATP-dependent 'molecular clamp' formation, acting as molecular chaperones that facilitate repair or degradation of denatured proteins and maintain the protein in its correctly folded state. This enables a range of client proteins to function in the principal signal transduction pathways involved in tumour cell survival and proliferation. The antitumour antibiotic geldanamycin, and derivatives such as 17-AAG are currently in phase I and II clinical trials. These bind HSP90 at the ATP-binding site on the N-terminal, leading to the degradation of client proteins as well as the accumulation of non-functioning denatured forms.

cycle, inhibition of oestrogen-induced cellular proliferation in hormone-dependent cancer and the induction of apoptosis. The first HSP90 inhibitor to be identified was geldanamycin, an ansamycin antibiotic isolated from *Streptomyces hygrocopicus*. The geldanamycin derivative 17-allylamino, 17-demethoxygeldanamycin (17-AAG, tanespimycin) showed increased biological activity, and when evaluated preclinically, was particularly effective in tumour cell lines with high levels of the oncogene *erb-b2*. Accordingly, 17-AAG has been evaluated in phase I clinical trials in advanced solid malignancies, although its formulation for human use has proved pharmaceutically

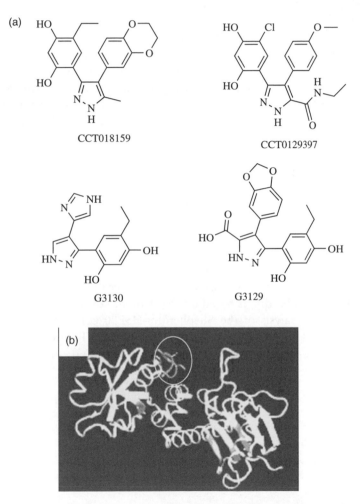

Figure 17.2 Structures of novel HSP90 inhibitors currently in preclinical development. These include the diarayl pyrapyrazole lead compound CCT018 159 and its derivative CCT0 129 397, discovered at the Institute of Cancer Research, the latter having been earmarked for further clinical development; the dihydroxyphenylpyrazoles G3130 and G3129, discovered at the Novartis Research Foundation in California, USA; and Shepherdin (b), a novel peptide mimetic, the interaction between the compound and the N-terminal is circled. Reproduced from Plescia *et al.* (2005) *Cancer Cell.* 7: 457–468, Elsevier.

challenging. Initial attempts were to dissolve the drug in large amounts of dimethyl sulfoxide, though a more practical formulation has now been developed. Phase II trials have now been initiated, including a recently reported trial evaluating the use of 17-AAG monotherapy in patients with metastatic papillary renal cell carcinoma (RCC) or metastatic clear cell RCC, although in this case there was no observable clinical response. Further phase II trials are also in progress targeting patients with other cancers, such as hormone-refractory metastatic prostate cancer and metastatic melanoma. Both 17-AAG and the second-generation geldanamycin 17-DMAG (alvespimycin) are licensed for development to Kosan Biosciences, who have initiated several phase I and II clinical trials. The downregulation of erb-b2/HER2 activity observed in preclinical studies has justified their clinical development as novel therapies for the treatment of HER2-positive breast cancers, and interim reports of significant clinical response in a phase II trial evaluating the use of 17-AAG in combination with trastuzumab in such patients are encouraging. Initial data coming from a phase I trial (reported in 2007) looking at a combination of 17-DMAG and trastuzumab in patients with HER-2 positive metastatic breast cancer and ovarian cancer have also proved promising, and a phase II trial is planned. There are several novel classes of HSP90 inhibitors in preclinical development (Figure 17.2a), which include the diarayl pyrapyrazole lead compound CCT018 159 and derivative CCT0 129 397, discovered at the Institute of Cancer Research using high throughput screening assays involving yeast HSP90 ATPase, the latter showing comparable activity to 17-AAG which has earmarked it for further clinical development. The structurally related dihydroxyphenylpyrazoles G3130 and G3129, lead compounds discovered at the Novartis Research Foundation in California, United States, may also yield derivatives with sufficient activity for further development. Another approach used for the development of HSP90 inhibitors has been to design peptide mimetics based on the sequence of HSP90 client proteins. One such compound, Shepherdin, is based on the structure of survivin, an anti-apoptotic protein. Structural analysis of the Shepherdin–HSP90 complex (Figure 17.2b) has demonstrated a dual action, where it inhibits the HSP90 ATPase at the N-terminal and the protein- protein interaction existing between HSP90 and survivin.

18

The proteasome

18.1 Introduction

The proteasome is a multi-enzyme catalytic complex located in the nucleus of
eukaryotic cells, which is responsible for the degradation of a range of target proteins,
such as signalling molecules, tumour suppressor proteins, cell cycle regulators, transcription factors and proteins that induce or inhibit apoptosis. The usual mechanism is
via conjugation with the protein ubiquitin, which is catalysed in a three-step pathway
(Figure 18.1) by the ubiquitin-conjugating enzymes E1 to E3, resulting in the covalent
linkage of the C-terminus of ubiquitin to a free amino acid group on the target protein.
The ubiquitylated protein is then recognized and degraded by the proteasome. The 26S
proteasome is a 2.4 MDa complex (Figure 18.2) consisting of two subunits-the 20S core
or catalytic particle, which contains the proteolytic active sites, and the 19S regulatory
particle, which regulates the function of the 20S particle. This subunit also processes the
substrate prior to proteolysis, controlling deubiquitylation, unfolding and translocation of the substrate, thereby controlling its access to the proteolytic core. The
proteasome, by regulating protein degradation, controls the level of a diverse number
of proteins involved in processes critical to cell proliferation and survival, and therefore
the molecular changes leading to malignant transformation and progression. Table 18.1
shows examples of critical proteasome substrates, where pharmacological interaction
with the proteasome function may result in the disruption of function of neoplastic
cells. The proteasome affects several cell cycle regulatory proteins, for example, the
cyclin-dependent protein kinases (CDKs) that control progression through the cell
cycle. CDKs are regulated by the endogenous CDK inhibitors p21 and p27, which are
themselves target substrates for the proteasome. Inhibition of proteasome function
consequently leads to increased CDK inhibition, resulting in cell cycle arrest and
apoptosis of tumour cells. Inhibition of the proteasome also causes rapid accumulation
of the tumour suppressor protein p53, which triggers cellular processes averse to
malignant progression such as differentiation, cell cycle arrest and DNA repair.
The transcription factor nuclear factor κB (NFκB) is integral to a number of
survival pathways, not only important for the control of cell cycle progression, but
also regulating the activation of growth factors, for example, interleukins, proteins

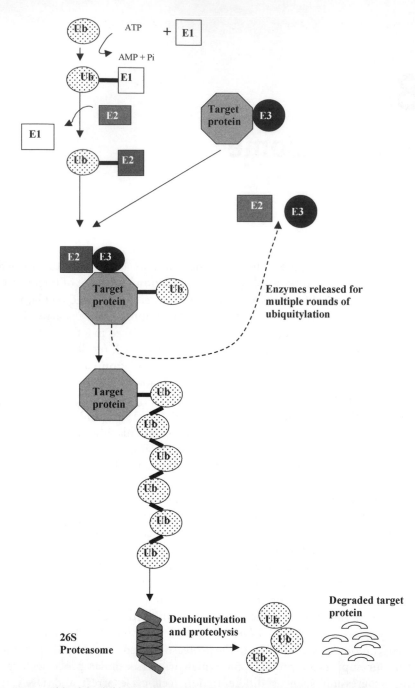

Figure 18.1 Ubiquitin (Ub) is activated by the ATP-dependent enzyme E1, forming a thiol bond. The activated ubiquitin is then transferred to the ubiquitin-conjugating enzyme E2. This complex is recognized by the E3 enzymes (consisting of HECT or RING families of ubiquitin ligases) which are substrate-specific and therefore ensure that ubiquitylation and subsequent proteolysis is specific to the target protein. Following transfer of ubiquitin to the substrate, enzymes are cleaved and the process repeated so that a polyubiquitylated substrate is formed, where ubiquitin chain elongation is catalysed by the enzyme E4. The target protein may then be recognized and degraded by the proteasome, where deubiquitylation takes place in the 19S subunit, followed by proteolytic degradation by the 20S subunit.

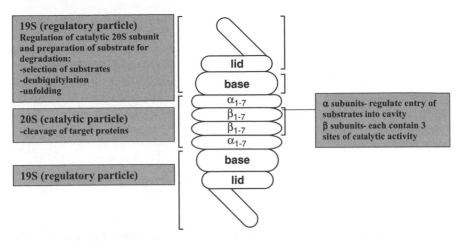

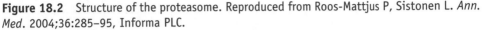

Figure 18.2 Structure of the proteasome. Reproduced from Roos-Mattjus P, Sistonen L. *Ann. Med.* 2004;36:285–95, Informa PLC.

important for cell to cell adhesion, for example, intracellular adhesion molecule-1 and vascular cell adhesion molecule-1), anti-apoptotic oncogenes, for example, bcl-2 and angiogenic factors. NFκB is itself regulated by the inhibitory protein IκB, which is degraded by the proteasome. Inhibition of the proteasome will therefore lead to increased NFκB inhibition and therefore downregulation of those processes advantageous to tumour growth and progression.

18.2 The proteasome as a target for novel drug strategies

Efforts to develop clinically useful proteasome inhibitors have led to the synthesis of the boronic acid peptide PS341, or bortezomib (Figure 18.3), a potent selective proteasome

Table 18.1 Examples of proteasome substrates

Protein class	Function
Cyclins and related proteins e.g. cyclins A, B, D, E, CDK	Cell cycle progression
Tumour suppressors, e.g. p53	Transcription factor
Oncogenes, e.g. *c-fos/c-jun*, *C-myc*, *N-myc*	Transcription factor
Pro-apoptotic proteins, e.g. Bax	Signalling proteins involved in the intrinsic (mitochondrial) apoptotic pathway
Anti-apoptotic protein, e.g. bcl2	
Inhibitory proteins, e.g. IκB	Inhibits survival promoting transcription factor NFκB
Oxygen-regulated transcription factor, e.g. HIF-1	Adaptation to hypoxia

HIF, hypoxia inducible factor.

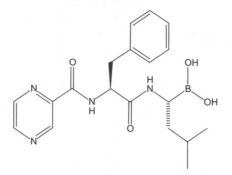

Figure 18.3 Bortezomib (Velcade).

inhibitor with promising activity in hematological malignancies, approved as the proprietary agent Velcade for the treatment of multiple myeloma in May 2003. Following phase II trials, for example, SUMMIT, and CREST, which examined the clinical efficacy of bortezomib in patients with relapsed and refractory myeloma, it was evaluated against high dose dexamethasone, was evaluated in a large scale international phase III trial, APEX (Assessment of Proteasome Inhibition for Extending Remission). Bortezomib is also, at the time of writing, undergoing a range of clinical studies in other haematological malignancies. These include phase I studies in patients with acute leukaemias, for example, in combination with idarubicin and cytarabine in patients with refractory acute myeloid leukaemia; and phase II studies in patients with Philadelphia chromosome-positive chronic myeloid leukaemia following treatment with imatinib (Gleevec). Phase II and III trials are also in progress in non-Hodgkin's, small lymphocytic, follicular and mantle cell lymphomas. Bortezomib is now undergoing clinical evaluation in solid tumours, where phase II studies are being carried out in combination with docetaxel in advanced non-small cell lung and prostate tumours, as well as tumours of the breast, head and neck, colon and kidney. Several phase I studies of refractory solid tumours of various types are examining the use of bortezomib-based regimens in combination with several classes of anticancer agent, such as irinotecan, doxorubicin and gemcitabine.

18.3 Ubiquitylation as a target

The E3 ubiquitin ligases, which transfer the target substrate to ubiquitin, show the greatest variability in the ubiquitin-proteasome pathway, and therefore offer the potential for specifically inhibiting the ubiquitylation and subsequent proteolytic degradation of a range of proteins involved in malignancy. There are two major families of E3 ubiquitin ligase, corresponding to those containing the 'homologous to E6-AP carboxy terminal' (HECT) and the amusingly named 'really interesting new gene' (RING) domains. Examples of each include E6-AP, the HECT domain containing E3 ligase that degrades the tumour suppressor gene p53 following infection with human papilloma virus (HPV), a viral carcinogen that leads to cancer of the cervix, and the RING domain containing E3 ligase MDM2, responsible for degradation of p53, overexpression of which will lead to p53 inactivation and subsequently increased

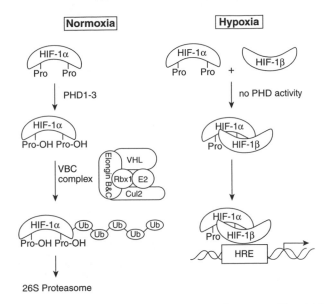

Figure 18.4 The role of the RING domain containing E3 ligase von Hippel-Lindau-Elongin BC (VBC) complex in the proteasomal degradation of HIF-1α in normoxic conditions. Reproduced from Roos-Mattjus P, Sistonen L. *Ann. Med.* 2004;36:285–95, Informa PLC.

cellular proliferation (see Section 4.3). Another example of a RING domain containing E3 ligase is the von Hippel–Lindau–Elongin BC (VBC) complex that mediates degradation of the hypoxia-inducible transcription factor HIF-1a (Figure 18.4), which takes place in normoxic conditions and so prevents induction of hypoxia- regulated genes such as the facilitative glucose transporters Glut-1 and Glut-3, the glycolytic enzymes and angiogenic growth factors.

Ubiquitin ligases may provide novel targets for anticancer strategies. In recent years, MDM2 has become one such target, where a number of strategies may be used to inhibit the inactivation of p53 by MDM2 (Figures 18.5 and 18.6). These include the use of

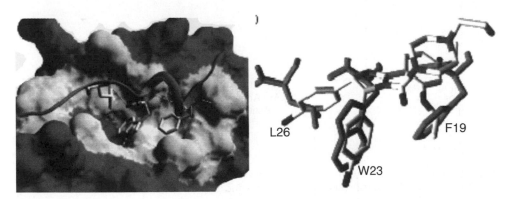

Figure 18.5 Nutlin 2 (right) binding to the human homologue of MDM2, HDM2, the complex sharing many characteristics with the p53/MDM2 complex (left). Reproduced from Fischer, P.M., Lane, D.P. *Trends Pharmacol. Sci.* 2004;25:343–6, Elsevier.

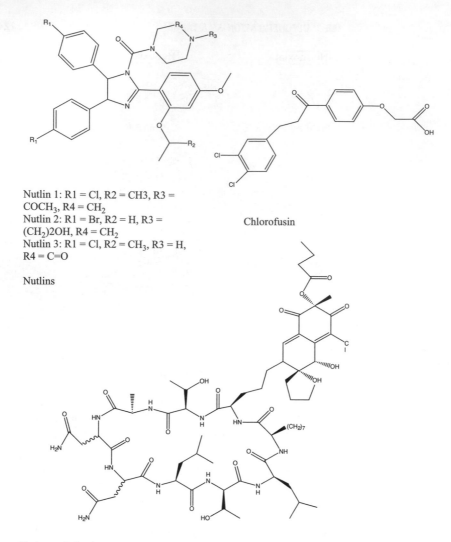

Nutlin 1: R1 = Cl, R2 = CH3, R3 = COCH₃, R4 = CH₂
Nutlin 2: R1 = Br, R2 = H, R3 = (CH₂)2OH, R4 = CH₂
Nutlin 3: R1 = Cl, R2 = CH3, R3 = H, R4 = C=O

Nutlins

Chlorofusin

Chalcone derivative

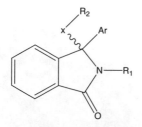

X=NH, O
Ar =Aromatic group
(substituted phenyl group)

Isoindolinone compounds

Figure 18.6 Strategies to inhibit the inactivation of p53 by Mdm2 include small molecule inhibitors of the p53–Mdm2 complex such as chalcone derivatives, chlorofusin, derived from the fungus *Fusarium*, and isoindolinone-based inhibitors. The most promising compounds, however, are peptide inhibitors mimicking the protein–protein interaction between p53 and MDM2 that are currently in development at Hoffman-La Roche in Nutley, New Jersey, and so have been given the nickname Nutlins.

antisense oligonucleotides, which decrease the level of MDM2 transcription in tumour cells, small molecule inhibitors of the enzymic activity of the ubiquitin ligase, and inhibitors of the p53–MDM2 complex, where release of p53 from MDM2 should activate the tumour suppressor function of p53. So far, most biological validation work has concentrated on characterizing the nature of the p53–MDM2 interaction, where structural analysis indicates the importance of three p53 residues which form a hydrophobic pocket into which MDM2 binds. Although small molecule inhibitors of this interaction are available, for example, chalcone derivatives, these lack potential as drug candidates due to their low potency, although the compound chlorofusin, which is derived from the fungus *Fusarium*, shows better activity. Isoindolinone-based inhibitors are another class of compounds undergoing evaluation in MDM2 amplified cell lines, after discovery of lead compounds using the National Cancer Institute drug screen. The most extensively studied and promising compounds, though, are peptide inhibitors that mimic the protein–protein interaction taking place between wild type p53 and MDM2 developed by Hoffman-La Roche in Nutley, New Jersey, and therefore nicknamed Nutlins. These compounds may prove useful not only as novel anticancer agents, where recent data showed around 90% tumour growth delay in mouse xenografts, but as a means of continuing characterization of the p53 tumour suppressor pathway, which may in turn reveal new targets for anticancer drug development. The development of MDM2 inhibitors involves the design of small molecule inhibitors of a protein–protein interface, which represents an important challenge in medicinal chemistry. For instance, it is generally accepted that factors such as bioavailability and permeability, which dictate uptake and accumulation in poorly vascularized tumours, limits the molecular weight of any potential new agents to below 500 Da, which is difficult when considering the large molecular weight of peptide chains. However, as novel targets emerge that target protein function in signal transduction pathways, rather than the classical strategy of targeting DNA, the experience gained overcoming these difficulties may prove useful in the future design of novel anticancer therapies.

19

Checkpoint protein kinases as novel targets – mammalian target of rapamycin (mTOR)

19.1 Mammalian target of rapamycin

Mammalian target of rapamycin (mTOR) is a large protein that has multiple domains and contains in excess of 2500 amino acids. It is analogous to the yeast genes *TOR1* and *TOR2*, discovered when screening for mediators of resistance to the immunosuppressant drug rapamycin (sirolimus), which binds mTOR as a complex with the cyclophilin FKBP12. The interest in mTOR, together with its upstream and downstream regulatory factors, as a novel target for anticancer drug design is gaining momentum due to its function as a signal for gene transcription and translation that are necessary to adjust the rate of cell growth and proliferation. This occurs in response to several metabolic stimuli, such as glucose, oxygen and amino acid levels, insulin and growth factors, but also upon exposure to DNA damaging agents (summarized in Figure 19.1). In doing so, mTOR-dependent pathways help integrate cellular metabolism by acting as a central microenvironmental sensor.

There are two major downstream targets of mTOR. One target is the S6Ks (S6K1 and S6K2), which are serine–threonine kinases implicated in mRNA translation, particularly of ribosomal proteins important in protein synthesis such as certain elongation factors. The other major target is the translational repressor protein 4E-BP1 (eukaryotic initiation factor 4E-binding protein), which is inactivated by mTOR, leading to increased rate of translation. Upstream of mTOR, the major factors determining its activation are the PKB/Akt pathway, which responds to insulin and growth factors, and the enzyme AMPK (5′ AMP kinase), which responds to fluctuations in ATP conferred by nutrient and/or severe oxygen deprivation. The role of hypoxia in the tumour microenvironment is intriguing, as although it may lead to decreased ATP which will suppress mTOR via reduced AMPK activity, there is evidence that mTOR itself regulates hypoxia-inducible transcription factor (HIF-1; see Chapter 12), where stabilization

Cancer Chemotherapy   Rachel Airley
© 2009 John Wiley & Sons, Ltd.

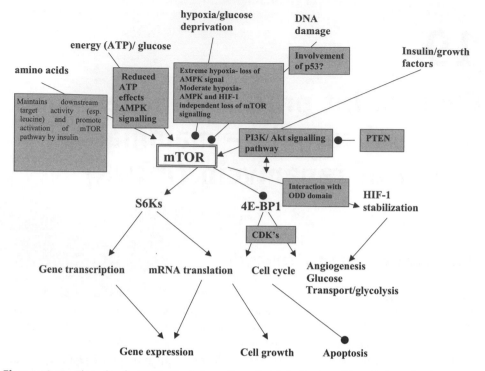

Figure 19.1 The role of mTOR in the integration of metabolic signalling. CDK, cyclin dependent kinases at cell cycle checkpoints must be activated for progression through cell cycle; ODD, oxygen degradation domain on HIF-1α; PI3K, phosphatidylinositol 3′ kinase; PTEN, phosphatase and tensin homologue deleted on chromosome 10; S6Ks, ribosomal protein kinases controlling translation; 4E-BP1, eukaryotic initiation factor 4E-binding protein, a translational repressor protein. Note the effect of hypoxia on mTOR signalling, which seems to be controlled by a number of discrete pathways and dependent upon the level of hypoxia. Whereas loss of ATP in hypoxic conditions may downregulate mTOR signalling to restrict proliferation in times of metabolic stress, mTOR is also believed to be instrumental in insulin, Akt and other pathways regulating HIF-1α stabilization, that will serve to upregulate certain proliferative and anti-apoptotic processes in tumour cells.

of the HIF-1 a subunit via an interaction with the ODD (oxygen degradation domain) promotes hypoxia-induced VEGF production and angiogenesis.

19.2 Structure and activation of mTOR

mTOR belongs to a family of phosphatidylinositol kinase-related enzymes, and may also be referred to as FRAP (FKB12 and rapamycin associated protein), RAFT1 (rapamycin and FKBP12 target 1) and RAPT1 (rapamycin target 1), due to its ability to act as a target for the immunosuppressive effects of the FKB12-rapamycin complex. The protein (Figure 19.2) consists of a catalytic kinase domain, FRB (FKBP12-rapamycin binding domain) and an auto-inhibitory domain that is thought to have a repressor

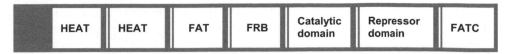

Figure 19.2   Structure of mTOR. Adapted from Hay and Sonenberg (2004).

function. There are also around 20 HEAT (Huntingtin, EF3, A subunit of PP2A and TOR) motifs at the N-terminus, which may assist protein–protein interactions and FAT (FRAP-ATM-TRRAP) and FATC (FAT C-terminus) domains, which may modulate the catalytic kinase activity of the protein. mTOR forms a scaffold complex with other proteins, which includes the regulatory associated protein of mTOR (RAPTOR). The possible role of RAPTOR is to link mTOR with its downstream effector proteins S6K1

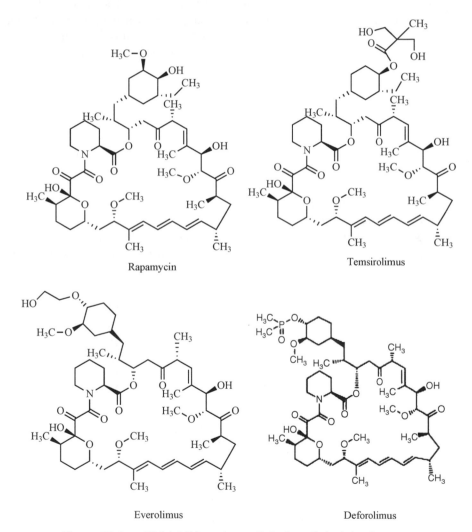

Figure 19.3   mTOR inhibitors in preclinical or clinical development.

and 4E-BP1. It is further suggested that RAPTOR acts as a sensor of the nutrient state of the cell, causing stimulation of mTOR in a nutrient deficient environment, an effect that is modulated by binding of the protein GβL.

19.3 Novel anticancer agents targeting mTOR

Efforts to target mTOR have focused on the production of water soluble, chemically and physically stable analogues of rapamycin (rapalogues) (Figure 19.3). Promising agents include the prodrug temsirolimus (Torisel, CCI-779), which was evaluated in phase II studies involving patients with advanced breast cancer, who had received prior chemotherapy (and second line) with anthracyclines and/or taxanes. Clinical benefit, that is, partial response or stable disease, was observed in 37% of patients enrolled into this trial. Temsirolimus was also evaluated in phase II clinical trials in patients with advanced renal cancer, showing promise when used in combination with interferon-α. This led to the initiation of a phase III study to compare this combination with interferon-α alone. Temsirolimus was approved by the FDA in summer 2007 for the treatment of patients with advanced renal carcinoma, and subsequently in the UK in late 2008. Phase I single agent studies have been carried out and demonstrated the clinical antitumour efficacy of the mTOR inhibitors RAD001 (everolimus) and AP23573 (deforolimus) in patients with tumours of the lung, cervix and uterus, as well as soft tissue sarcoma and astrocytoma. In preclinical studies, everolimus has proved effective in combination with cytotoxics such as paclitaxel, gemcitabine and doxorubicin, as well as some of the modern signal transduction or tyrosine kinase inhibitors such as imatinib (Glivec) and gefitinib (Iressa). One phase I study evaluating the use of a combination of everolimus and gemcitabine showed significantly increased risk of myelosuppression, however, it is anticipated that a phase 1 study to evaluate the use of everolimus in combination with imatinib will be initiated in patients with imatinib-resistant gastro-intestinal stromal tumours.

20

Telomerase

Eukaryotic chromosomes are linear and independent, which confer the advantage of enabling recombination and chromosomal shuffling during meiosis, leading to greater genetic diversity. However, the linear nature of chromosomes leads to two problems. First, free DNA ends are vulnerable to degradation by nucleases and the risk of ligation with other free DNA ends. Second, the mechanism of DNA replication leads to a conundrum referred to as the 'end replication problem', which is associated with the synthesis of DNA at the ends of chromosomes. The replication of DNA uses both strands of the chromosome as templates. However, because DNA synthesis always occurs in one direction, that is, from the 5′ to 3′ end, the replicating chromosomes form a leading strand, where DNA is formed in one continuous strand, and the lagging strand, where smaller strands of DNA, or Okazaki fragments are formed. In this case, polymerization originates from several RNA primers, which are eventually degraded and replaced by these short DNA sequences, leaving gaps that are filled by extension of the adjacent Okazaki fragment. Problems arise because there is no template for the last Okazaki fragment beyond the 5′ end of the chromosome, so that one strand of DNA cannot be synthesized to the very end (Figure 20.1). This results in the progressive shortening of chromosomes at the 3′ ends through successive cell cycles, where around 50 base pairs are lost due to incomplete replication of the lagging strand. Ultimately, this phenomenon determines the rate of ageing and therefore the mortality of normal cells. To maintain chromosomal stability, the ends of chromosomes are furnished with telomeres, the position of which is shown in Figure 20.2. These consist of a DNA component and several protein components. The DNA component incorporates a set of repeating sequences, which varies according to species, but in humans, is the hexanucleotide 5′-TTAGGG-3′. There are approximately 1000–2000 repeats of this sequence, which amounts to 6000–6012 000 base pairs. Sequence-specific DNA-binding proteins, such as TRF1 and TRF2, specifically recognize and attach to DNA sequences, which stabilize the telomere and regulate its length. In human chromosomes, telomeres are joined centromerically by the subtelomeric region, which is derived from degnerated telomeric DNA sequences and unique repeats. The DNA component of telomeres is synthesized via the enzyme telomerase, which is a reverse

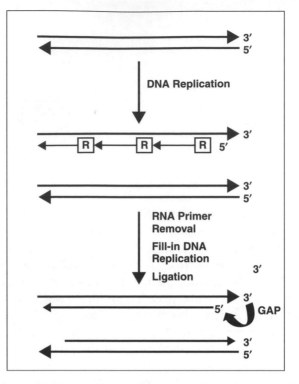

Figure 20.1 The end replication problem, where progressive shortening of the chromosome at the 3′ end is caused by there being no template for the last Okazaki fragment beyond the 5′ end of the chromosome. Reproduced from Meyerson, M. *J. Clin. Oncol.* 2000;18:2626–34, American Society of Clinical Oncology.

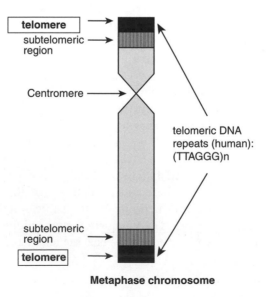

Figure 20.2 Structure of the metaphase chromosome showing position of the telomeres. Reproduced with permission from Dahse, R., Fiedler, W., Ernst, G. *Clin. Chem.* 1997;43:708–14, American Association for Clinical Chemistry.

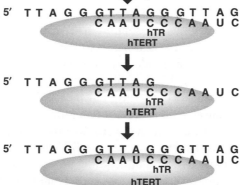

Figure 20.3 Telomerase binds to telomere repeat sequences, allowing the addition of deoxynucleotides to the 3′ end of the telomere. This maintains chromosomal length and prevents chromosomal shortening. The subunit hTERT synthesizes new telomeric GGTTAG repeat sequences, which are complementary to the sequence CCCUAA in the subunit hTR. Reproduced from Meyerson, M. *J. Clin. Oncol.* 2000;18:2626–34, American Society of Clinical Oncology.

transcriptase composed of an RNA subunit that acts as a template for telomere addition to the chromosome, and a protein subunit that catalyses telomere synthesis. The human telomerase, which consists of the RNA subunit hTR (human telomerase RNA) and the protein subunit hTERT (human telomerase reverse transcriptase) has been cloned and has a molecular mass of more than 300 kDa (Figure 20.3). The function of telomerase is to bind to telomere repeat sequences, which facilitates the addition of deoxynucleotides to the 3′ end of the telomere, therefore maintaining chromosomal length and preventing the chromosomal shortening that is thought to limit the number of possible mitotic cell divisions and therefore the life span of the cell. The interest in telomerase shown by those involved in cancer therapeutics lies in the increased telomerase activity that arises in malignant cells relative to normal somatic cells. Ordinarily, only cells with unlimited replicative capacity, such as male germ cells, lymphocytes and stem cells express telomerase, where telomerase activity in other cells is switched off following embryonic differentiation. Immortalized cells in culture show increased telomerase activity, which contributes to a loss of control of cell proliferation and oncogenesis. Further, overexpression of hTERT *in vitro* induces telomerase activity and extends the lifespan of the cells. Telomerase activity is detectable in a wide range of tumour types, and may be used as an indicator of malignancy and poor prognosis, measured using techniques such as the TRAP (telomerase repeat amplification protocol) assay, for example, telomerase activity is associated with tumours of the lung, breast and bladder. The development of telomerase as a novel therapeutic target is ongoing. It must be considered, though, that the mode of action of these agents is dependent upon the longer-term erosion of telomeres, and therefore the eventual shortening of the lifespan of the tumour cell, which may or may not impact on the rate of tumour regrowth after conventional therapy. As a result, clinical response may not be immediate if the agents are used as single line therapy, and in any case, treatment would necessitate clinical monitoring of telomerase activity and telomere length. One strategy makes use of the means by which the telomerase subunit hTR uses the 11-basepair sequence 5′-CUAACCCUAAC-3′ to bind the telomere, employing the use of oligonucleotide-based inhibitors. Traditionally, the mode of action of therapeutic oligonucleotides is to act as antisense inhibitors, that is, they contain DNA bases that are able to form complexes with mRNA, which are then cleaved by the enzyme Rnase H. These have had a measure of success in clinical trials, as is the case for the oligonucleotides Formivirsen, now an approved drug for the treatment of cytomegalovirus retinitis. In the treatment of cancer, Genasense, which targets the oncogene Bcl2, is currently in phase III trials; and ISIS 3521, which targets H-Ras, is undergoing phase II trials in pancreatic, colon and skin cancers. Experience with these agents shows that delivery of oligonucleotides to their target within a tumour is possible in terms of pharmacokinetics.

Small molecule telomerase inhibitors in preclinical and clinical development are shown in Figure 20.4. The design of oligonucleotide telomerase inhibitors has taken a slightly different direction, in that cleavage of the target hTR by Rnase H and therefore the formation of a DNA–RNA complex are unnecessary. Consequently, binding of these agents to hTR becomes more analogous to that of competitive inhibitors binding to the active site of an enzyme. For this reason, the most promising agents consist of chemically modified bases that show high affinity binding to complementary sequences within hTR, and unlike conventional antisense oligonucleotides, may be as short as eight bases. So far, the class of agents most likely to undergo clinical development as telomerase inhibitors is based on 2′-O-alkyl RNA, for example, 2′-O-methoxyethyl RNA and 2′-O-methyl RNA, which are relatively non-toxic in humans, have good bioavailability and are amenable to large-scale synthesis.

Another approach is to use non-nucleosidic small molecule telomerase inhibitors. The identification of drug candidates generally involves high throughput TRAP assay, bolstered by direct assays that measure telomerase inhibition, and cellular cytotoxicity. Emerging compounds include the BIBR class of compounds, for example, BIBR 1532, originally developed at Boehringer–Ingelheim, which through the induction of telomere dysfunction are able to produce a senescent phenotype in tumour cells, which is more analogous to that seen in normal cells. In fact, microarray technology has revealed a magnitude of transcriptional changes exerted by long-term treatment with this class of telomerase inhibitor. These changes seem to be related to the genetic changes seen in ageing cells, such as cell cycle control proteins, for example, the cyclins and cyclin-dependent kinases, and proteins involved in mitosis, DNA synthesis, DNA synthesis and replication, as well as the production of DNA repair proteins. BIBR 1532 shows activity against many tumour types *in vitro*, such as prostate, breast and latterly, leukaemias, as well as significant growth delay *in vivo* in fibrosarcoma xenograft models. Promising avenues include the use of small-molecule telomerase inhibitors based upon nucleoside analogues such as the reverse transcriptase inhibitor zidovudine, for example, dideoxyguanosine triphosphate (ddGTP). However, these agents tend to

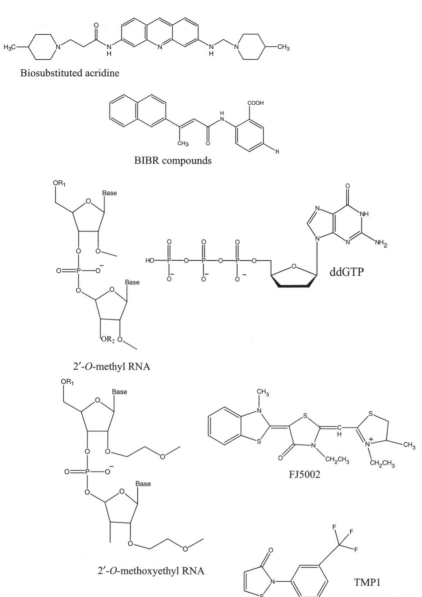

Figure 20.4 Telomerase inhibitors in preclinical and clinical development, including the 2'-*O*-alkyl RNA oligonucleotides 2'-*O*-methoxyethyl RNA and 2'-*O*-methyl RNA; the BIBR class of compounds; nucleoside analogues of the reverse transcriptase inhibitor zidovudine, for example, dideoxyguanosine triphosphate (ddGTP); the isothiazolone derivative TMPI and the rhodocyanine FJ5002.

interact with other polymerases. Agents that target telomerase more specifically include the bisubstituted acridines, which bind selectively to a G-rich quadruplex within the telomere, blocking the interaction with telomerase and the addition of the sequences necessary to elongate the telomere. Other agents shown to induce cell death by telomere shortening include the isothiazolone derivatives TMPI and the rhodocyanine FJ5002. The rhodacyanines resulted from the identification of the alkaloid berberine as a weak inhibitor of telomerase during a disease-oriented screening programme; and further analysis of compounds with similar activity led to the identification of the rhodacyanine derivative MKT077, and consequently, the close derivative FJ5002.

21
Histone deacetylase: an epigenetic drug target

21.1 Introduction

The *epigenome* is concerned with the outcomes of gene transcription that are not directly linked to the genetic code. Instead, the *epigenetic code* is determined by a combination of mechanisms that serve to fine tune the genetic code and therefore the precise nature of the downstream protein product, which may be structural, an enzyme or have a role in multiple signal transduction processes. Epigenetic factors include the extent of DNA methylation, where the addition of a methyl group to the C5 position of cytosine is catalysed by DNA methyl transferase (DNMT), processes such as gene silencing, for example, RNA interference (described in Section 10.2.2) and the production of mRNA splice variants. Histone modifications catalysed by histone deacetylases (HDAC) and histone acetyl transferase (HAT) also influence transcriptional processes by regulating the extent of DNA condensation as well as the binding and functionality of transcription factors. There are a range of exploitable epigenetic targets, to which there has been significant progress in the design and development of therapeutic inhibitors. DNMT inhibitors, such as 5-azacytidine (azacitidine) and 5-aza-2′-deoxycytidine (decitabine), are approved by the FDA for the treatment of myelodysplastic syndrome. Others, such as 5-fluoro-2′−deoxycytidine, are in phase I/II trials (reviewed by Mack in the *Journal of the National Cancer Institute*, Vol. 98, No. 20, 2006). The focus of this chapter, however, will be histone deacetylase (HDAC), where major progress in this area has resulted in a number of HDAC inhibitors in clinical trial (depsipeptide, benzamidine, valproic acid), and the approval of vorinostat (Zolinza).

21.2 HDAC and DNA packaging

The packaging of DNA into chromosomes depends upon the action of histones, of which there are 5 main types, H1, H2A, H2, H3 and H4. These proteins are highly basic, and by virtue of their high lysine and arginine content have a large number of positively charged side chains that are able to bind to DNA, itself negatively charged as a result of the phosphate element of the nucleotide units. Histones bind DNA at an approximate weight for weight ratio of 1 : 1 to form chromatin. Such packaging of DNA by histones (Figure 21.1) is found in a number of forms which determine the extent of DNA condensation arising in the nucleus during cellular processes such as mitosis. The first level of packaging is the 'beads on a string' formation, where the 'beads' or nucleosomes,

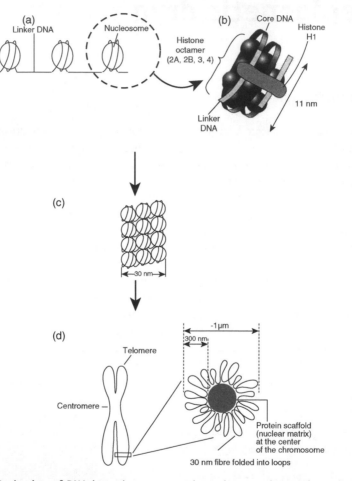

Figure 21.1   Packaging of DNA into chromosomes depends upon the condensation of chromatin, formed when DNA is bound by histones. Chromatin condensation occurs at a number of levels- the first level (a) referred to as the 'beads on a string' structure, where the 'beads' are nucleosomes consisting of the DNA double helix wound 1.8 times round a histone octamer (histones H2A, H2B, H3 and H4) (b), and the 'string' is linker DNA; the second (c), is the 30 nM fibre, or 'solenoid', formed when nucleosomes are pulled together by the binding of linker DNA by histone H1; and the third level of packaging apparent in chromosomes is the formation of radial loops (d), where the 30 nM fibre is arranged on a central protein scaffold by attachment at certain multiple locations. Adapted from Hames and Hooper, *Instant Notes Biochemistry* (2nd edition) Bios Scientific Publishers, Oxford, 2000.

consist of a 146 base pairs length of DNA wrapped 1.8 times round a histone octamer in a left-handed supercoil. The histone octamer is a complex of two molecules each of H2A, H2B, H3 and H4 subunits. The nucleosomes are joined by linker DNA, the 'string', which is usually around 55 base pairs long, but may vary between organisms. At this stage, the packing ratio, or the ratio of the lengths of linear and condensed DNA, is around 7. The next level of chromatin condensation is the formation of 30 nM fibres, where linker DNA adjacent to each side of the nucleosome bead is bound by H1 histones. Forces between H1 subunits are thought to pull the DNA into a helix three nucleosomes wide and with six nucleosomes per turn – a solenoid structure with a packing ratio of around 40. At metaphase, DNA is at its most condensed in preparation for alignment along the mitotic spindle and segregation, ranging in size from 1.3 to 10 μm in length. Here, chromosomes may be observed, where DNA has been condensed even further by the arrangement of the 30 nM fibre in radial loops around a central protein scaffold or nuclear matrix, giving a packing ratio of between 10^2 and 10^3.

Condensation of DNA by histones depends largely upon their positive charge, which is conferred by deacetylation of lysine residues in the amino acid tails of the histone molecules within the nucleosomal core. The extent of histone acetylation depends upon the opposing functions of the enzyme HDAC, which catalyses the removal, and histone acetyl transferase (HAT), which catalyses the addition of acetyl groups. There are currently 18 known isoforms of HDAC, the most well characterized being arranged into classes I, II and III according to their homology to the yeast HDACs. These differ in terms of molecular weight, number of catalytic sites and dependence on the enzyme co-factor NAD. At the time of writing, there are limited data available on the prognostic effects of the HDAC isoforms in tumours, though immunohistochemical analysis of colorectal carcinoma samples has revealed higher levels of HDAC1 relative to normal colonic mucosa (Ishihama *et al.* (2007), see Further reading). Bioinformatic methods, however, such as SAGE tags (serial analysis of gene expression, Velculescu *et al.*, 1995), have provided preliminary data on the distribution of HDAC isoforms across normal tissue and tumour types (Table 21.1). Such biochemical properties, as well as the subcellular location, tumour specificity and substrate specificity of the HDACs ultimately influence their use as drug targets and the activity of HDAC inhibitors. Inhibition of HDAC through molecular interventions carried out in tumour models, or through the action of novel anticancer agents, has a number of effects on a range of genes and tumorigenic processes, summarized in Figure 21.2. Briefly, HDAC inhibitors are thought to exert their effect by inhibiting the removal of acetyl groups. Hyper-acetylated histones carry positive charge which is required for the condensation of negatively charged DNA molecules. Consequently, DNA in cells exposed to HDAC inhibitor is less tightly packaged and therefore accessible to the transcription machinery necessary for the expression of genes involved in pathways that run contrary to tumorigenesis and suppress tumour growth. For instance, exposure of tumour cell lines to HDAC inhibitors such as sodium butyrate, trichostatin A and trapoxin lead to differentiation, apoptosis and cell cycle arrest. More recent progress in the character-ization and functional analysis of HDAC isoforms has shown that, as well as determin-ing the extent of DNA condensation and therefore physical access to the DNA molecule during transcription, HDAC itself interacts with proteins involved with transcriptional

Table 21.1 Classification of HDACs by isoform, biochemical properties and normal tissue and tumour specificity

HDAC isoform	Biochemical properties	Average overall normal tissue/tumour expression (calculated using SAGE data)		Normal tissue/tumour type with highest level of expression (calculated using SAGE data) (Average number of hits per 100 000 tags)	
		Normal	Tumour	Normal	Tumour
Class I					
HDAC 1	Homology with yeast RPD3 deacetylase	1.4	1.75	Ovary (4.1)	Ovary (2.6)
HDAC 2		3.0	4.1	Kidney (11.9)	Neuroblastoma (9.1)
HDAC 3	MW 22–55 kDa	1.85	1.95	Ovary (5.2)	Pancreas (3.0)
HDAC 8		0.2	0.55	Kidney (0.9)*	Pancreas (1.5)
Class II					
HDAC 4	Homology with yeast HDA1 deacetylase.	0.01	0.19	ND*	Brain (6.1)
HDAC 5		0.42	3.4	Heart (9.5)*	Neuroblastoma (8.5)
HDAC 7	MW 120–135 kDa	2.2	2.15	Ovary (9.3)	Breast (3.2)
HDAC 9		0.55	1.0	Ovary (2.1)*	Colon (2.6)
Class III					
Sir 2 family (hSirt 1–7)	Require NAD. Not inhibited by class I and II HDAC inhibitors. Histones not primary substrate	ND		ND	
HDAC 6	Class IIb, 2 catalytic sites	4.5	5.5	Breast (8.6)	Breast (8.9)
HDAC 10		1.15	1.3	Prostate (5.2)	Breast (4.3)
HDAC 11	Class IV – catalytic core has elements of both class I and II HDACs	ND		ND	

Data describing normal tissue and tumour specificity are reproduced from a review by Annemieke et al. (2003) *Biochem. J.* 370, 737–749. Here, the authors carried out a preliminary bioinformatic study where SAGE (serial analysis of gene expression) tags, which are unique to the gene in question, were obtained from the NCBI SAGE database (http://www.ncbi.nlm.nih.gov/UniGene/) and compared with data from normal and tumour tissues found in the Human Transcriptome Map (www.amc.uva.nl). A range of normal tissue (brain, breast colon, kidney, ovary, pancreas, prostate, heart) and tumour (brain, breast, colon, neuroblastoma, ovary, pancreas, prostate, heart) types were included in the study. For values marked * expression data from three or more normal tissue/tumour types were missing.
NAD, nicotinamide adenine dinucleotide.

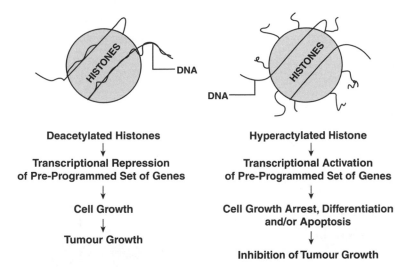

Figure 21.2 HDAC as an anticancer drug target. The binding of histones to DNA depends to a large extent upon the presence of positively charged lysine residues on the amino acid tails of histones in the nucleosome cores. By removing acetyl groups from these lysine residues, HDAC restores positive charge and the DNA is condensed, repressing transcription of certain genes that may inhibit cellular proliferation and tumour growth. Inhibition of HDAC, however, leads to an accumulation of hyperacetylated histones, which have the opposite effect, inhibiting tumour growth by activating the transcription of genes that induce cell cycle arrest, differentiation and/or apoptosis. Reprinted with permission from Reproduced from Marks *et al.* (2000) *J. Natl. Cancer Inst.* 92:1210–6, Oxford University Press.

regulation at DNA sequences that may silence certain genes. Typically, a three-component repressor complex is formed when a DNA-binding protein, such as Mad or E2F, recruits a corepressor such as Sin3 or rb, which in turn leads to the recruitment of HDAC. Mechanisms occurring independently of HDAC catalytic activity have also been shown; where HDAC forms a complex with and therefore prevents binding of the dephosphorylating enzyme protein phosphatase (PP1) to both the signal transduction protein AkT/protein kinase B (PKB) and the transcription factor cAMP response element binding protein (CREB). Dephosphorylation deactivates these proteins, impacting on the expression of downstream genes. This is normally kept in check by complexation and inactivation of PP1 activity by HDAC. However, upon exposure to HDAC inhibitor, PP1 is released from the HDAC/PP1 complex, leading to increased dephosphorylation and consequently deactivation of Akt/PKB and CREB. Therapeutic inhibition of HDAC is now believed to disrupt the expression of genes mediated by these pathways, causing both activation and deactivation of genes critical to tumour progression pathways (Figure 21.3). The large number of non-histone HDAC substrates extends to the androgen and oestrogen receptors; signalling mediators for example, stat3, B-catenin and IRS-1; DNA repair enzymes for example, ku 70 and WRN; the molecular chaperone HSP90 (see Chapter 17); the structural protein α tubulin; inflammatory mediators for example, HMGB1; and the viral proteins, for example, T antigen, E1A and human immunodeficiency virus Tat. HDAC is also known to

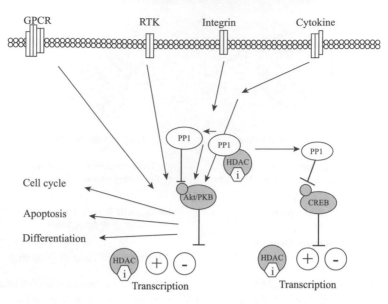

Figure 21.3 HDAC inhibitors have histone deacetylation-independent pharmacological effects. In normal conditions, HDAC forms a complex with the protein phosphatase PP1, preventing binding and dephosphorylation of both AkT/PKB and CREB. HDAC inhibitor therefore induces dephosphorylation and therefore deactivation of these proteins, disrupting expression of downstream genes that may be critical to tumour progression. GPCR, G-Protein coupled receptor; RTK, receptor tyrosine kinase. Reproduced with permission from Kostrouchova *et al.* (2007) *Folia Biologica* (*Praha*) 53: 37–49, Charles University in Prague, 1st Faculty of Medicine.

include among its substrates the transcription factors p53, nuclear factor-κB, hypoxia inducible factor-1 (HIF-1), YY1 and c-Myc. Consequently, numerous pathways are impacted upon exposure to HDAC inhibitors (Figure 21.4). For instance, disruption of HIF-1- mediated transcription by HDAC inhibitor leads to the downregulation of the hypoxia-inducible angiogenic growth factor VEGF and the VEGF receptor. This occurs through a number the mechanisms. These may be direct- where disrupting the association between class II HDACs and HIF-1α renders the latter vulnerable to degradation; and indirect- where HDAC inhibitor blocks the function of the protective chaperone protein HSP90 and therefore also promotes degradation of the hypoxia-regulated HIF-1α subunit. HDAC inhibitors also increases the expression of FIH (factor inhibiting HIF-1), which inhibits the transactivation of HIF-1 and therefore its function as a transcription factor. Another important group of pathways affected by HDAC inhibition induce cell death, where, for instance, both the extrinsic and intrinsic apoptosis pathways are activated (see Section 2.3.1). The extrinsic pathway involves the activation of caspase 8 via stimulation of death receptors such as Fas (CD95) or tumour necrosis factor receptor (TNFR-1) by drugs or ligands such as FasL and TNF. HDAC inhibitors induce apoptosis by upregulating both the death receptors and their ligands. The intrinsic pathway, however, is mediated by mitochondrial proteins, where the production of cytochrome C triggers apoptosis via caspase 9. HDAC inhibitors

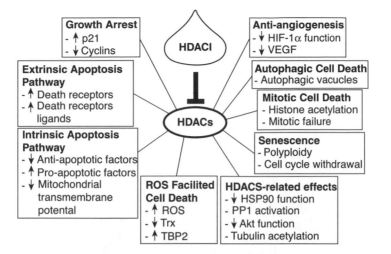

Figure 21.4 A summary of pathways impacted by the effect of HDAC inhibition on a wide range of histone and non-histone targets, including transcription factors, DNA repair enzymes and proteins involved in signalling and cell death mechanisms. Reproduced from Xu *et al.* (2007) *Oncogene* 26, 5541–52, Nature Publishing Group.

induce this pathway by increasing production of cytochrome C and activating caspase 9, but also by decreasing the levels of antiapoptotic proteins such as the bcl-2 family.

21.3 HDAC inhibitors

There are several classes of HDAC inhibitor at various stages of preclinical and clinical development (Figure 21.5) such as: (a) hydroximates, for example, trichostatin A, SAHA (vorinostat); (b) cyclic peptides, for example, FK-228 (depsipeptide); (c) aliphatic acids, for example, valproic acid (2-propylpentanoic acid); and (d) benzamides, for example, MS-275 (benzamidine). The structure of the catalytic core of HDAC, or the deacetylase core, is common to all isoforms, and its characterization by X-ray crystallography has helped to form an understanding of how HDAC inhibitors bind and exert their inhibitory action (Figure 21.6). The accumulation of H3 histones versus acetyl H3 histones is used as a surrogate marker of HDAC inhibition in preclinical and clinical studies of novel HDAC inhibitors.

Hydroximates include the natural lead product trichostatin A, originally an antifungal agent; as well as its analogue SAHA (vorinostat), licensed to Merck in 2007 under the brand name of Zolinza for the treatment of the rare cutaneous manifestations of T-cell lymphoma (CTCL), which lead to pruritus and complications such as breakdown of the skin and systemic infection. At the time of writing, vorinostat is also in phase I/II clinical trials for solid malignancies, in combination with carboplatin and paclitaxel for advanced solid malignancies.

Depsipeptide (FK-228) has been evaluated in a Childrens Oncology Group administered phase I trial in children with refractory or recurrent solid tumours

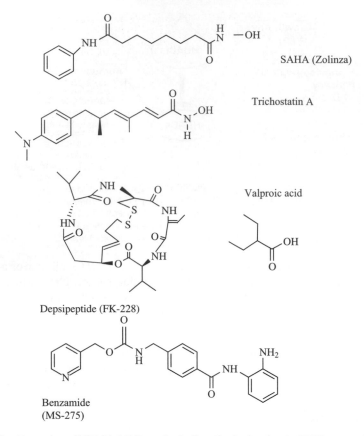

Figure 21.5 Examples of HDAC inhibitors, including the hydroximate SAHA, an analogue of the earlier agent trichostatin A; the cyclic peptide depsipeptide (FK-228); the aliphatic valproic acid and the benzamide MS-275.

(Fouladi *et al.*, 2006), which included paediatric tumour types such as Ewing's sarcoma, osteosarcoma, medulloblastoma, rhabdomyosarcoma and nephroblastoma. Dose-limiting toxicity mainly presented as electrocardiogram abnormalities, such as asymptomatic T-wave inversions, alongside the more generalized adverse effects of myelosuppression and gastrointestinal effects. Although no tumour response was observed, three of the 23 patients receiving the treatment experienced prolonged disease stabilization.

The teratogenicity of valproic acid, a drug approved for the treatment of all forms of epilepsy as well as bipolar disorder, by virtue of its pharmacological potentiation of the neurotransmitter gamma-aminobenzoic acid, carries an increased risk of neural tube defects, for example, spina bifida, if used in pregnancy. The study of these adverse effects may offer a clue as to its potential use as an anticancer agent via a pharmacological link with mechanisms that block cellular proliferation and differentiation, and certain developmental processes. Although the toxicity profile of valproic acid is well characterized due to clinical experience gained from around 30 years of use as an

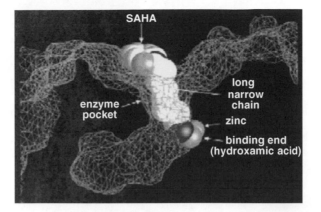

Figure 21.6 SAHA (suberoylanilide hydroxamic acid) binds to the pocket of the catalytic site of a histone deacetylase-like protein, schematically represented by the netting. SAHA makes contact with residues at the rim, walls and bottom of the pocket (enzyme pocket). The hydroxamic acid moiety of SAHA binds to the zinc at the bottom of the pocket. Reproduced from Marks *et al.* (2000) *J. Natl. Cancer Inst.* 2000;92:1210–6, Oxford University Press.

antiepileptic agent, the change in benefit versus risk when proposing an alternative use as an anticancer agent dictated the need for a new dose escalation study carried out in patients with refractory advanced cancers. In fact, the starting dose in this trial (30 mg/ kg infused over 1 h) approximated to the standard maintenance dose (15–30 mg/kg/ day) used in the treatment of epilepsy. The maximum tolerated dose, however, proved to be 60 mg/kg/day; higher doses preceding the onset of dose-limiting neurotoxicity. Valproic acid is currently in phase I clinical trial in combination with the topoisomerase II inhibitor epirubicin in patients with advanced solid tumours, and in a separate phase I trial, in combination with the DNMT inhibitor decitabine in patients with acute myeloid leukaemia.

Benzamide (MS-275) is currently in phase I/II trials, a dose escalation phase I trial having been carried out in refractory or relapsed haematological malignancies. Further phase I trials have been carried out in solid tumours and lymphomas, and in one trial, in combination with 13-*cis*-retinoic acid. Phase II trials have been initiated in patients with metastatic melanoma, and in combination with the DNMT inhibitor azacytidine in patients with recurrent advanced non-small cell lung carcinoma. Two further trials are in progress aiming to evaluate the use of azacytidine in combination with benzamide for the treatment of myelodysplastic syndrome, chronic myeloid leukaemia or acute myeloid leukaemia.

22

Pharmaceutical problems in cancer chemotherapy

22.1 Manifestation of toxicity

Usually anticancer agents are most toxic to rapidly dividing cells. The tissues that are typically affected include mucous membranes, skin, hair, bone marrow and the gastrointestinal tract. There are also adverse drug reactions that are specific to a particular anticancer agent. Toxicity may be graded according to criteria set out by the World Health Organization (WHO) or the National Cancer Institute (NCI), ranging from Grade 1 (mild adverse event) to grade 5 (death related to adverse event) (Figure 22.1).

Toxicity to chemotherapy can be acute, occurring within hours or a few days of drug administration, or chronic, where the adverse events may occur weeks, months or even years after treatment (Figure 22.2).

- *Mucous membranes:* Patients receiving chemotherapy are frequently affected by stomatitis, or inflammation of the oral mucosa, for example, 5-fluorouracil and methotrexate. Symptoms include erythema, pain, dry mouth, ulceration and bleeding. Prophylactic mouth care regimes are important in this case, where patients are often prescribed antiseptic mouthwashes. Pain may be severe, sometimes requiring opioid analgesics, and in severe cases, a decreased drug dose may be necessary.

- *Dermatological:* Occurs where there is damage to cells or structures within the skin, for example, damage to hair-producing cells results in alopecia after administration of many cytotoxic drugs. There may also be skin changes such as dryness and photosensitivity with 5-fluorouracil and methotrexate.

- *Bone marrow suppression:* Dose-related, the most frequently occurring dose-limiting side effect of chemotherapy. There are several types – neutropenia (decreased leukocytes), thrombocytopenia (decreased platelets) and, though not as common, anaemias. These effects may be alleviated by the addition of granulocytic colony

Cancer Chemotherapy   Rachel Airley
© 2009 John Wiley & Sons, Ltd.

Common Terminology Criteria for Adverse Events v3.0 (CTCAE)
Publish Date: December 12, 2003

Quick Reference

The NCI Common Terminology Criteria for Adverse Events v3.0 is a descriptive terminology which can be utilized for Adverse Event (AE) reporting. A grading (severity) scale is provided for each AE term.

Components and Organization

CATEGORY

A CATEGORY is a broad classification of AEs based on anatomy and/or pathophysiology. Within each CATEGORY, AEs are listed accompanied by their descriptions of severity (Grade).

Adverse Event Terms

An AE is any unfavorable and unintended sign (including an abnormal laboratory finding), symptom, or disease temporally associated with the use of a medical treatment or procedure that may or may not be considered related to the medical treatment or procedure. An AE is a term that is a unique representation of a specific event used for medical documentation and scientific analyses. Each AE term is mapped to a MedDRA term and code. AEs are listed alphabetically within CATEGORIES.

Short AE Name

The 'SHORT NAME' column is new and it is used to simplify documentation of AE names on Case Report Forms.

Supra-ordinate Terms

A supra-ordinate term is located within a CATEGORY and is a grouping term based on disease process, signs, symptoms.

or diagnosis. A supra-ordinate term is followed by the word 'Select' and is accompanied by specific AEs that are all related to the supra-ordinate term. Supra-ordinate terms provide clustering and consistent representation of Grade for related AEs. Supra-ordinate terms are not AEs, are not mapped to a MedDRA term and code, cannot be graded and cannot be used for reporting.

REMARK

A 'REMARK' is a clarification of an AE.

ALSO CONSIDER

An 'ALSO CONSIDER' indicates additional AEs that are to be graded if they are clinically significant.

NAVIGATION NOTE

A 'NAVIGATION NOTE' indicates the location of an AE term within the CTCAE document. It lists signs/symptoms alphabetically and the CTCAE term will appear in the same CATEGORY unless the 'NAVIGATION NOTE' states differently.

Grades

Grade refers to the severity of the AE. The CTCAE v3.0 displays Grades 1 through 5 with unique clinical descriptions of severity for each AE based on this general guideline:

Grade 1   Mild AE
Grade 2   Moderate AE
Grade 3   Severe AE
Grade 4   Life-threatening or disabling AE
Grade 5   Death related to AE

A Semi-colon indicates 'or' within the description of the grade.

An 'Em dash' (—) indicates a grade not available.

Not all Grades are appropriate for all AEs. Therefore, some AEs are listed with fewer than five options for Grade selection.

Grade 5

Grade 5 (Death) is not appropriate for some AEs and therefore is not an option.

The DEATH CATEGORY is new. Only one Supra-ordinate term is listed in this CATEGORY: 'Death not associated with CTCAE term - Select' with 4 AE options: Death NOS; Disease progression NOS; Multi-organ failure; Sudden death.

Important:

- Grade 5 is the only appropriate Grade
- This AE is to be used in the situation where a death
    1. cannot be reported using a CTCAE v3.0 term associated with Grade 5, or
    2. cannot be reported within a CTCAE CATEGORY as 'Other (Specify)'

Contents

Cancer Therapy Evaluation Program, Common Terminology Criteria for Adverse Events, Version 3.0, DCTD, NCI, NIH, DHHS
March 31, 2003 (http://ctep.cancer.gov). Publish Date: December 12, 2003

Figure 22.1 The National Cancer Institute Common Terminology Criteria for Adverse Events (CTCAE) is a periodically updated dictionary of adverse drug reactions used to standardise the reporting of toxicities observed during NCI-sponsored clinical evaluation of novel anti-cancer regimens. Adverse events (AEs) are defined according to grade, describing the severity of the AE from grade 1 (mild AE) to 5 (death); and category, where AEs are grouped according to the specific pathology diagnosed or changes in clinical biochemistry. These are systematically catalogued (introductory page shown here), examples of categories including allergic or immune reactions, e.g. hypersensitivity to the agent – grade 1 representing transient flushing and grade 4 anaphylaxis; blood/bone marrow events, e.g. neutropenia, grade 1 representing a neutrophil count of $<1500/mm^3$ and grade 4 a neutrophil count of $<500/mm^3$; and dermatological events, e.g. rash (desquamation), where grade 1 is defined as a macular or popular eruption or erythema without associated symptoms and grade 4 as a generalized exfoliative, ulcerative, or bullous dermatitis. Reproduced with permission from http://ctep.cancer.gov/forms/CTCAEv3.pdf.

stimulating factor, for example, lenograstim (Granocyte). Examples of anticancer agents causing bone marrow suppression include carmustine, cytarabine, paclitaxel and the anthracyclines (doxorubicin, adriamycin). Amifostine, which protects against oxygen-based free radicals and electrophilic reactive drugs, is used to reduce neutropenia-associated infection in patients with ovarian carcinoma treated with cyclophosphamide and cisplatin.

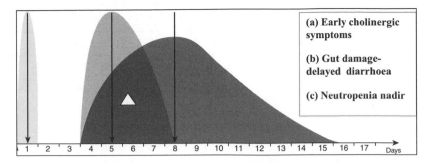

Figure 22.2 Timeframe of adverse drug reactions after chemotherapy. Adapted from Allwood *et al.* (2002).

- *Gatrointestinal:* Manifests as nausea, vomiting, diarrhoea and/or constipation. Severe vomiting may result in dehydration, electrolyte disturbances and oesophageal tears. Adverse effects may be severe enough to warrant discontinuation of therapy. Vomiting may be acute, delayed or anticipatory that is, the patient is affected by vomiting before administration of chemotherapy having experienced side effects upon previous exposure. A combination of the emetogenicity of the agent or combination of agents, dose, route of administration and patient characteristics influences the occurrence of nausea and vomiting. The emetogenic potential of an anticancer agent describes the likelihood and extent of nausea and vomiting it may induce. This varies widely between drugs and is graded on a scale of 1–5 (Table 22.1).

- *Renal and hepatic:* Signs include elevated serum creatinine, elevated BUN (blood urea nitrogen, a measure of renal capacity to eliminate urea) and electrolyte abnormalities; which are adverse effects of agents such as cisplatin, ifosphamide, methotrexate. Small doses of amifostine may be used to alleviate nephrotoxic events. Hepatotoxicity may be revealed by liver function tests, in some cases leading to jaundice and hepatitis: for example, asparaginase, cytarabine, 6-mercaptopurine, methotrexate.

- *Neurotoxicity:* May occur with systemic or intrathecal (spinal) therapy, and may be dose-limiting, reversible or irreversible. Chemotherapy-induced neuropathies may be autonomic, for example, gait disturbances (vincristine) and loss of deep tendon reflexes (vincristine, taxanes), or peripheral, giving rise to numb hands and feet. High dose cytarabine may cause loss of hand–eye coordination, patients receiving platinum-based drugs are at risk of ototoxicity. Further risks include confusion, dizziness and headaches (fluorouracil) and encephalopathy (asparaginase, ifosfamide). Arachnoiditis may result from intrathecal administration of cytarabine or methotrexate, and accidental intrathecal administration of vincristine leads to fatal neurotoxicity.

- *Hypersensitivity:* This constitutes type I anaphylaxis, (immunoglobulin G-mediated) which may be life threatening if not treated promptly and correctly, for example, asparaginase, platinum, etoposide, paclitaxel. Symptoms include localized or generalized

Table 22.1   Emetogenic potential of single and combination anticancer agents

EMETOGENIC POTENTIAL OF ANTINEOPLASTIC AGENTS

High Risk (>90% frequency without antiemetics)

- AC combination: Doxorubicin (Adriamycin) or Epirubicin (Ellence) + Cyclophosphamide (Cytoxan, Neosar)
- Altretamine (HMM, Hexalen)
- Carmustine (BCNU, BiCNU) >250 mg/m^2
- Cisplatin (CDDP, Platinol, Platinol-AQ) $\geq$50 mg/m^2

- Cyclophosphamide (CTX, Cytoxan, Neosar) >1,500 mg/m^2
- Dacarbazine (DTIC, DTIC-Dome)
- Mechlorethamine (Mustargen)
- Procarbazine (Matulane) *oral*
- Streptozocin (Zanosar)

Moderate Risk (30–90% frequency without antiemetics)

- Aldesleukin (IL-2, Proleukin) >12–15 million units/m^2
- Amifostine (Ethyol) >300 mg/m^2
- Arsenic trioxide (As$_2$O$_3$, Trisenox)
- Azacitidine (Vidaza)
- Busulfan (Busulfex) high dose >4 mg/d
- Carboplatin (Paraplatin)
- Carmustine (BCNU, BiCNU) $\leq$250 mg/m^2
- Cisplatin (CDDP, Platinol, Platinol-AQ) <50 mg/m^2
- Cyclophosphamide (CTX, Cytoxan, Neosar) $\leq$1,500 mg/m^2
- Cyclophosphamide (CTX) *oral*
- Cytarabine (ARA-C, Cytosar-U) >1 g/m^2
- Dactinomycin (actinomycin D, Cosmegen)
- Daunorubicin (Cerubidine, Daunomycin)

- Doxorubicin (Adriamycin)
- Epirubicin (Ellence)
- Etoposide (VP-16, VePesid) *oral*
- Idarubicin (Idamycin)
- Ifosfamide (Ifex)
- Imatinib (Gleevec) *oral*
- Irinotecan (CPT-11, Camptosar)
- Lomustine (CCNU, CeeNU)
- Melphalan (L-PAM, Alkeran) >50 mg/m^2 *IV*
- Methotrexate (MTX) 250 to >1,000 mg/m^2
- Oxaliplatin (Eloxatin) >75 mg/m^2
- Temozolomide (Temodar) *oral*
- Vinorelbine (Navelbine) *oral*

Low Risk (10–30% frequency without antiemetics)

- Amifostine (Ethoyl) $\leq$300 mg
- Bexarotene (Targretin)
- Capecitabine (Xeloda) *oral*
- Cetuximab (C225, Erbitux)
- Cytarabine (ARA-C, Cytosar-U) $\leq$1 g/m^2
- Docetaxel (Taxotere)
- Doxorubicin liposomal (Doxil)
- Etoposide (VP-16, Etopophos, VePesid) *IV*
- Fludarabine (Fludara) *oral*

- Fluorouracil (5-FU)
- Gemcitabine (Gemzar)
- Methotrexate (MTX) >50 mg/m^2 to <250 mg/m^2
- Mitomycin (MTC, Mitozytrex, Mutamycin)
- Mitoxantrone (DHAD, Novantrone)
- Paclitaxel (Taxol)
- Paclitaxel albumin (Abraxane)
- Pemetrexed (Alimta)
- Topotecan (Hycamtin)

Minimal Risk (<10% frequency without antiemetics)

- Alemtuzumab (Campath)
- Asparaginase (Elspar)

- Hydroxyurea (Hydrea) *oral*
- Interferon alpha (IFN-alpha, Intron A)

Table 22.1 *(Continued)*

EMETOGENIC POTENTIAL OF ANTINEOPLASTIC AGENTS	
• Bevacizumab (Avastin)	• Lenalidomide (Revlimid)
• Bleomycin (Blenoxane)	• Melphalan (L-PAM, Alkeran) low dose *oral*
• Bortezomib (Velcade)	• Methotrexate (MTX) $\leq$50 mg/m^2
• Busulfan (Busulfex)	• Nelarabine (Arranon)
• Chlorambucil (Leukeran) *oral*	• Pentostatin (Nipent)
• Cladribine (2-CdA, Leustatin)	• Rituximab (Rituxan)
• Dasatinib (Sprycel)	• Sorafenib (Nexavar)
• Decitabine (Dacogen)	• Sunitinib (Sutent)
• Denileukin diftitox (Ontak)	• Thalidomide (Thalomid)
• Dexrazoxane (Totect, Zinecard)	• Thioguanine (6-TG, Tabloid) *oral*
• Erlotinib (Tarceva)	• Trastuzumab (Herceptin)
• Fludarabine (Fludara) *IV*	• Vinblastine (VLB)
• Gefitinib (Iressa)	• Vincristine (VCR)
• Gemtuzumab ozogamicin (Mylotarg)	• Vinorelbine (Navelbine) *IV*

*Daily use of antiemetics is not recommended based on clinical experience.
Adapted from:
1. Kris MG, Hesketh PJ, Somerfield MR, et al. American Society of Clinical Oncology Guideline for Antiemetics in Oncology: Update 2006. J Clin Oncol 2006;24:2932–2947.
2. National Comprehensive Cancer Network. NCCN Clinical Practice Guidelines in Oncology; v.1.2007: Antiemesis.
Available at: http://www.nccn.org/professionals/physician_gls/PDF/antiemesis.pdf. Accessed August 2008.

itching, flushing, shortness of breath, agitation, local or facial oedema, tightness of chest, dizziness, light-headedness, tachycardia, hypotension and sometimes flu-like symptoms and violent shaking. Administration of dexamethasone prior to and following treatment may be used as a preventative strategy.

• *Chills and fever:* This effect may occur after administration of agents such as bleomycin, trastazumab and liposomal doxorubicin.

• *Infertility:* may be temporary or permanent, for example, cyclophosphamide, chlorambucol, melphalan.

22.2 Regimen-related toxicity

Some adverse drug reactions are less predictable and are specific to certain anticancer drugs. These include the onset of haemorrhagic cystitis after administration of cyclophosphamide or ifosfamide (and less commonly with etoposide and busulphan) which presents as lower abdominal pain, urinary urgency and frequency, and haematuria. The complication is a result of irritation of the bladder mucosa by drug metabolites such as acrolein. Treatment includes aggressive hydration, and administration of the acrolein binder Mesna. Pulmonary toxicity for example, bleomycin, busulphan, carmustine and mitomycin C, is generally irreversible and may be life threatening. Signs and symptoms include shortness of breath, non-productive cough and low-grade fever. Cardiotoxicity is associated with the use of anthracyclines and mitoxantrone, and may be acute or chronic. Acute effects may be detectable as transient electrocardiogram abnormalities and may not be clinically significant, whereas chronic effects may manifest as irreversible congestive cardiac failure. Attempts to limit cardiotoxicity include the co-administration of cardioprotective agents such as the iron chelator dexrazoxane.

22.3 Secondary malignancies

Secondary malignancies may arise as a long-term consequence of cancer chemotherapy. The increased survival rates associated with improvements in cancer treatment mean that patients may be at risk of recurrence, either of the primary disease, or from an unrelated tumour that may have arisen after exposure to certain anticancer drugs. Drug-induced malignancy may be hard to distinguish from malignancies caused by biological factors that may also have caused the primary disease, such as deregulated expression of oncogenes and chromosomal defects. Nevertheless, secondary malignancies are most likely to take the form of therapy-related leukaemia (TRL), the commonest form being an acute myeloid leukaemia (t-AML) most likely to occur 2.5–7 years after treatment of a primary malignancy. The risk of developing TRL correlates with cumulative dose of anticancer agent received, as well as concurrent treatment such as radiotherapy, and has occurred in patients following treatment for non-Hodgkin's lymphoma, soft tissue sarcomas, brain, small cell lung and ovarian tumours. They are also associated with the treatment of childhood cancers such as neuroblastoma, acute lymphoblastic leukaemia and Wilms' tumour. Secondary malignancies in children are an unfortunate consequence of the vast improvements in the treatment of these diseases that in the first half of the twentieth century were almost always fatal, a stunning example being the survival rates of young patients with acute lymphoblastic leukaemia. The early age of onset, however, necessitates careful long-term follow up. A greater risk of secondary malignancy is associated with the use of drugs with leukaemogenic potential, such as alkylating agents, etoposide and doxorubicin, and is thought to stem from ineffective or inappropriate DNA repair, which may permanently disrupt DNA replication and transcription, ultimately leading to carcinogenesis. Certain patients may have a genetic predisposition to treatment-related secondary malignancies. For example, those with germ-line mutations of the tumour suppressor gene *p53* are prone to developing t-AML after exposure to alkylating agents. Inter-patient variation in metabolic activation or elimination, caused by genetic polymorphisms in the expression of drug metabolizing enzymes, may increase the leukaemogenic potential of a drug. This may impact on the elimination of toxic intermediates associated with quinones such as mitomycin C, where polymorphic expression of the enzyme NADPH: quinone oxidoreductase (NQO1) leads to reductase activity, and with defective metabolism of 6-mercaptopurine, a genetic polymorphism that leads to reduced thiopurine methyltransferase

(TPMT) activity. Other therapy-related secondary malignancies that may arise after treatment with chemotherapy and/or radiotherapy include tumours of the central nervous system, osteosarcomas and melanomas, and these are also particularly associated with the treatment of childhood cancers.

22.4 Drug resistance

There are several mechanisms by which chemoresponse or chemosensitivity to certain anticancer agents or groups of agents may be reduced. These may be due to tumour or patient characteristics, and largely depend upon the pharmacodynamic and pharma-cokinetic properties of the drug.

22.4.1 Multiple drug resistance

This type of drug resistance is mediated by the expression and activity of drug efflux transporters found on the plasma membrane of tumour cells, which pump drug out of the tumour cell, therefore reducing intracellular accumulation of drug to levels that may be below those which are therapeutically useful. They are large transmembrane glycoproteins ($\sim$170 kDa), which are classed as ABC type transporters, that is, the transporter is characterized by the presence of an ATP-binding casette, so that the level of activity is dependent upon the presence of ATP. There are several types of multi-drug resistance transporter, including p-glycoprotein, which is regulated by the *MDR1* gene, multi-drug resistance associated protein (MRP), breast cancer resistance protein (BCRP) and lung cancer resistance protein (LRP). Drug resistance mediated by multi-drug resistance transporters may be intrinsic, that is, determined by gene expression, or acquired, where exposure of tumour cells to certain anticancer agents may cause selection of multiply resistant mutants. Multi-drug resistance can arise in most tumour types, at all stages of disease, and presents a problem when treating with drugs that are substrates for multi-drug resistance transporters, for example, daunorubicin, the taxanes and the vinca alkaloids. One novel anticancer strategy aims to use p-glycoprotein inhibitors (Figure 22.3) to improve the activity of anticancer agents where multi-drug resistance is a problem. The anti-arrhythmic drug verapamil and ciclosporin A are inhibitors of p-glycoprotein, although phase III trials in combination with chemotherapy vulnerable to p-glycoprotein-dependent resistance failed to show a significant improvement in clinical outcome. Since then, however, there has been an assortment of second generation p-glycoprotein inhibitors, such as the ciclosporin A derivative PSC-833 (Valspodar), VX-710 (Biricodar) and MS-209 (Dofequidar), which are showing promise in preclinical and clinical development.

22.4.2 Enhanced DNA repair

This mode of resistance is mediated via DNA repair enzymes that repair DNA crosslinks. For instance, the enzyme O6-alkylguanine-DNA alkyltransferase (AGT) catalyses direct repair of DNA damage exerted by agents that alkylate DNA at the *O6*

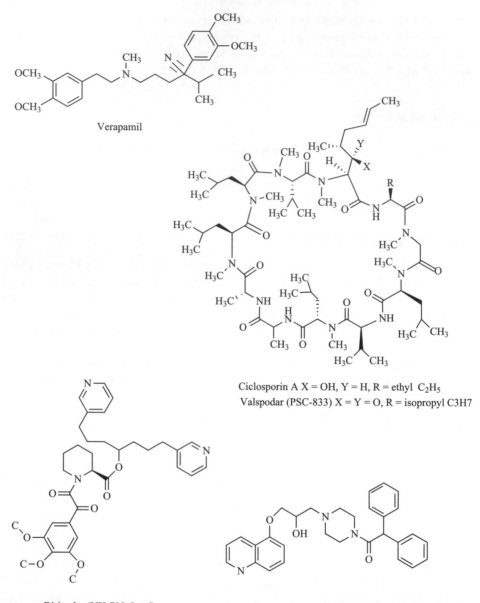

Verapamil

Ciclosporin A X = OH, Y = H, R = ethyl C₂H₅
Valspodar (PSC-833) X = Y = O, R = isopropyl C3H7

Biricodar (VX-710, Incel)   Doefequidar (MS-209).

Figure 22.3 p-glycoprotein inhibitors. Reproduced from Atadja, P., Watanabe, T., Xu, H., Cohen, D. *Cancer Metastasis Rev.* 1998;17:163–8, Springer.

position of guanine, that is, the chloroethylating mustards carmustine and lomustine and the methylating agents temozolomide, dacarbazine, procarbazine and streptozotocin. Other DNA repair enzymes are involved in base excision repair, where alkylated DNA bases are removed, for example by the repair enzyme DNA glycosylase, and the resulting gaps are ligated through the activation of enzyme complexes such as XRCC1 and ligase III-α complex. These are recruited by a further repair enzyme PARP-1, one of a family of PARP (poly (ADP-ribose) polymerase) enzymes that catalyse the addition of repeating units of ADP-ribose to protein or DNA via reduction of NAD^+. Novel anticancer agents that target DNA repair enzymes are currently in development, with the aim of using them to improve chemoresponse to alkylating agents. O6-Benzyl-guanine (O6-BG), an analogue of O6 alkyl guanine, is currently in development as an AGT inhibitor. AGT is able to repair damaged guanine residues by removing a range of alkyl groups from guanine and transferring them to a cysteine residue at its active site. If alkylating agents are co-administered with O6-BG, AGT will preferentially transfer and form a complex with the aromatic R group on O6-BG (Figure 22.4a), resulting in benzylation and therefore inhibition of the enzyme (Figure 22.4b). O6-BG has been evaluated in two separate phase I clinical trials in combination with temozolamide and with carmustine in children with brain tumours, and in phase II trials also in combination with carmustine in patients with multiple myeloma and advanced soft tissue sarcoma. Efforts to develop inhibitors of PARP-1 (Figure 22.5) are also underway; building on earlier work carried out in the 1980s involving the use of 3-amino-benzamide to potentiate the cytotoxic effects of radiotherapy; and the antibiotic benadrostin, produced by the microorganism *Streptomyces flavovirens*. More potent PARP-1 inhibitors include the quinazolinones, for example, NU-1025 (8-hydroxy-2-methyl-quinazolin-4-[3H]one); and the tricyclic benzimidazole lead compound AG14361, which have been investigated in preclinical studies in combination with

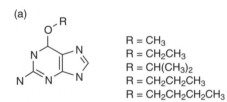

(a)

R = CH₃
R = CH₂CH₃
R = CH(CH₃)₂
R = CH₂CH₂CH₃
R = CH₂CH₂CH₂CH₃

O^6-**Alkylated Guanine**

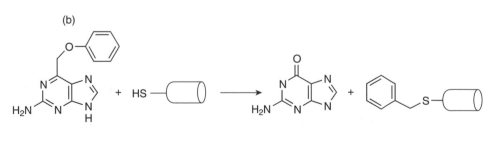

(b)

O^6-**Benzylguanine**   **AGT**   **Guanine**   **Benzylated AGT**

Figure 22.4 The DNA repair enzyme O6-alkylguanine-DNA alkyltransferase (AGT) confers chemoresistance, reversing DNA damage by removing alkyl groups (R) from O6 alkyl guanine residues (a) formed after exposure to alkylating anti-cancer agents. This effect may be overcome by addition of the O6-guanine antimetabolite O6-benzylguanine (O6-BG), which acts as an AGT inhibitor (b). Reproduced from Rabik *et al. Cancer Treat. Rev.* 2006;32:261–276, Elsevier.

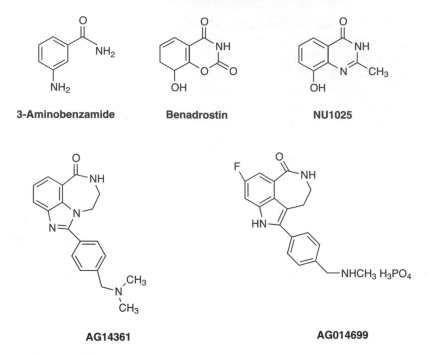

3-Aminobenzamide   **Benadrostin**   **NU1025**

AG14361   **AG014699**

Figure 22.5   Poly (ADP-ribose) polymerase-1 (PARP-1) inhibitors that have been the subject of preclinical studies include 3-aminobenzamide, benadrostin, NU1025 and the tricyclic benzimidazole lead compound AG14361. The tricyclic indole AG014699 is currently being evaluated in phase II clinical trials in combination with temazolamide in patients with malignant melanoma. Adapted from Miwa and Masutani (2007).

temazolamide and with the topoisomerase I inhibitors camptothecin and topotecan. After a promising phase I clinical trial completed in 2005, the tricyclic indole AG014699 is currently being evaluated in phase II clinical trials in combination with temazolamide in patients with malignant melanoma.

22.4.3 Alteration of drug targets

The action of anticancer agents may depend upon the activation or inhibition of enzymes or receptors. Resistance may be mediated via reduction in the level of expression of these drug targets. One example of this phenomenon is the evolution of methotrexate resistance caused by a decreased number of membrane-bound folate receptors, which significantly reduces uptake of the drug into the tumour cells.

22.5 Pharmaceutical complications

Administration of anticancer agents carries the risk of extravasation, phlebitis and venous irritation. The risk of these complications necessitates strict monitoring procedures, comprehensive clinical protocols and specialized training of health personnel.

22.5.1 Extravasation

Extravasation is caused by the inappropriate or accidental administration of chemotherapy into the tissues surrounding a vein, causing pain, erythema, inflammation and discomfort. Any delay in the treatment of extravasation may have dangerous consequences, ultimately leading to necrosis and functional loss of tissue. Damage may be inflicted upon structures such as nerves, tendons and joints, sometimes continuing months after the extravasation incident. For this reason, hospitals treating cancer patients generally have guidelines on site, which describe the correct course of action in the event of an extravasation incident. Extravasation risk may be associated with drug or patient characteristics. The mode of drug administration may increase extravasation risk, such as the device used and the location of the cannula. Risks associated with individual anticancer drugs depend upon their ability to bind DNA directly, their cytotoxicity to replicating cells and their ability to cause vascular dilatation. The physical properties of the drug and its formulation also determine extravasation risk, where increased risk is associated with high injection volumes, a pH outside the range 5.5–8.5, osmolality greater than that of plasma (290 mosmol/L) and formulation excipients such as alcohol, polyethylene glycol and surfactants for example, the Tweens. Drugs may be classified according to potential to cause necrosis with extravasation as follows (see also Table 22.2):

Group 1   Vesicants: cause pain, inflammation and blistering of local skin and underlying structures, leading to tissue necrosis.

Group 2   Exfoliants: cause inflammation and shedding of the skin, but necrosis is unlikely.

Group 3   Irritants: cause inflammation and irritation, in rare circumstances followed by tissue breakdown.

Group 4   Inflammatory agents: may see mild to moderate inflammatory response in local tissues.

Group 5   Neutrals: 'inert' drugs that do not have deleterious effects on tissue.

  Patient factors that determine extravasation risk include the nature of the disease, for example, the presence of lymphoedema; underlying conditions such as diabetes and peripheral circulatory disease; and previous radiotherapy. Extravasation risk also depends upon the use of concurrent medication that might ultimately exacerbate injury caused by extravasated anticancer drugs, as defined by the Joshua Index. These include anticoagulant, antiplatelet and antifibrinolytic drugs, which may exacerbate extravasation by increasing risk of local bleeding; vasodilators and diuretics, which can increase local blood flow and therefore extend the area of damage; and hormonal therapies and steroids, which have vasodilatory properties. Antihistamines, by their action as vasoconstricting agents, can worsen the effects of extravasation by causing ischaemic injury; and patients receiving both topical and centrally acting analgesics should be monitored closely as these medicines may shield the symptoms of

Table 22.2 Classification of anticancer agents according to potential to cause necrosis with extravasation.

Group 1 Vesicants	Group 2 Exfoliants	Group 3 Irritants	Group 4 Inflammatory agents	Group 5 Neutrals
Amsacrine	Aclarubicin	Carboplatin	Etoposide phosphate	Asparaginase
Carmustine	Cisplatin	Etoposide	5-Fluorouracil	Bleomycin
Dacarbazine	Liposomal daunorubicin	Irinotecan	Methotrexate	Cladribine
Dactinomycin	Docetaxel	Teniposide	Raltotrexed	Cyclophosphamide
Daunorubicin	Liposomal doxorubicin			Cytarabine
Doxorubicin	Floxuridine (FUDR)			Fludarabine
Epirubicin	Mitoxantrone			Gemicitabine
Idiarubicin	Oxaliplatin			Ifosfamide
Mitomycin C	Topotecan			Interleukin-2
Mustine				Melphalan
Paclitaxel				Pentostatin
Streptozocin				Thiotepa
Treosulphan				α-Interferons
Vinblastine				
Vincristine				
Vindesine				
Vinorelbine				

Reproduced with permission from *Cytotoxics Handbook* (4th edition) edited by Michael Allwood, Andrew Stanley and Patricia Wright, Radcliffe Publishing, 2002, Slough, UK.

extravasation and therefore lead to delayed reporting. Intravenous antibiotics, which themselves carry a risk of vascular thrombosis, may compound the effects of extravasation, as may any drugs that have previously elicited a hypersensitivity reaction. The treatment of extravasation injury is dependent upon the class of drug administered and includes the initial use of steroids to limit local tissue inflammation, followed by hyaluronidase or normal saline to disperse or dilute the drug over a large area, so that the local concentration of drug is limited. This strategy will be used alongside elevation of the limb and the cold or warm compresses.

22.5.2 Green card reporting

The National Extravasation Information Service carries web-based information on risks, diagnosis and treatment of extravasation (www.extravasation.org.uk). In addition, the organization collates statistics from oncology health professionals who have reported extravasation incidents using their Green Card Scheme (Figure 22.6), with the aim of carrying out research into the types and causes of extravasation most

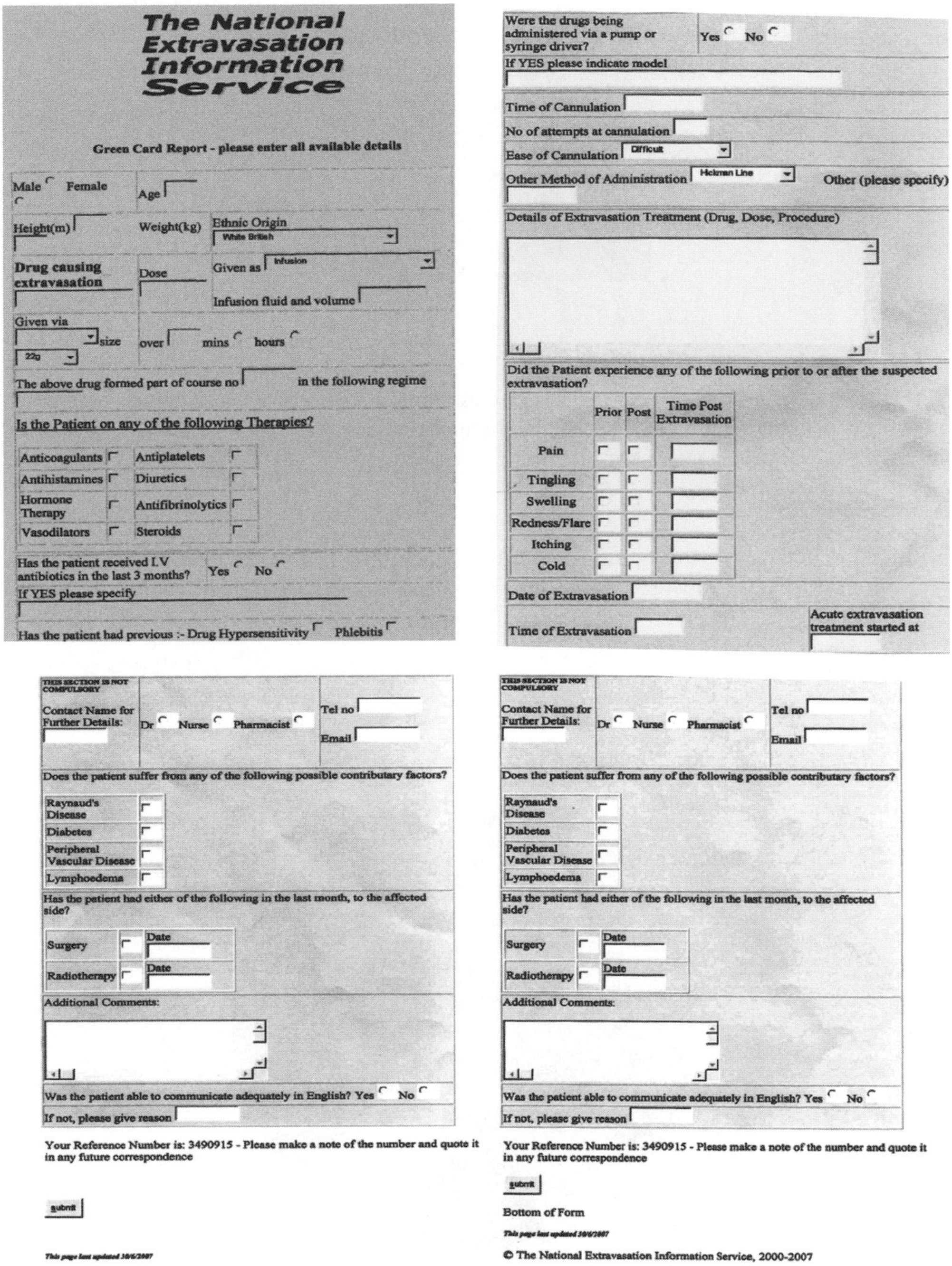

The National Extravasation Information Service

Green Card Report - please enter all available details

Male Female

Age

Height(m) Weight(kg) Ethnic Origin [White British]

Drug causing extravasation

Dose

Given as [Infusion]

Infusion fluid and volume

Given via

size [22g] over mins hours

The above drug formed part of course no in the following regime

Is the Patient on any of the following Therapies?

Anticoagulants	☐	Antiplatelets	☐
Antihistamines	☐	Diuretics	☐
Hormone Therapy	☐	Antifibrinolytics	☐
Vasodilators	☐	Steroids	☐

Has the patient received I.V antibiotics in the last 3 months? Yes No

If YES please specify

Has the patient had previous :- Drug Hypersensitivity Phlebitis

Were the drugs being administered via a pump or syringe driver? Yes No

If YES please indicate model

Time of Cannulation

No of attempts at cannulation

Ease of Cannulation [Difficult]

Other Method of Administration [Hickman Line] Other (please specify)

Details of Extravasation Treatment (Drug, Dose, Procedure)

Did the Patient experience any of the following prior to or after the suspected extravasation?

	Prior	Post	Time Post Extravasation
Pain	☐	☐	
Tingling	☐	☐	
Swelling	☐	☐	
Redness/Flare	☐	☐	
Itching	☐	☐	
Cold	☐	☐	

Date of Extravasation

Time of Extravasation

Acute extravasation treatment started at

THIS SECTION IS NOT COMPULSORY

Contact Name for Further Details: Dr Nurse Pharmacist Tel no Email

Does the patient suffer from any of the following possible contributary factors?

Raynaud's Disease	☐
Diabetes	☐
Peripheral Vascular Disease	☐
Lymphoedema	☐

Has the patient had either of the following in the last month, to the affected side?

Surgery	☐	Date
Radiotherapy	☐	Date

Additional Comments:

Was the patient able to communicate adequately in English? Yes No

If not, please give reason

Your Reference Number is: 3490915 - Please make a note of the number and quote it in any future correspondence

submit

This page last updated 30/6/2007

THIS SECTION IS NOT COMPULSORY

Contact Name for Further Details: Dr Nurse Pharmacist Tel no Email

Does the patient suffer from any of the following possible contributary factors?

Raynaud's Disease
Diabetes
Peripheral Vascular Disease
Lymphoedema

Has the patient had either of the following in the last month, to the affected side?

Surgery Date
Radiotherapy Date

Additional Comments:

Was the patient able to communicate adequately in English? Yes No

If not, please give reason

Your Reference Number is: 3490915 - Please make a note of the number and quote it in any future correspondence

submit

Bottom of Form

This page last updated 30/6/2007

Figure 22.6 The Green Card Report available on the National Extravasation Information Service web site www.extravasation.org.uk allow the reporting of extravasation incidents by doctors, nurses and pharmacists involved in the prescribing, compounding and administration of cytotoxics.

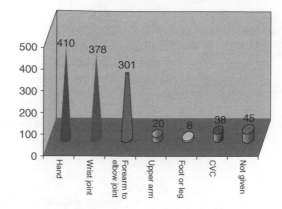

Figure 22.7   Area of body affected by extravasation. CVC (central venou catheter). Reproduced with permission from Dr Andrew Stanley, National Extravasation Information Service website www.extravasation.org.uk (August 2008).

likely to occur, in order to improve outcome. Figures 22.7–22.9, provided by this web site, show that the most frequent site of extravasation is the hand, wrist and elbow, and that it is most likely to have occurred with the administration of the group 4 inflammatory agent 5-fluorouracil.

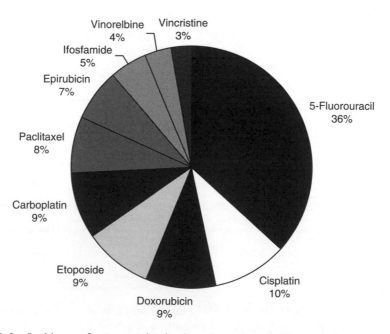

Figure 22.8   Incidence of extravasation by drug. Reproduced with permission from Dr Andrew Stanley, National Extravasation Information Service website www.extravasation.org.uk (August 2008).

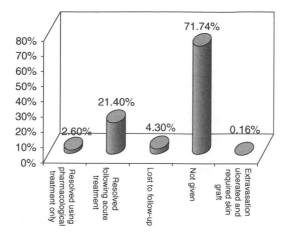

Figure 22.9 Outcome of extravasation incident drug. Reproduced with permission from Dr Andrew Stanley, National Extravasation Information Service website www.extravasation. org.uk (August 2008).

22.6 Phlebitis and venous irritation

This effect manifests as a transient but pronounced inflammation along the line of the vein, and may occur alongside or be part of the effects of extravasation syndrome. Reactions are confined to the venous compartment, and are related to the chemical properties of anticancer drugs such as pH, the type of excipient, the effect of the drug on vascular tone, drug concentration and the presence of impurities in the formulation.

22.7 Health and safety

Anticancer agents may be toxic to pharmacy personnel involved in the handling and compounding of these medicines, and are subject to cytotoxic handling and waste disposal guidelines. All pharmacists and pharmacy technicians working in cytotoxic compounding units therefore receive specialized training. Parenteral chemotherapy is prepared in a cytotoxic isolator, which ensures product and user protection. Procedures also include the use of luer lock fittings on syringes, and the use of a negative pressure technique when withdrawing medication from the vial. Exposure to anticancer agents presents a risk of carcinogenesis, therefore there should be biological monitoring of personnel. This includes the use of urine mutagenicity testing, which monitors mutations in bacterial cells, and sister chromatid exchange testing, which detects reciprocal exchanges between chromatids that are caused by low levels of mutagenic substances.

22.8 National guidance on the safe administration of intrathecal chemotherapy

Accidental intrathecal administration of vincristine, which should be given intravenously, has resulted in the paralysis or death of 13 patients since 1985. Building upon the publication of the NHS policy document 'An Organization with a Memory' and the later publication of the report 'Building a Safer NHS for Patients', published in 2001, the government agreed to set a target of reducing the number of deaths or serious injuries resulting from wrongly administered vincristine to zero. The guidance covering the implementation of this target was set out according to recommendations made by two reports made in 2001: one investigating the death of a teenager in Nottingham and the other a review of clinical policy dealing with the prevention of such chemotherapy administration errors. A summary of the guidance and recommendations defining the prescription, dispensing, checking and administration of cancer chemotherapy, and the implications to the health professionals involved, is as follows:

- A register of designated personnel that have been trained to work with intrathecal chemotherapy must be established.

- An induction programme for all new staff involved in cancer chemotherapy should be provided.

- Regular training programmes for staff on the intrathecal chemotherapy register.

- All chemotherapy staff should be provided with a written protocol describing national guidance and local amendments to chemotherapy guidelines.

- Intrathecal chemotherapy must only be prescribed by a consultant or specialist registrar.

- Patients receiving intrathecal chemotherapy must have a purpose-designed chart.

- Intrathecal chemotherapy must only be issued or received by designated staff.

- Intrathecal drugs should be kept in a lockable, designated refrigerator if not to be used immediately.

- Intravenous drugs should be given before intrathecal drugs are issued, unless to a child under general anaesthesia.

- Intrathecal chemotherapy must be administered in a designated, separate area within normal working hours and intravenous drugs should not be stored in this area.

- Checks should be made by medical, nursing and pharmacy staff throughout the process.

- Drugs with life-threatening consequences must be clearly labelled, with positive, rather than negative instructions that is, 'For intravenous use only – fatal if given by other routes' rather than 'Not for intrathecal use'.

- Dilutions of intravenous chemotherapy drugs must be standardized.

23

Oncology pharmacy at home and abroad

The following web sites provide useful information on oncology pharmacy and related clinical oncology organizations abroad.

International

ISOPP (International Society for Oncology Pharmacy Practitioners) www.isopp.org

European Union

BOPA (British Oncology Pharmacy Association) www.bopa-web.org
ESOP (European Society of Oncology Pharmacists) www.esop.li
DGOP (Deutsche Gesellschaft für Onkologische Pharmazie) www.dgop.org

United States

HOPA (Hematology Oncology Pharmacy Association) www.hoparx.org
ASCO (American Society of Clinical Oncology) www.asco.org
GOG (The Gynecology Oncology Group) www.gog.org

The National Cancer Institute (National Institutes of Health) www.cancer.gov has web pages aimed at the general public, scientists and oncology health professionals. The NCI web site is also a good source of information on clinical trials currently in progress.

BPS (The Board of Pharmaceutical Specialties) www.bpsweb.org

To practice as an oncology pharmacist in the United States it is necessary to pass a certification examination set by the BPS Specialty Council on Oncology. The examination makes the assessment by testing knowledge and skills in four domains:

Cancer Chemotherapy Rachel Airley
© 2009 John Wiley & Sons, Ltd.

(1) Collaboration with other health professionals in pursuing optimal drug therapy for patients with cancer. This requires that the oncology pharmacist collect and interpret pertinent clinical data, and assume personal responsibility for successful drug therapy outcomes (such as through the recommendation, design, implementation, monitoring and modification of pharmacotherapeutic plans for the patient).

(2) Interpretation, generation and/or dissemination of knowledge in oncology as it applies to oncology pharmacy practice.

(3) In collaboration with other professionals, patients, and the public, recommendation, design, implementation, monitoring, and modification of systems and policies to optimize the use of drugs inpatients with cancer.

(4) Collaborate with other professionals and the public in addressing public health issues (e.g. risk factors, prevention, screening, cancer survivorship) as they relate to oncology pharmacy practice.

Canada

CAPHO (The Canadian Association of Pharmacy in Oncology) www.capho.org

Provides HOPE (helping oncology pharmacists through e-learning) online education packages which are useful for the CPD needs of oncology pharmacists.

CCO (Cancer Care Ontario) www.cancercare.on.ca

Australia

The Australian Regulatory Group www.tga.gov.au

Similar to the Medicines and Healthcare products Regulatory Agency in the United Kingdom, provides data on clinical trials and regulatory affairs, but is not specifically aimed at providers of cancer therapy.

COSA (Clinical Oncology Society of Australia) www.cosa.org.au

COSA has a Pharmacy Group, which is made up pharmacists practising in a variety of oncology settings including medical oncology, haematology, palliative care, and cytotoxic preparation services. The group provides a national multidisciplinary forum for pharmacists working in cancer services and aims to facilitate training, education and research within pharmacy and cancer services whilst ensuring that pharmacists have an input into key national policy documents and clinical guidelines.

24

Practice exam questions

Below are some worked examples of structured essay questions and marking schemes of the type that might appear on undergraduate examinations in core pharmacology or elective cancer chemotherapy modules. For pharmacy undergraduates at least, there is usually an essay question on cancer chemotherapy somewhere in the third or fourth year that everyone tries to avoid, as I did as a pharmacy student. Some general advice, though, is to include references to background reading. This demonstrates interest in a subject that, after all, the lecturer marking your examination paper is passionate about, and likely to be spending long hours researching in the laboratory between setting your exams. Although this might seem daunting with the demanding workload of the pharmaceutical, medical or allied health courses, I have found that if students prioritize reading to the two or three topics that they found the most interesting in lectures, snippets of background knowledge are retained a lot more easily, and just like with certain GCSE English Literature texts, become more interesting once the formal teaching is over! Pay attention to the percentage mark allocation, as it gives a reliable clue as to the amount of time that should be spent on each part of the question, in what depth to write and the extent of detail that should be included. For example, if 5% is awarded for describing an anticancer agent, a very brief description is usually all that is required; whereas if this part of the question has a 70% mark allocation, the response should probably include a precise description along with appropriate diagrams on points such as, depending upon the wording of the question, chemical structure, mode of action, clinical use and toxicology.

Questions

1. (a) Define and describe the cell cycle. (40)

   (b) Indicate where in the cell cycle the anticancer agents methotrexate, cyclophosphamide and vincristine act, and in doing so, describe their mode of action. (30)

   (c) Briefly describe two novel agents in preclinical and/or clinical development. How do these influence progression through the cell cycle? (30)

Cancer Chemotherapy   Rachel Airley
© 2009 John Wiley & Sons, Ltd.

2 (a) Define angiogenesis and describe its role in tumour progression. (40)

  (b) Giving three examples of anti-angiogenic agents, describe how angiogenesis might be targeted by anticancer agents. Your answer may include those that have been recently approved or are currently being developed. (40)

  (c) How might anti-angiogenic agents be used in the clinic? (20)

3 With reference to the research and development of the tyrosine kinase inhibitors, describe the process by which a novel anticancer agent is discovered and approved for clinical use. Include in your answer references to *in vitro* drug screening, *in vivo* tumour models and clinical trials.

4 (a) Describe how cancer chemotherapy is administered and scheduled and explain the role of the different health professionals involved in this process. (60)

  (b) Give two examples of clinically used cancer chemotherapy regimens and the type of cancer they are used to treat. (20)

  (c) With reference to current or recently reported clinical trials, discuss the current and future role of the histone deacetylase inhibitors. (20)

5 (a) Define biomarker and describe how they may contribute to the diagnosis and treatment of cancer? (30)

  (b) Give three examples of tumour biomarkers and explain the biological basis of their expression in tumours. (50)

  (c) How is a tumour biomarker validated clinically? (20)

6 (a) Describe the histology and physiological conditions existing in the tumour microenvironment (40)

  (b) Describe how response to chemotherapy may be adversely affected by the tumour microenvironment (30)

  (c) How are bioreductive drugs used to exploit this feature of tumours? (30)

7 (a) Define the term antitumour antibiotic (10)

  (b) Describe the mode of action of the following:

      1. Adriamycin
      2. Geldanamycin
      3. Trabectedin (60)

  (c) Giving examples of specific cancer types, briefly describe the clinical role of antitumour antibiotics. (30)

8 (a) Describe the role of proteasomal degradation and the mechanism by which it takes place. (60)

  (b) Describe the pharmacodynamics and clinical development of two groups of novel anticancer agents that target proteasomal degradation. (40)

9 (a) Explain the role of tubulins in tumour cell proliferation. (50)

  (b) Describe the chemistry, pharmacology and clinical use of anticancer agents that inhibit the synthesis and/or function of tubulins. (50)

10 (a) Describe the mechanisms by which tumours develop resistance to anticancer agents. (30)

  (b) How might these resistance mechanisms be overcome pharmacologically? (40)

  (c) Explain the terms *primary tumour*, *metastasis*, *local recurrence* and *secondary malignancy*. (30)

Model answers

1 (a) A diagram of the cell cycle should be included here and would constitute a significant proportion of the mark allocation. Quickly setting a diagram to paper will also provide an *aide memoir* and a springboard for your written explanation. A diagram, as in Figure 8.1 is suitable.

A description should include the following:

- G1, S, G2 and M phase: in summary, synthesis of DNA replication machinery (G1), DNA synthesis and replication (S), synthesis of cellular components, for example, ribosomes (G2) and mitosis (M). A common mistake I saw when setting a question like this was confusion between the phases of the cell cycle and the phases of mitosis, that is, interphase, metaphase, anaphase, telophase, and so on. Only two phases are considered by the cell cycle: m-phase, which corresponds to the whole of the mitotic process, and interphase, which is made up of G1, S and G2 phase. Also consider G0 phase, when cells are not cycling (quiescent or in resting phase).

- Checkpoints, which determine transition into successive phases of the cell cycle, including the G1 restriction point, the S replication point, and the G2 and M checkpoints (Table 4.1).

  (b) Mark on the diagram of the cell cycle where the respective anticancer agents act. The correct response is:

- Methotrexate acts at S phase. An antimetabolite, it is an analogue of folic acid and an inhibitor of the enzyme dihydrofolate reductase. This results in inhibition of the synthesis of purine synthesis, a constituent of DNA.

- Cyclophosphamide is an alkylating agent. Their effect on DNA is to disrupt its structure and therefore function, rather than to inhibit its synthesis. The correct response is therefore any phase apart from S-phase, for example, G1 phase.

- Vincristine acts at M-phase. This is an antimitotic agent that binds tubulin subunits.

(c) This is a very open question and the response can include anything from novel anthracyclines to monoclonal antibodies targeting a range of extracellular receptors. It also presents an opportunity to demonstrate background knowledge obtained from the relevant journals. The cell cycle itself is a source of novel targets, described very well in a review paper by Malumbres (see Further reading), such as the cyclin-dependent kinases, mitotic kinases and microtubule motor proteins. Of course, if a drug targets cell cycle progression at a certain point, its activity must be dependent upon the presence of tumour cells that are currently in that precise phase of the cell-cycle. In general, when considering a drug in development, first consider whether the mode of action of the drug depends upon whether cells are cycling (in G1, S, G2 and M phases) or non-cycling (G0, or quiescent). Cells in G0 phase are usually refractory to treatment as they are not actively undergoing the cellular processes targeted by most anticancer agents. Therefore, tumours with a high G0 fraction, or a high proportion of cells in G0 phase, are less responsive to chemotherapy. The activity of anticancer drugs in development specifically aimed at slow growing tumours may show less cell-cycle dependency. Examples of classic anticancer agents in this bracket are the cytotoxics: for example, cisplatin, the nitrogen mustards and the alkylating agents. These may also be used to 'debulk' tumours, a process that reduces the size of the tumour and knocks remaining quiescent cells back into the cell cycle; in doing so increasing their sensitivity to phase-specific anticancer drugs. Novel cytotoxics in development include satraplatin, a platinum based agent; glufosfamide, which is glucose conjugate of the mustard ifosfamide; and the hypoxia-dependent bioreductive alkylating agents such as tirapazamine and AQ4N. Phase-specific drugs target tumour cells in certain phases of the cell-cycle, which is determined by their mode of action. Agents such as the vinca alkaloids and the taxanes target tubulins and therefore mitosis, so are strongly M-phase-specific. Accordingly, novel tubulin inhibitors such as the epothilones and vinflunine will show M-phase-dependent activity, whereas novel antimetabolites such as clofarabine target DNA synthesis and are therefore likely to be S-phase specific. Predicting the cell-cycle specificity of anticancer agents that target specific genes, proteins or signal transduction mechanisms is more difficult. Consider firstly which cells within the tumour are targeted, for example, if it is an angiogenesis inhibitor, determine whether it targets the endothelial cells of tumour vasculature or the production of angiogenic growth factors by tumour cells. If the drug targets the production or activity of certain enzymes or growth factors think about the phase in the cell cycle where this is likely to be most influential. If the drug targets a signal transduction pathway that regulates apoptosis or proliferation, again, it is likely to be most active against highly proliferative cells. Also worth considering is that a lot of anticancer agents themselves modulate the cell cycle, for example, causing cell cycle arrest at various points within the cell cycle; this having a knock-on effect on the use of further phase-dependent drugs. This may have a knock on effect when evaluating novel anticancer agents clinically, as this is often carried out in association with established treatments.

2 (a) Angiogenesis is the process by which new blood vessels are formed. In the case of tumours, vasculature is initially host-derived, but as the tumour mass increases, tumour cells trigger the production of angiogenic growth factors and enzymes that initiate the growth of tumour-derived blood vessels. A diagram to illustrate the interaction between the tumour vasculature, tumour cells and other cells within the tumour matrix or stroma would generate a significant proportion of the 40% mark allocation, as would a diagram to illustrate angiogenesis at the cellular level, showing the function of matrix metalloproteinases, integrins, growth factor receptors and endothelial cell morphology.

(b) A diagram such as Figure 13.4 summarizes the modes of action of the major classes of anti-angiogenic agents currently in development. This question also has a 40% mark allocation which warrants a comprehensive answer and evidence of background reading. Angiogenesis remains a major focus of cancer research, which has culminated in the approval of bevacizumab (Avastin), a monoclonal antibody inhibitor of vascular endothelial growth factor (VEGF); closely followed by sunitinib (Sutent), a mixed tyrosine kinase inhibitor that exerts its anti-angiogenic affect by the receptors VEGFR (1, 2 and 3), platelet-derived growth factor receptor (PDGFR), stem-cell factor receptor and Fms-like tyrosine kinase receptor 3. Angiostatic agents such as endostatin and angiostatin may also be described, as the isolation of these agents were critical for much of the basic research carried out in the initial stages of angiogenesis research to assess the affect of interfering with tumour vasculature and the merit of angiogenesis as a therapeutic target. There have been some disappointments in the development of angiogenesis inhibitors, such as the adverse effects observed in clinical trials of the broad spectrum TIMPs, for example, marimastat; and some surprises, such as the re-emergence of thalidomide (Thalomid) as an inhibitor of VEGF and fibroblast growth factor (FGF) secretion, and its subsequent approval, swiftly followed by its analogue lenalidomide (Revlimid), for the treatment of multiple myeloma. The integrins, in particular $\alpha v \beta 3$, are also targets for anti-angiogenic agents currently undergoing development, such as cilengitide and Vitaxin, both having undergone a range of phase II clinical trials.

(c) Preclinical models of angiogenesis include *in vitro* cell culture methods such as the use of endothelial cell lines, for example, HUVEC, in endothelial cell migration assays using Matrigel basement membrane matrix, a methodology described in Figure 10.13. *In vivo* assays include the hollow fibre assay, the window chamber assay and the corneal micropocket assay. Additionally, imaging of angiogenesis maybe carried out using radiographic means such as PET and MRI, along with tracers designed to detect targets such as VEGF or integrins. Vascularity may also be measured as an end-point in the evaluation of response to anti-angiogenic agents, for example, using technologies such as dynamic MRI and Doppler ultrasonography, which enable analysis of blood flow.

3 To select this type of 'long answer' essay question, one should be either very confident or very interested in drug development and/or tyrosine kinase inhibitors, as the mark allocation is entirely open-ended. These types of questions do appear though, and it is tempting to try and waffle through them. To avoid this, the best way to tackle them is to spend five minutes or so constructing an essay plan. This will help divide the essay into stages where the question fails to do so; and will help focus the response so that it includes all the relevant information but in a logical sequence. A sample essay plan might be written as in Figure 24.1.

4 (a) The 60% mark allocation for this part of the question may be roughly divided into two parts. Firstly, define the different stages of chemotherapy, that is, induction, consolidation/intensification, and neoadjuvant/adjuvant che-motherapy. Also define the role of maintenance and salvage chemotherapy, which may also be given in some types of cancers under certain conditions. The aims and objectives of each stage of chemotherapy should be stated in terms of clinical response, expressed in terms of complete or partial response, stable disease or progression. There should be a reference to chemotherapy scheduling, where chemotherapy may be pulsed or administered in cycles. There should also be an appreciation of the fact that chemotherapy is often given in combination, where the relative scheduling of two or more drugs is precisely determined to achieve the best chemoresponse, which takes into account factors such as drug resistance and synergy. The second part of (a) should be a description of the health professionals involved in the diagnosis and treatment of cancer. These should include the various medical specialities, such as medical oncologists, surgical oncologists, radiologists, radiotherapists and also the medical specialities asso-ciated with the cancer site, for example, patients with head and neck cancers are under the care of maxillofacial surgeons.

(b) There are many chemotherapy regimens to choose from and some are used more frequently and have been used for many more years than others. Each che-motherapy regimen has been evaluated in a clinical trial and sometimes a new indication will be approved as a result of a clinical trial involving patients with a different type of cancer. Some examples of classic chemotherapy regimens are described in Table 8.1, such as CAP (cyclophosphamide, doxorubicin and cisplatin) for head and neck cancer; CMF (cyclophosphamide, methotrexate and 5-fluorouracil) for breast cancer and CHOP (cyclophosphamide, mitoxan-trone, vincristine and prednisolone) for non-Hodgkin's lymphoma. Providing

a) Research and development

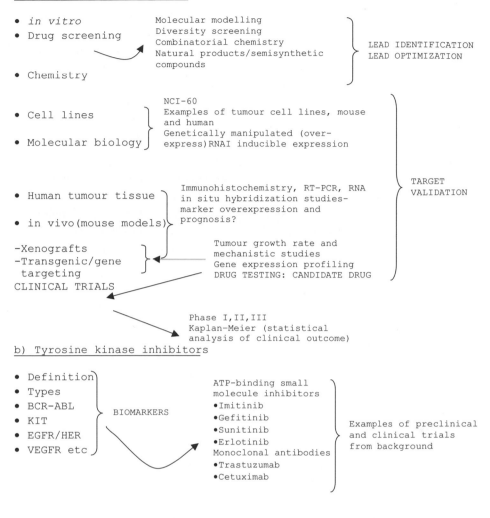

- *in vitro*
- Drug screening

Molecular modelling
Diversity screening
Combinatorial chemistry
Natural products/semisynthetic
compounds

LEAD IDENTIFICATION
LEAD OPTIMIZATION

- Chemistry

- Cell lines
- Molecular biology

NCI-60
Examples of tumour cell lines, mouse
and human
Genetically manipulated (overexpress)RNAI inducible expression

TARGET
VALIDATION

- Human tumour tissue
- in vivo(mouse models)

Immunohistochemistry, RT-PCR, RNA
in situ hybridization studies-
marker overexpression and
prognosis?

-Xenografts
-Transgenic/gene
 targeting
CLINICAL TRIALS

Tumour growth rate and
mechanistic studies
Gene expression profiling
DRUG TESTING: CANDIDATE DRUG

Phase I,II,III
Kaplan-Meier (statistical
analysis of clinical outcome)

b) Tyrosine kinase inhibitors

- Definition
- Types
- BCR-ABL
- KIT
- EGFR/HER
- VEGFR etc

BIOMARKERS

ATP-binding small
molecule inhibitors
- Imitinib
- Gefitinib
- Sunitinib
- Erlotinib
Monoclonal antibodies
- Trastuzumab
- Cetuximab

Examples of preclinical
and clinical trials
from background

- Diagram - receptor showing subunits with pharmacological
  intervention

Figure 24.1 Sample essay plan suitable for a 'long answer' essay like Question 3.

additional detail, such as dosage and route of administration may get additional credit in this type of question.

(c) This part of the question is designed to test if knowledge of the clinical role of established chemotherapy regimens may be applied to the projected use of a novel anti-cancer agent that may have been approved recently and/or is still in clinical trial for certain other cancer types. HDAC inhibitors are a good example, as although one, vorinostat, is currently approved for skin manifestations of T-cell lymphoma, there are others in various stages of clinical trial for a range of cancer types, including vorinostat itself, for solid tumours; depsipeptide, for paediatric cancers; and benzamide, for haematological malignancies, non-small cell lung carcinoma and melanoma. When a new anticancer agent is developed and evaluated in a clinical trial, it is usually given in combination with standard treatments so that a new chemotherapy regimen is evaluated and may be adopted into clinical practice. These may be picked up by background reading of the literature and are sometimes announced in mainstream clinical publications such as the *British Medical Journal*, *The Lancet* and *The Pharmaceutical Journal*.

5 (a) A biomarker is a biological characteristic that may provide diagnostic information on malignancy, tumour aggressiveness, treatment sensitivity and prognosis (likelihood of metastasis, local recurrence and disease-free survival). Inclusion of a diagram such as Figure 7.2 would explain how the detection of biomarkers at diagnosis or following treatment, by analysis of either biopsy or surgically resected material, may be used to select the best treatment for a patient.

   (b) Table 7.1 shows examples of biomarkers that may be detected by analysis of tissue material or in some cases serum proteins and metabolites. For the 50% mark allocation stated here, diagrams illustrating the appropriate molecular pathways should be included. For example, for the use of cyclins as a prognostic indicator, a diagram of the cell cycle which illustrates the role of cyclins in progression through the checkpoints may be used (Figure 8.1). The oncogenes *Ras*, a GTPase involved in signal transduction, and bcl-2, an anti-apoptotic protein, have a role in cellular proliferation and suppression of apoptosis. An example of a diagram that may be used to illustrate the role of Ras is Figure 15.1, which illustrates how the Ras protein complex, upon activation of tyrosine kinase receptors, induces transcription factors via activation of the proteins PI3K, MEKK and MEK. The role of bcl-2 in the suppression of apoptosis is shown in Figure 2.3. Although covered elsewhere, diagnostic imaging methods such as MRI and PET might also yield data on biomarker expression, for example, FDG-PET can be used to assess the volume, metabolic status and chemoresponse of a tumour before and after treatment. Specific tracers may also be used to identify suitable candidates for treatment with novel anticancer agents, for example, RGD (Arg-Gly-Asp) peptide-based probes for the imaging of integrin-positive tumours and monoclonal antibodies to tyrosine kinase receptors such as VEGFR may be used to rationally select patients for treatment with the respective anti-angiogenic agents.

   (c) A tumour biomarker will be validated clinically by carrying out studies in human subjects, where biomarker expression is found to be statistically linked with malignancy and/or prognosis. These studies may be retrospective, where archival material collected from routine biopsy specimens of patients that were treated over a certain time period are analysed. Studies should also be carried out prospectively, where patients are especially recruited to a study with a view to analysing their tumour material for biomarker expression. If the results of these studies are statistically sound, as determined, for example, by Kaplan–Meier analysis, a biomarker may be used to rationally select patients for more aggressive cancer treatment, or to receive a novel treatment that targets that particular biomarker. To validate a biomarker for this purpose, a phase III clinical trial may be carried out to compare the outcome of patients treated according to or independently of biomarker expression. For completeness, this response should also include an appreciation of the factors that make a biomarker suitable for use in the clinic, that is, it should be non-invasive, non-toxic, not compromise treatment and so on. There are also numerous biomarker validation studies available in the literature, which may be revealed by a PUBMED or MEDLINE search with the keywords 'prognosis' and 'cancer'. Familiarity with a couple of these studies could be advantageous.

6 (a) Malignant and non-malignant tissues have specific histological differences, which may be illustrated by a diagram such as Figure 2.1. These include changes in cell differentiation and specialization, leading to distinct differences in cell morphology. In tumour tissue, there is also an absence of a basement membrane and organized cell to cell communication. In this question, histological characteristics are distinct from physiological characteristics, which refer to the conditions existing within the tissue, such as oxygenation, pH and nutrient levels. These physiological conditions are dependent upon factors such as tumour volume, the rate of cellular proliferation and cell death, and blood supply. These can all influence gene expression in the tumour tissue, determining tumour aggressiveness, for example, likelihood of metastasis and treatment sensitivity. To illustrate the physiological tumour microenvironment, a diagram such as Figures 12.1 and 12.3 or elements of Figure 12.2 may be used, which show the existence of tumour 'nests' within extracellular matrix, or stroma, consisting of cells such as fibroblasts and often carrying tumour-derived capillaries. The text and diagrams should demonstrate how oxygen gradients are formed, and how these lead to hypoxia, necrosis, decreased pH, increased glucose metabolism and areas of high vascular density within tumour tissue. The adverse architecture of this tumour-derived blood supply, that is, the lack of organization and poor vasomotor control should also be shown.

(b) There are three major mechanisms by which the tumour microenvironment may adversely affect chemoresponse, and for a 30% mark allocation roughly 10% may be devoted to each. First, the poorly vascularized, hypoxic tumour presents a physical barrier to chemotherapy, where the lack of an efficient blood supply hinders distribution of anticancer agents throughout the tumour tissue and therefore exposure of tumour cells to their toxic effects. For this reason, small molecule agents that are able to diffuse freely through tumour cells may be favoured. Second, hypoxia induces several molecular changes which decrease sensitivity to many classic anticancer agents. These include cell cycle changes, where hypoxic cells tend to be in G0 phase, rendering them resistant to cell cycle-phase-specific drugs. In addition, hypoxia also induces changes in gene expression that decrease chemosensitivity by increasing the expression of resistance proteins such as the multi-drug resistance efflux transporters; decreasing the level of target proteins, for example, topoisomerases; and by increasing the level of anti-apoptotic proteins, problematic as anticancer agents often cause tumour cell death by apoptosis. Finally, many anticancer agents depend upon the presence of oxygen for their chemical activation, for example, bleomycin.

(c) Bioreductive drugs are prodrugs activated by tumour-specific enzymes, that is, enzymes that are expressed at high levels in tumours relative to normal tissue. Hypoxia-selective bioreductive drugs are also activated by tumour-specific enzymes but are designed to be activated in hypoxic conditions whilst remaining inactive in normoxic tissue; therefore achieving tumour specificity by exploiting hypoxia as a physiological feature that is rarely found in non-malignant tissue. A suitable diagram to illustrate this is Figure 12.5, which shows the activation of the hypoxia-selective bioreductive drugs tirapazamine and AQ4N. Whilst accurate representation of the chemical structures in an examination deserves credit, it would be more important in this case to demonstrate an understanding of the bioreduction process, which involves electron transfer and the generation of intermediate products; and ultimately the active cytotoxic compound. The pharmacological effects of the activated prodrugs should be described, where the active tirapazamine radical acts as a DNA strand breaking agent and the active intermediate of AQ4N, AQ4, inhibits topoisomerase I. The mode of enzymatic activation should also be described in terms of the level of tumour-specific expression of these enzymes. Also relevant is the fact that these prodrugs are small molecules, enabling distribution throughout the hypoxic areas of a tumour. Their place in the clinic in combination with classical anticancer agents more effective in normoxic tissue may be demonstrated by referring to the regimens used in clinical trials involving hypoxia-selective bioreductive agents, for example, where tirapazamine is used in combination with cisplatin to exert a synergistic action.

7 (a) An antitumour antibiotic usually refers to an anticancer drug that is either produced by a micro-organism or is a semi-synthetic derivative. These are classically intercalating agents; however more recently discovered antitumour antibiotics may work by alternative means.

(b) (i) Adriamycin, along with similar compounds such as daunorubicin and epirubicin, is an anthracycline anticancer agent that has several modes of action:
- *Intercalating agents*. This group of drugs slot between adjacent pairs of DNA bases and disrupt the double helix structure. Their planar, aromatic structure, and how this facilitates intercalation between the DNA bases,

should be discussed. Intercalation lengthens the double helix, interfering with DNA replication and transcription via inhibition of DNA polymerase and DNA-dependent RNA polymerase. Figure 8.14, which shows the action of intercalating agents, would be a suitable diagram to illustrate this effect.

- *Free radical production.* Anthracyclines also exert their action by producing cytotoxic free radicals which alkylate DNA. Anthracyclines are actually bioreductive quinones that are reduced intracellularly by reductase enzymes such as cytochrome P450 reductase and xanthine oxidase to produce a semi-quinone radical which is oxidized to reactive intermediates that causes strand scission. This may be illustrated by using a diagram such as Figure 8.15.

- *Topoisomerase II inhibitors.* Anthracyclines inhibit the enzyme topoisomerase II, which in normal conditions cleaves DNA so that it can be reoriented and then resealed about the replication fork, facilitating replication. Inhibition of topoisomerase II stabilizes a DNA–enzyme intermediate preventing resealing.

- *Cross-linking agents.* A further mode of action of the anthracyclines is the formation of anthracycline-DNA adducts, which leads to cross-linking of DNA strands. The mechanism by which this occurs is suitably represented by Figure 8.16.

If presented with a question like this, it might be worthwhile allocating more exam time (and more marks) to this part of the question as the pharmacology of anthracyclines is so complex.

(ii) Geldanamycin is a novel antitumour antibiotic currently in preclinical and clinical development that acts as an inhibitor of HSP90. HSP90 is a stress protein produced in response to heat, nutrient deprivation and oxidative stress, but its importance as a drug target relates to its role as a molecular chaperone to client proteins involved in signal transduction in tumour proliferative and regulatory processes, such as the oncogenes Src and HER2; the signal transduction kinase MEK; the transcription factor HIF-1; and cyclin-dependent kinases. Binding of these client proteins by HSP90 maintains the protein in its folded state, mediates repair or degradation of partially denatured protein and initiates refolding of misfolded proteins – thus preventing denaturation of the protein in stress conditions. Inhibition of HSP90 will prevent this process, leading to defective client protein functionality and increased treatment sensitivity. A suitable diagram to explain this would be Figure 17.1, which shows the structure of HSP90 and how it binds client proteins. For completeness, it might also be useful in a question like this to include a diagram summarizing the role of an example client protein, such as in Figure 15.1, which shows the role of MEK, and Figure 14.1, which shows the role of Src in tumour biology. There are some good diagrams or images of the HSP90–geldanamycin complex available in the literature, such as those shown in the Stebbins paper (Stebbins *et al.*, 1997), which comprehensively described the crystal structure of the complex. Simplified versions of these may be included as relevant diagrams in this part of the question.

(iii) Trabectedin is a tetrahydro-isoquinoline alkaloid with three subunits, where subunits A and B recognize and bind DNA and subunit C remains unbound, protruding from the minor groove. Trabectedin binding disrupts the DNA helix, bending it towards the major groove and widening the minor groove, where its structure and mode of action may be illustrated using a simplified version of Figure 8.26.

(c) There are several standard drug regimens as well as novel combinations in clinical trial that include the antitumour antibiotics. These may be discussed in a similar fashion to Question 4c. It is worth reading the relevant chapter of the British National Formulary (Cytotoxic antibiotics), as there is an informative introduction at the start on the clinical uses of currently used drugs that may be useful for a question such as this one that asks about specific cancer types. Regarding accurate drawing of chemical structures, the antitumour antibiotics, being originally derived from natural products, are notoriously complicated and therefore difficult to memorize. Part (b) of the question carries 60% of the marks distributed over three parts, therefore prioritize this mark allocation to showing a diagram of the pharmacology. For instance, showing the position of DNA cross-links for the anthracyclines, or groove binding by distamycin – accompanied by explanatory text – may prove to be preferable to using up all the time allocation trying to perfectly reproduce these complex molecules.

8 (a) A description of the mechanism by which proteasomal degradation takes place may be in two parts, discussing firstly the ubiquitylation step, where the substrate is conjugated with the protein ubiquitin via covalent bonds linking the C-terminus of ubiquitin to a free amino acid group on the target protein. This process is catalysed by the ubiquitin ligase family of enzymes, E1, E2 and E3. After conjugation with the substrate, elongation of the ubiquitin is catalysed by the ubiquitin ligase E4, producing the polyubiquitylated substrate. The second step is the recognition of the ubiquitylated substrate by the proteasome itself, a process made possible by the substrate specificity of the E3 enzyme. The regulatory 19S subunit processes the substrate, mediating deubiquitylation, unfolding and eventually the translocation of the substrate to the proteolytic core contained in the 20S catalytic subunit. Refer to examples of proteasomal substrates, the ones described in Table 18.1 are the cyclin-dependent kinases and the cyclins A, B, D and E; the oncogenes bcl2, myc and fos/jun; the tumour suppressor p53; the pro-apoptotic protein bax; and the inhibitory protein IκB, which inhibits the action of the transcription factor NFκB, a transcriptional mediator of tumour survival and the activation of several growth factors. There are several diagrams suitable for inclusion in this question which may

accumulate about a half of the 60% mark allocation. A useful diagram to introduce the topic would be an illustration of the 26S proteasome complex as in Figure 18.2, showing the two subunits – the 20S subunit, containing the catalytic core; and the 19S subunit, the regulatory component that processes the substrate prior to proteolysis. The initial ubiquitylation step may be illustrated using Figure 18.1, which shows the generalized process. For the purpose of showing substrate specific ubiquitylation, Figure 18.4 represents the ubiquitylation step of the transcription factor subunit HIF-1α, where substrate specificity is determined by the von Hippel–Lindau (VHL) E3 ligase complex.

(b) The mechanism of proteasomal degradation, as discussed in part (a), consists of two processes: ubiquitylation and proteasomal degradation. Each offer new drug targets and have stimulated the development of novel anticancer agents. This is an example of how an examination question should be read very carefully – if the question asked for a description of anticancer agents that inhibited the *proteasome*, inhibitors of ubiquitylation may be irrelevant. However, this question asked for inhibitors of *proteasomal degradation*, so it could be argued that inhibitors of the ubiquitylation process and the regulatory and catalytic activity of the proteasome itself are both relevant for discussion here. Therefore, the 40% mark allocation may be divided between the development of proteasome inhibitors such as the boronic acid peptide PS-341, or bortezomib, and the development of ubiquitin ligase inhibitors, such as the Nutlins, which inhibit the interaction between p53 and Mdm2. Where possible, cite examples of preclinical and clinical studies. Bortezomib (Velcade), approved for the treatment of multiple myeloma in May 2003, underwent phase II trials – for example, SUMMIT, and CREST, which evaluated the use of bortezomib in patients with relapsed and refractory myeloma; and the large scale international phase III trial APEX (Assessment of Proteasome Inhibition for Extending Remission). This was followed by the initiation of further phase II and III trials in other haematological malignancies and a range of solid tumours. At the time of writing, the Nutlins are not yet in clinical trial; however, as with all the novel agents discussed in this book, background reading of the current journals may reveal changes in status as they happen. Further examples of E3 ligase inhibitors that may be described here are small molecule inhibitors such as the chalcone derivatives, for example, chlorofusin, as well as the isoindolinone-based inhibitors (Figure 18.6).

9 (a) Tubulins are constituents of the mitotic spindle formed during metaphase of mitosis, where mitosis is the process by which nuclear material is replicated and transferred to two daughter cells during cell proliferation. The mitotic process should be summarized, including a diagram such as Figure 8.33 to show clearly the gross structure of a mitotic spindle. The fine structure of the mitotic spindle may be illustrated using a diagram such as Figure 8.34, accompanied by text describing the microtubule polymerization process. This is initiated by the

formation of α and β tubulin heterodimers (8 nm) that form a microtubule nucleus. The nucleus is then elongated at each end to form a cylinder 24 nm in diameter, consisting of 13 protofilaments, which appear as parallel arrangements of tubulin heterodimers laid end to end, where the (+) end is made up of β-tubulin units, and the (−) end α-tubulin units. The role of microtubule dynamics should also be explained, perhaps by using an adaptation of Figure 8.35, where the stability of a microtubule is determined by the rate of polymerization versus depolymerization of tubulin heterodimers. Microtubule stability impacts on the functionality of microtubules in the mitotic spindle, which depends upon the changes in length taking place during chromosomal segregation.

(b) It is useful here to summarize the pharmacology of tubulin inhibitors by marking on a diagram of tubulin formation the site of binding and inhibition by each class of agent, as in Figure 8.37. The tubulin inhibitors are typically complex molecules derived from plants. These include the vinca alkaloids and the more recently developed taxanes. There are also more novel agents in development, such as the epothilones and vinflunine, a semisynthetic vinca alkaloid. The tubulin inhibitors typically target microtubule dynamics by interfering with the equilibrium that exists between the polymerization and depolymerization of tubulins that affords the changes in length necessary for microtubule function. The vinca alkaloids bind tubulin dimers at the (+) end of the microtubule, whereas the taxanes bind the microtubule on the interior surface of the cylindrical structure. As in the antitumour antibiotics, these compounds are derived from natural products so can be chemically complex. If the chemistry is specifically asked for in the question, as it is here, attempt to represent an example of a tubulin inhibitor, obviously the taxanes are the most difficult to remember! However, there are other points about the chemistry, such as their natural or semi-synthetic origin, which should be worth some marks. The clinical uses of vinca alkaloids are well established in the treatment of haematological malignancies, for example, PVD (prednisolone/vincristine/asparaginase), for the treatment of paediatric acute lymphoblastic leukaemia; and the taxanes are used in breast, lung and ovarian cancers, for example, CT (cisplatin/Taxol), for the treatment of epithelial tumours of the ovary. Clinical trials are usually in progress to evaluate the use of these agents either in combination with novel anticancer agents or to investigate the effect of changes in scheduling, their efficacy in other cancer types, or the effect of substituting two similar drugs, for example, the ERASME 3 study (Radaideh and Sledge, 2007), a phase III trial comparing doxorubicin and docetaxel versus doxorubicin and paclitaxel in metastatic breast cancer. Clinical trials taking place to evaluate the novel tubulin inhibitors may also be cited, for example, the phase II trial evaluating the novel taxane milataxel and the phase III trial carried out by Thomas *et al.* (2007) comparing ixabepilone (an epothilone) plus capecitabine versus capecitabine alone in anthracycline and taxane-resistant metastatic breast cancer.

10 (a) Resistance to chemotherapy may develop through the mechanisms discussed in Section 22.4:

- *Multiple drug resistance.* The expression of multi-drug resistance efflux transporters, such as p-glycoprotein, MRP (multi-drug resistance associated protein), BCRP (breast cancer resistance protein) and LRP (lung cancer resistance protein) after prolonged exposure to anticancer agents leads to the cell actively pumping the drug out of the cell and therefore reduces intracellular accumulation to sub-clinical levels.

- *Enhanced DNA repair.* DNA repair enzymes such as O6-alkylguanine-DNA alkyltransferase (AGT) mediate direct repair of DNA-cross links caused by anticancer agents such as the platinum-based compounds. DNA glycosylase and Poly (ADP-ribose) polymerase-1 (PARP-1) catalyse steps in base excision repair, where damaged bases are removed from the DNA double helix and repaired. Figure 22.4a may be used to illustrate the O6 alkylated guanine bases that are substrates for AGT.

- *Alteration of drug targets.* Downregulation of target receptor or enzyme, for example, methotrexate resistance caused by reduced expression of the enzyme dihydrofolate reductase (DHFR).

Chemoresistance may also be an effect of hypoxia (Chapter 12), where poor oxygenation is linked with a high G0 fraction (cells in G0 are not cycling and therefore refractory to cell-cycle specific anticancer agents); show disorganized vasculature, which adversely effects the distribution of larger drug molecules throughout the tumour; and inhibits the activation of several drugs, for example, bleomycin and methotrexate. Hypoxia also induces the expression of certain resistance genes, such as MRP, and downregulates pro-apoptotic proteins such as Bax, where anticancer agents may exert their effect by causing apoptosis of tumour cells.

(b) Strategies to overcome chemoresistance include the following:
- p-glycoprotein inhibitors – verapamil and the ciclosporins were evaluated in combination with chemotherapy in phase II trials but there was no significant improvement in clinical response.

- Novel inhibitors of the p-glycoprotein, for example, VX-710 (Biricodar) and PSC-833 (Valspodar) (Figure 22.3) are currently in clinical trial. Inhibition of p-glycoprotein will increase the intracellular accumulation of anticancer drugs vulnerable to the effects of multi-drug resistance, for example, daunorubicin, the taxanes and the vinca alkaloids. They may also prove useful if high levels of multi-drug resistance genes or proteins are detected in the tumours of individual patients at biopsy or after surgery.

- Novel inhibitors of DNA repair enzymes, for example, O6-benzylguanine (O6-BG), an analogue of O6-alkyl guanine that inhibits AGT (this may be illustrated using a diagram such as Figure 22.4b).

- Several PARP inhibitors have been in preclinical and clinical development, for example, AG014699 and AG14361, in phase II trials with temozolomide for malignant melanoma, where the chemical structure is shown in Figure 22.5.

(c) A primary tumour is at the site where the tumour first arose. For instance, a primary bone tumour first arose in the bone, for example, osteosarcoma. This is distinct from a bone metastasis that may be the result of disseminated cells reaching the bone via the circulatory systems from a primary tumour elsewhere, for example, a breast carcinoma. A metastasis is sometimes referred to as a distant recurrence, and likely sites are the lymph nodes, the brain and the liver as well as in bone. A local recurrence, however, is a regrowth of the tumour at the primary site. Both these types of recurrence may be detected by imaging techniques such as MRI and PET, either at the original diagnosis, or after treatment to observe clinical outcome. The detection of metastasis or local recurrence after treatment may lead to a diagnosis of disease progression. A secondary malignancy should not be confused with a metastasis. In fact, this is a cancer that might arise as a result of treating a tumour with anticancer agents that are themselves carcinogenic, for example, alkylating agents, etoposide and doxorubicin, and are therefore a long term risk of cancer chemotherapy. A good example of a secondary malignancy is therapy-related leukaemia (TRL), most commonly t-AML, an acute myeloid leukaemia that has occurred in patients previously treated for non-Hodgkin's lymphoma, soft tissue sarcomas, brain, small cell lung and ovarian tumours. Owing to the improved survival rates of children with cancer, especially with acute lymphoblastic leukaemia (ALL), secondary malignancies have also become an issue in childhood cancers, hence the need for long term follow up.

25
Bibliography and further reading

Epidemiology

Armstrong, B.K., Kricker, A.and English, D.R. (1997) Sun exposure and skin cancer. *Australasian Journal of Dermatology*, **38** (Suppl. 1), S1–S6.

Su, S.J., Yeh, T.M., Lei, H.Y. and Chow, N.H. (2000) The potential of soybean foods as a chemoprevention approach for human urinary tract cancer. *Clinical Cancer Research*, **6** (1), 230–236.

Clinical oncology

Akhtar, S. (2002) Pharmacogenomics: are pharmacists ready for genotyped prescribing? *Pharmaceutical Journal*, **268**, 296–299.

American Pharmaceutical Association (1999–2000) *Drug Information Handbook for Oncology* (eds D.A. Solimando, L.R. Bressler, P.E. Kintzel and M.C. Geraci), Lexi-Comp Inc., Ohio, USA.

Anon (2003) How genetics could change pharmacy (news item). *Pharmaceutical Journal*, **270**, 508–509.

Govindan, R. (2002) *Washington Manual of Oncology*, 1st edn, Lippincott Williams & Wilkins, NY, USA.

Johnson, M. and Henke Yarbro, C. (1981) Principles of oncology nursing, in *Cancer Medicine*, 6th edn (eds R.C. Bast, D.W. Kufe, R.E. Pollock, R.R. Weichselbaum, J.F. Holland, E.F. Freiand T.S. Gansler), BC Decker Inc., Ontario, Canada.

Lee, W., Lockhart, A.C., Kim, R.B. and Rothenberg, M.L. (2005) Cancer pharmacogenomics: powerful tools in cancer chemotherapy and drug development. *Oncologist*, **10**, 104–111.

Molecular biology of cancer

Bertram, J.S. (2000) The molecular biology of cancer. *Molecular Aspects of Medicine*, **21**, 167–223.

Bos, J.L. (1989) Ras oncogenes in human cancer: a review. *Cancer Research*, **49**, 4682–4689.

Cancer Chemotherapy   Rachel Airley
© 2009 John Wiley & Sons, Ltd.

Bryan, J.T. (2007) Developing an HPV vaccine to prevent cervical cancer and genital warts. *Vaccine*, **25**, 3001–3006.

Butel, J.S. (2000) Viral carcinogenesis: revelation of molecular mechanisms and etiology of human disease. *Carcinogenesis*, **21**, 405–426.

Callahan, R. and Smith, G.H. (2000) MMTV-induced mammary tumorigenesis: gene discovery, progression to malignancy and cellular pathways. *Oncogene*, **19**, 992–1001.

Chowdhury, I., Tharakan, B. and Bhat, G.K. (2006) Current concepts in apoptosis: the physiological suicide program revisited. *Cellular & Molecular Biology Letters*, **11**, 506–525.

Coates, P.J. (2007) p53 and Mdm2: not all cells are equal. *Journal of Pathology*, **213**, 357–359.

Corcoran, C.A., Huang, Y. and Sheikh, M.S. (2004) The p53 paddy wagon: COP1, Pirh2 and MDM2 are found resisting apoptosis and growth arrest. *Cancer Biology & Therapy*, **3**, 721–725.

Damia, G. and Broggini, M. (2004) Improving the selectivity of cancer treatments by interfering with cell response pathways. *European Journal of Cancer*, **40**, 2550–2559.

Degterev, A., Huang, Z., Boyce, M. *et al.* (2005) Chemical inhibitor of nonapoptotic cell death with therapeutic potential for ischemic brain injury. *Nature Chemical Biology*, **1**, 112–119.

Degterev, A., Hitomi, J., Germscheid, M. *et al.* (2008) Identification of RIP1 kinase as a specific cellular target of necrostatins. *Nature Chemical Biology*, **4**, 313–321.

Drake, J.W. and Baltz, R.H. (1976) The biochemistry of mutagenesis. *Annual Review of Biochemistry*, **45**, 11–37.

Fink, S.L. and Cookson, B.T. (2005) Apoptosis, pyroptosis, and necrosis: mechanistic description of dead and dying eukaryotic cells. *Infection and Immunity*, **73**, 1907–1916.

Gallagher, S.J., Kefford, R.F. and Rizos, H. (2006) The ARF tumour suppressor. *International Journal of Biochemistry & Cell Biology*, **38**, 1637–1641.

Gasparini, P., Sozzi, G. and Pierotti, M.A. (2007) The role of chromosomal alterations in human cancer development. *Journal of Cellular Biochemistry*, **102**, 320–331.

Golstein, P. and Kroemer, G. (2007) A multiplicity of cell death pathways. Symposium on apoptotic and non-apoptotic cell death pathways. *EMBO Reports*, **8**, 829–833.

Guilford, P. (2000) The inherited susceptibility to cancer. *Cellular and Molecular Life Sciences*, **57**, 589–603.

Hecht, J.L. and Aster, J.C. (2000) Molecular biology of Burkitt's lymphoma. *Journal of Clinical Oncology*, **18**, 3707–3721.

Hodgson, S. (2008) Mechanisms of inherited cancer susceptibility. *Journal of Zhejiang University. Science B*, **9**, 1–4.

Hoppe-Seyler, F. and Butz, K. (1995) Molecular mechanisms of virus-induced carcinogenesis: the interaction of viral factors with cellular tumor suppressor proteins. *Journal of Molecular Medicine (Berlin, Germany)*, **73**, 529–538.

Houston, A. and O'Connell, J. (2004) The Fas signalling pathway and its role in the pathogenesis of cancer. *Current Opinion in Pharmacology*, **4**, 321–326.

Hu, X., Han, W. and Li, L. (2007) Targeting the weak point of cancer by induction of necroptosis. *Autophagy*, **3**, 490–492.

Hu, X. and Xuan, Y. (2008) Bypassing cancer drug resistance by activating multiple death pathways – a proposal from the study of circumventing cancer drug resistance by induction of necroptosis. *Cancer Letters*, **259**, 127–137.

Joerger, A.C. and Fersht, A.R. (2007) Structural Biology of the tumor suppressor p53 and cancer-associated mutants. *Advances in Cancer Research*, **97**, 1–23.

Kaelin, W.G. Jr. (1999) The p53 gene family. *Oncogene*, **18**, 7701–7705.

Kaelin, W.G. Jr. (2004) The von Hippel–Lindau tumor suppressor gene and kidney cancer. *Clinical Cancer Research*, **10**, 6290S–6295S.

Kim, W.Y. and Kaelin, W.G. (2004) Role of VHL gene mutation in human cancer. *Journal of Clinical Oncology*, **22**, 4991–5004.

Kim, Y.S., Morgan, M.J., Choksi, S. and Liu, Z.G. (2007) TNF-induced activation of the Nox1 NADPH oxidase and its role in the induction of necrotic cell death. *Molecular Cell*, **26**, 675–687.

King, R.J. (2000) *Cancer Biology*, 2nd edn, Prentice Hall, New Jersey, USA.

Kumar, V., Abbas, A.K. and Fausto, N. (eds) (2005) *Robbins and Coltran Pathologic Basis of Disease*, 7th edn, Elsevier Saunders, London.

Maeda, T., Hobbs, R.M., Merghoub, T. *et al.* (2005) Role of the proto-oncogene Pokemon in cellular transformation and ARF repression. *Nature*, **433**, 278–285.

Maeda, T., Hobbs, R.M. and Pandolfi, P.P. (2005) The transcription factor Pokemon: a new key player in cancer pathogenesis. *Cancer Research*, **65**, 8575–8578.

Makin, G. and Hickman, J.A. (2000) Apoptosis and cancer chemotherapy. *Cell and Tissue Research*, **301**, 143–152.

Malumbres, M. (2006) Therapeutic opportunities to control tumor cell cycles. *Clinical and Translational Oncology*, **8**, 399–408.

McIntosh, J., Sturpe, D.A. and Khanna, N. (2008) Human papillomavirus vaccine and cervical cancer prevention: practice and policy implications for pharmacists. *Journal of the American Pharmaceutical Association*, **48**, e1–e13.

McLaughlin-Drubin, M.E. and Munger, K. (2008) Viruses associated with human cancer. *Biochimica et Biophysica Acta*, **1782**, 127–150.

Meek, D.W. (2004) The p53 response to DNA damage. *DNA Repair*, **3**, 1049–1056.

Mignotte, B. and Vayssiere, J.L. (1998) Mitochondria and apoptosis. *European Journal of Biochemistry*, **252**, 1–15.

Parthasarathy, R. and Fridey, S.M. (1986) Conformation of O6-alkylguanosines: molecular mechanism of mutagenesis. *Carcinogenesis*, **7**, 221–227.

Pecorino, L. (2005) *Molecular Biology of Cancer: Mechanisms, Targets and Therapeutics*, Oxford University Press, Oxford, UK.

Pulciani, S., Santos, E., Long, L.K. *et al.* (1985) Ras gene amplification and malignant transformation. *Molecular and Cellular Biology*, **5**, 2836–2841.

Shah, M.A. and Schwartz, G.K. (2001) Cell cycle-mediated drug resistance: an emerging concept in cancer therapy. *Clinical Cancer Research*, **7**, 2168–2181.

Schuler, M. and Green, D.R. (2001) Mechanisms of p53-dependent apoptosis. *Biochemical Society Transactions*, **29**, 684–688.

Schwartz, G.K. and Shah, M.A. (2005) Targeting the cell cycle: a new approach to cancer therapy. *Journal of Clinical Oncology*, **23**, 9408–9421.

Silvius, J.R. (2002) Mechanisms of Ras protein targeting in mammalian cells. *Journal of Membrane Biology*, **190**, 83–92.

Sperandio, S., de Belle, I. and Bredesen, D.E. (2000) An alternative, nonapoptotic form of programmed cell death. *Proceedings of the National Academy of Sciences of the United States of America*, **97**, 14376–14381.

Tannock, I.F., Hill, R.P., Bristow, R.G. and Harrington, L. (eds) (2005) *The Basic Science of Oncology*, 4th edn, McGraw Hill, New York, USA.

Van Cruchten, S. and Van Den Broeck, W. (2002) Morphological and biochemical aspects of apoptosis, oncosis and necrosis. *Anatomia, Histologia, Embryologia*, **31**, 214–223.

Vogt, P.K. (1993) Cancer genes. *Western Journal of Medicine*, **158**, 273–278.

Vose, C.W., Coombs, M.M. and Bhatt, T.S. (1981) Co-carcinogenicity of promoting agents. *Carcinogenesis*, **2**, 687–689.

Wogan, G.N., Hecht, S.S., Felton, J.S. *et al.* (2004) Environmental and chemical carcinogenesis. *Seminars in Cancer Biology*, **14**, 473–486.

Zimmermann, K.C., Bonzon, C. and Green, D.R. (2001) The machinery of programmed cell death. *Pharmacology & Therapeutics*, **92**, 57–70.

Biomarkers

Bendardaf, R., Lamlum, H. and Pyrhönen, S. (2004) Prognostic and predictive molecular markers in colorectal carcinoma. *Anticancer Research*, **24**, 2519–2530.

Conley, B.A. and Taube, S.E. (2004) Prognostic and predictive markers in cancer. *Disease Markers*, **20**, 35–43.

Coradini, D. and Daidone, M.G. (2004) Biomolecular prognostic factors in breast cancer. *Current Opinion in Obstetrics & Gynecology*, **16**, 49–55.

Diamandis, E.P. (1998) Prostate-specific antigen: its usefulness in clinical medicine. *Trends in Endocrinology and Metabolism*, **9**, 310–316.

Gontero, P., Banisadr, S., Frea, B. and Brausi, M. (2004) Metastasis markers in bladder cancer: a review of the literature and clinical considerations. *European Urology*, **46**, 296–311.

Goonewardene, T.I., Sowter, H.M. and Harris, A.L. (2002) Hypoxia-induced pathways in breast cancer. *Microscopy Research and Technique*, **59**, 41–48.

Holdenrieder, S. and Stieber, P. (2004) Apoptotic markers in cancer. *Clinical Biochemistry*, **37**, 605–617.

Nadiminty, N., Lou, W., Lee, S.O. *et al.* (2006) Prostate-specific antigen modulates genes involved in bone remodeling and induces osteoblast differentiation of human osteosarcoma cell line SaOS-2. *Clinical Cancer Research*, **12**, 1420–1430.

Nishi, M., Miyake, H., Takeda, T. *et al.* (1998) The relationship between homovanillic/vanillylmandelic acid ratios and prognosis in neuroblastoma. *Oncology Reports*, **5**, 631–633.

Riley, R.D., Abrams, K.R., Sutton, A.J. *et al.* (2003) Reporting of prognostic markers: current problems and development of guidelines for evidence-based practice in the future. *British Journal of Cancer*, **88**, 1191–1198.

Ross, J.S., Jennings, T.A., Nazeer, T. *et al.* (2003) Prognostic factors in prostate cancer. *American Journal of Clinical Pathology*, **120** (Suppl.), S85–S90.

Scartozzi, M., Galizia, E., Freddari, F. *et al.* (2004) Molecular biology of sporadic gastric cancer: prognostic indicators and novel therapeutic approaches. *Cancer Treatment Reviews*, **30**, 451–459.

Classic anticancer agents

Adjei, A.A. (2004) Pemetrexed (ALIMTA). A novel multitargeted antineoplastic agent. *Clinical Cancer Research*, **10**, 4276s–4280s.

Agarwala, S.S. and Kirkwood, J.M. (2000) Temozolomide, a novel alkylating agent with activity in the central nervous system, may improve the treatment of advanced metastatic melanoma. *Oncologist*, **5**, 144–151.

Albright, C.F., Graciani, N., Han, W. *et al.* (2005) Matrix metalloproteinase-activated doxorubicin prodrugs inhibit HT1080 xenograft growth better than doxorubicin with less toxicity. *Molecular Cancer Therapeutics*, **4**, 751–760.

Anon, (2004) Nanomedicines in action (editorial). *Pharmaceutical Journal*, 485–488.

Campone, M., Cortes-Funes, H., Vorobiof, D. *et al.* (2006) Vinflunine: a new active drug for second-line treatment of advanced breast cancer. Results of a phase II and pharmacokinetic study in patients progressing after first-line anthracycline/taxane-based chemotherapy. *British Journal of Cancer*, **95**, 1161–1166.

Chen, J. and Stubbe, J. (2005) Bleomycins: towards better therapeutics. *Nature Reviews Cancer*, **5**, 102–112.

Cohen, M.H., Johnson, J.R., Massie, T. *et al.* (2006) Approval summary: nelarabine for the treatment of T-cell lymphoblastic leukemia/lymphoma. *Clinical Cancer Research*, **12**, 5329–5335.

Cortes, J. and Baselga, J. (2007) Targeting the microtubules in breast cancer beyond taxanes: the epothilones. *Oncologist*, **12**, 271–280.

Cozzi, P. (2000) Recent outcome in the field of distamycin-derived minor groove binders. *Il Farmaco*, **55**, 168–173.

Cummings, J., Spanswick, V.J., Tomasz, M. and Smyth, J.F. (1998) Enzymology of mitomycin C metabolic activation in tumour tissue: implications for enzyme-directed bioreductive drug development. *Biochemical Pharmacology*, **56**, 405–414.

Dervieux, T., Meshkin, B. and Neri, B. (2005) Pharmacogenetic testing: proofs of principle and pharmacoeconomic implications. *Mutation Research*, **573**, 180–194.

D'Incalci, M., Erba, E., Damia, G. *et al.* (2002) Unique features of the mode of action of ET-743. *Oncologist*, **7**, 210–216.

Eggermont, A.M.M. and Kirkwood, J.M. (2004) Re-evaluating the role of dacarbazine in metastatic melanoma: what have we learned in 30 years? *European Journal of Cancer*, **40**, 1825–1836.

Faderl, S., Gandhi, V., Keating, M.J. *et al.* (2005) The role of clofarabine in hematologic and solid malignancies – development of a next-generation nucleoside analog. *Cancer*, **103**, 1985–1995.

Faithfulla, S. and Deery, P. (2004) Implementation of capecitabine (Xeloda) into a cancer centre: UK experience. *European Journal of Oncology Nursing*, **8**, S54–S62.

Farrugia, D.C., Ford, H.E.R., Cunningham, D. *et al.* (2003) Thymidylate synthase expression in advanced colorectal cancer predicts for response to raltitrexed. *Clinical Cancer Research*, **9**, 792–801.

Fayette, J., Coquard, I.R., Alberti, L. *et al.* (2006) ET-743: a novel agent with activity in soft-tissue sarcomas. *Current Opinion in Oncology*, **18**, 347–353.

Fayette, J., Coquard, I.R., Alberti, L. *et al.* (2005) ET-743: a novel agent with activity in soft-tissue sarcomas. *Oncologist*, **10**, 827–832.

Fortune, J.M. and Osheroff, N. (2000) Topoisomerase II as a target for anticancer drugs: when enzymes stop being nice. *Progress in Nucleic Acid Research and Molecular Biology*, **64**, 221–253.

Galmarini, C.M., Mackey, J.R. and Dumontet, C. (2002) Nucleoside analogues and nucleobases in cancer treatment. *Lancet Oncology*, **3**, 415–424.

Gandhi, V., Keating, M.J., Bate, G. and Kirkpatrick, P. (2006) Nelarabine. *Nature Reviews. Drug Discovery*, **5**, 17–18.

Gewirtz, D.A. (1999) A critical evaluation of the mechanisms of action proposed for the antitumor effects of the anthracycline antibiotics adriamycin and daunorubicin. *Biochemical Pharmacology*, **57**, 727–741.

Giannakakou, P., Gussio, R., Nogales, E. *et al.* (2000) A common pharmacophore for epothilone and taxanes: molecular basis for drug resistance conferred by tubulin mutations in human cancer cells. *Proceedings of the National Academy of Sciences of the United States of America*, **97**, 2904–2909.

Goodin, S., Kane, M.P. and Rubin, E.H. (2004) Epothilones: mechanism of action and biologic activity. *Journal of Clinical Oncology*, **22**, 2015–2025.

Graham, M.L. (2003) Pegaspargase: a review of clinical studies. *Advanced Drug Delivery Reviews*, **55** (10), 1293–1302.

Hande, K.R. (1998) Clinical applications of anticancer drugs targeted to topoisomerase II. *Biochimica et Biophysica Acta*, **1400**, 173–184.

Hande, K.R. (2006) Topoisomerase II inhibitors. *Update on Cancer Therapeutics*, **1**, 3–15.

Hood, K.A., West, L.M., Rouwé, B. *et al.* (2002) Peloruside A, a novel antimitotic agent with paclitaxel-like microtubule stabilizing activity. *Cancer Research*, **62**, 3356–3360.

Ismael, G.F., Rosa, D.D., Mano, M.S. and Awada, A. (2008) Novel cytotoxic drugs: old challenges, new solutions. *Cancer Treatment Reviews*, **34**, 81–91.

Jordan, M.A. and Wilson, L. (2004) Microtubules as a target for anticancer drugs. *Nature Reviews. Cancer*, **4**, 253–265.

Jung, K. and Reszka, R. (2001) Mitochondria as subcellular targets for clinically useful anthracyclines. *Advanced Drug Delivery Reviews*, **49**, 87–105.

Kamath, K. and Jordan, M.A. (2003) Suppression of microtubule dynamics by epothilone b is associated with mitotic arrest. *Cancer Research*, **63**, 6026–6031.

Kaufmann, R., Spieth, K., Leiter, U. *et al.* (2005) Temozolomide in combination with interferon-alfa versus temozolomide alone in patients with advanced metastatic melanoma: a randomized, phase III, multicenter study from the Dermatologic Cooperative Oncology Group. *Journal of Clinical Oncology*, **23**, 9001–9007.

Komiyama, K. (1992) Antitumour antibiotics and their producing microorganisms. *World Journal of Microbiology & Biotechnology*, **8** (Suppl. 1), 77–78.

Kopka, M.L., Yoon, C., Goodsell, D. *et al.* (1985) The molecular origin of DNA-drug specificity in netropsin and distamycin. *Proceedings of the National Academy of Sciences of the United States of America*, **82**, 1376–1380.

Kowalski, R.J., Giannakakou, P. and Hamel, E. (1997) Activities of the microtubule-stabilizing agents epothilones A and B with purified tubulin and in cells resistant to paclitaxel (Taxol). *Journal of Biological Chemistry*, **272**, 2534–2541.

Kratz, F., Warnecke, A., Schmid, B. *et al.* (2006) Prodrugs of anthracyclines in cancer chemotherapy. *Current Medicinal Chemistry*, **13**, 477–523.

Li, Q., Boyer, C., Lee, J.Y. and Shepard, H.M. (2001) A novel approach to thymidylate synthase as a target for cancer chemotherapy. *Molecular Pharmacology*, **59**, 446–452.

Liu, Y., Miyoshi, H. and Nakamura, M. (2007) Nanomedicine for drug delivery and imaging: A promising avenue for cancer therapy and diagnosis using targeted functional nanoparticles. *International Journal of Cancer*, **120**, 2527–2537.

Lombó, F., Menéndez, N., Salas, J.A. and Méndez, C. (2006) The aureolic acid family of antitumor compounds: structure, mode of action, biosynthesis, and novel derivatives. *Applied Microbiology and Biotechnology*, **73**, 1–14.

Lorusso, V., Manzione, L. and Silvestris, N. (2007) Role of liposomal anthracyclines in breast cancer. *Annals of Oncology*, **18** (Suppl. 6), vi70–vi73.

Low, J.A., Wedam, S.B., Lee, J.J. *et al.* (2005) Phase II clinical trial of ixabepilone (BMS-247550), an epothilone B analog, in metastatic and locally advanced breast cancer. *Journal of Clinical Oncology*, **23**, 2726–2734.

Mansour, A.M., Drevs, J., Esser, N. *et al.* (2003) A new approach for the treatment of malignant melanoma: enhanced antitumor efficacy of an albumin-binding doxorubicin prodrug that is cleaved by matrix metalloproteinase 2. *Cancer Research*, **63**, 4062–4066.

McClendona, A.K. and Osheroff, N. (2007) DNA topoisomerase II, genotoxicity, and cancer. *Mutation Research*, **623**, 83–97.

Montero, A., Fossella, F., Hortobagyi, G. and Valero, V. (2005) Docetaxel for treatment of solid tumours: a systematic review of clinical data. *Lancet Oncology*, **6**, 229–239.

Narta, U.K., Kanwar, S.S. and Azmi, W. (2007) Pharmacological and clinical evaluation of l-asparaginase in the treatment of leukemia. *Critical Reviews in Oncology/Hematology*, **61**, 208–221.

Nelson, S.M., Ferguson, L.R. and Denny, W.A. (2007) Non-covalent ligand/DNA interactions: minor groove binding agents. *Mutation Research*, **623**, 24–40.

Ngan, V.K., Bellman, K., Hill, B.T. *et al.* (2001) Mechanism of mitotic block and inhibition of cell proliferation by the semisynthetic vinca alkaloids vinorelbine and its newer derivative vinflunine. *Molecular Pharmacology*, **60**, 225–232.

Odin, E., Wettergren, Y., Nilsson, S. *et al.* (2003) Altered gene expression of folate enzymes in adjacent mucosa is associated with outcome of colorectal cancer patients. *Clinical Cancer Research*, **9**, 6012–6019.

Okouneva, T., Hill, B.T., Wilson, L. and Jordan, M.A. (2003) The effects of vinflunine, vinorelbine, and vinblastine on centromere dynamics. *Molecular Cancer Therapeutics*, **2**, 427–436.

O'Neil, B.H. and Goldberg, R.M. (2005) Chemotherapy for advanced colorectal cancer: let's not forget how we got here (until we really can). *Seminars in Oncology*, **32**, 35–42.

Peterson, J.K., Tucker, C., Favours, E. *et al.* (2005) In vivo evaluation of ixabepilone (BMS247550), a novel epothilone B derivative, against pediatric cancer models. *Clinical Cancer Research*, **11**, 6950–6958.

Pizzolato, J.F. and Saltz, L.B. (2003) The camptothecins. *Lancet*, **361**, 2235–2242.

Pommier, Y. (2006) Topoisomerase I inhibitors: camptothecins and beyond. *Nature Reviews. Cancer*, **6**, 789–802.

Quintieri, L., Geroni, C., Fantin, M. *et al.* (2005) Formation and antitumor activity of PNU-159682, a major metabolite of nemorubicin in human liver microsomes. *Clinical Cancer Research*, **11**, 1608–1617.

Radaideh, S.M. and Sledge, G.W. (2007) Taxane vs. taxane: is the duel at an end? A commentary on a phase-III trial of doxorubicin and docetaxel versus doxorubicin and paclitaxel in metastatic breast cancer: results of the ERASME 3 study. *Breast Cancer Research and Treatment*, **111** (2), 203–208.

Ramanathan, R.K., Picus, J., Raftopoulos, H. *et al.* (2008) A phase II study of milataxel: a novel taxane analoguein previously treated patients with advanced colorectal cancer. *Cancer Chemotherapy and Pharmacology*, **61**, 453–458.

Reid, J.M., Kuffel, M.J., Miller, J.K. *et al.* (1999) Metabolic activation of dacarbazine by human cytochromes P450: the role of CYP1A1, CYP1A2, and CYP2E1. *Clinical Cancer Research*, **5**, 2192–2197.

Rinaldi, D.A., Kuhn, J.G., Burris, H.A. *et al.* (1999) A phase I evaluation of multitargeted antifolate (MTA, LY231514), administered every 21 days, utilizing the modified continual reassessment method for dose escalation. *Cancer Chemotherapy and Pharmacology*, **44**, 372–380.

Rivera, E. (2003) Liposomal anthracyclines in metastatic breast cancer: clinical update. *Oncologist*, **8** (Suppl. 2), 3–9.

Saleem, A., Brown, G.D., Brady, F. *et al.* (2003) Metabolic activation of temozolomide measured in vivo using positron emission tomography. *Cancer Research*, **63**, 2409–2415.

Sampath, D., Discafani, C.M., Loganzo, F. *et al.* (2003) MAC-321, a novel taxane with greater efficacy than paclitaxel and docetaxel in vitro and in vivo. *Molecular Cancer Therapeutics*, **2**, 873–884.

Sampath, D., Greenberger, L.M., Beyer, C. *et al.* (2006) Preclinical pharmacologic evaluation of MST-997, an orally active taxane with superior in vitro and in vivo efficacy in paclitaxel- and docetaxel-resistant tumor models. *Clinical Cancer Research*, **12**, 3459–3469.

Sansom, C. (1999) Temozolomide presents breakthrough in glioblastoma multiforme treatment. *Pharmaceutical Science & Technology Today*, **4**, 131–133.

Schellens, J.H.M. (2007) Capecitabine. *Oncologist*, **12**, 152–155.

Secrist, J.A. (2005) Nucleosides as anticancer agents: from concept to the clinic. *Nucleic Acids Symposium Series (Oxford)*, **49**, 15–16.

Sessa, C., Valota, O. and Geroni, C. (2007) Ongoing phase I and II studies of novel anthracyclines. *Cardiovascular Toxicology*, **7**, 75–79.

Sessa, C., Zucchetti, M., Ghielmini, M. *et al.* (1999) Phase I clinical and pharmacological study of oral methoxymorpholinyl doxorubicin (PNU 152243). *Cancer Chemotherapy and Pharmacology*, **44**, 403–410.

Socinski, M.A., Stinchcombe, T.E. and Hayes, D.N. (2005) The evolving role of pemetrexed (Alimta) in lung cancer. *Seminars in Oncology*, **32** (Suppl. 2), S16–S22.

Spanswick, V.J., Cummings, J. and Smyth, J.F. (1998) Current issues in the enzymology of mitomycin C metabolic activation. *General Pharmacology*, **31**, 539–544.

Takeda, K., Takifuji, N., Negoro, S. *et al.* (2007) Phase II study of amrubicin, 9-amino-anthracycline, in patients with advanced non-small-cell lung cancer: a West Japan Thoracic Oncology Group (WJTOG) study. *Investigational New Drugs*, **25**, 377–383.

Tarnowski, G.S., Mountain, I.M. and Stock, C.C. (1970) Combination therapy of animal tumors with L-asparaginase and antagonists of glutamine or glutamic acid. *Cancer Research*, **30**, 1118–1122.

Teicher, B.A. (2008) Next generation topoisomerase I inhibitors: rationale and biomarker strategies. *Biochemical Pharmacology*, **75**, 1262–1271.

Thomas, E.S., Gomez, H.L., Li, R.K. *et al.* (2007) Pilone plus capecitabine for metastatic breast cancer progressing after anthracycline and taxane treatment. *Clinical Oncology*, **25**, 5210–5217.

Walko, C.M. and Lindley, C. (2005) Capecitabine: a review. *Clinical Therapeutics*, **27**, 23–44.

Waud, W.R., Gilbert, K.S., Shepherd, R.V. *et al.* (2003) Preclinical antitumor activity of 4¢-thio-b-D-arabinofuranosylcytosine (4¢-thio-ara-C). *Cancer Chemotherapy and Pharmacology*, **51**, 422–426.

Woynarowski, J.M. (2002) Targeting critical regions in genomic DNA with AT-specific anticancer drugs. *Biochimica et Biophysica Acta*, **1587**, 300–308.

Yana, T., Negoro, S., Takada, M. *et al.* (2007) Phase II study of amrubicin in previously untreated patients with extensive-disease small cell lung cancer: West Japan Thoracic Oncology Group (WJTOG) study. *Investigational New Drugs*, **25**, 253–258.

Yuan, S., Zhang, X., Lu, L. *et al.* (2004) Anticancer activity of methoxymorpholinyl doxorubicin (PNU 152243) on human hepatocellular carcinoma. *Anti-Cancer Drugs*, **15**, 641–646.

Zelek, L., Yovine, A., Brain, E. *et al.* (2006) A phase II study of Yondelis (trabectedin, ET-743) as a 24-h continuous intravenous infusion in pretreated advanced breast cancer. *British Journal of Cancer*, **94**, 1610–1614.

Zeman, S.M., Phillips, D.R. and Crothers, D.M. (1998) Characterization of covalent adriamycin–DNA adducts. *Proceedings of the National Academy of Sciences of the United States of America*, **95**, 11561–11565.

Zhao, R., Gao, F., Hanscom, M. and Goldman, I.D. (2004) A prominent low-pH methotrexate transport activity in human solid tumors: contribution to the preservation of methotrexate pharmacologic activity in HeLa cells lacking the reduced folate carrier. *Clinical Cancer Research*, **10**, 718–727.

Zhao, R., Hanscom, M., Chattopadhyay, S. and Goldman, I.D. (2004) Selective preservation of pemetrexed pharmacological activity in HeLa cells lacking the reduced folate carrier: association with the presence of a secondary transport pathway. *Cancer Research*, **64**, 3313–3319.

Zhuang, S.H., Agrawal, M., Edgerly, M. *et al.* (2005) A Phase I clinical trial of ixabepilone (BMS-247550), an epothilone B analog, administered intravenously on a daily schedule for 3 days. *Cancer*, **103**, 1932–1938.

Hormonal agents

Bentel, J.M. and Tilley, W.D. (1996) Androgen receptors in prostate cancer. *Journal of Endocrinology*, **151**, 1–11.

Cook, T. and Sheridan, W.P. (2000) Development of GnRH antagonists for prostate cancer: new approaches to treatment. *Oncologist*, **5**, 162–168.

Debruyne, F.M. (2004) Gonadotropin-releasing hormone antagonist in the management of prostate cancer. *Reviews in Urology*, **6** (Suppl. 7), S25–S32.

Debruyne, F., Bhat, G. and Garnick, M.B. (2006) Abarelix for injectable suspension: first-in-class gonadotropin-releasing hormone antagonist for prostate cancer. *Future Oncology*, **2**, 677–696.

Frasor, J., Danes, J.M., Komm, B. *et al.* (2003) Profiling of estrogen up- and down-regulated gene expression in human breast cancer cells: insights into gene networks and pathways underlying estrogenic control of proliferation and cell phenotype. *Endocrinology*, **144**, 4562–4574.

Gillatt, D. (2006) Antiandrogen treatments in locally advanced prostate cancer: are they all the same? *Journal of Cancer Research and Clinical Oncology*, **132** (Suppl. 1), S17–S26.

Howell, A. and Abram, P. (2005) Clinical development of fulvestrant ('Faslodex'). *Cancer Treatment Reviews*, **31** (Suppl. 2), S3–S9.

Lønning, P.E. (2002) The role of aromatase inactivators in the treatment of breast cancer. *International Journal of Clinical Oncology/Japan Society of Clinical Oncology*, **7**, 265–270.

Shetty, Y.C., Chakkarwar, P.N., Acharya, S.S. and Tammela, T. (2004) Endocrine treatment of prostate cancer. *Journal of Steroid Biochemistry and Molecular Biology*, **92**, 287–295.

Shetty, Y.C., Chakkarwar, P.N., Acharya, S.S. and Rajadhyaksha, V.D. (2007) Exemestane: a milestone against breast cancer. *Journal of Postgraduate Medicine*, **53**, 135–138.

Stokes, Z. and Chan, S. (2006) Principles of cancer treatment by hormone therapy. *Surgery (Oxford)*, **24**, 59–62.

Drug development process

Bernard, P.S. and Wittwer, C.T. (2002) Real-time PCR technology for cancer diagnostics. *Clinical Chemistry*, **48**, 1178–1185.

Blagosklonny, M. (2004) Analysis of FDA approved anticancer drugs reveals the future of cancer therapy. *Cell Cycle*, **3**, 1035–1042.

Espinosa, E., Zamora, P., Feliu, J. and González Barón, M. (2003) Classification of anticancer drugs – a new system based on therapeutic targets. *Cancer Treatment Reviews*, **29**, 515–523.

Knox, K. and Kerr, D.J. (2004) Establishing a national tissue bank for surgically harvested cancer tissue. *British Journal of Surgery*, **91**, 134–136.

Newell, D.R. (2005) How to develop a successful cancer drug – molecules to medicines or targets to treatments? *European Journal of Cancer*, **41**, 676–682.

Sausville, E.A. and Holbeck, S.L. (2004) Transcription profiling of gene expression in drug discovery and development: the NCI experience. *European Journal of Cancer*, **40**, 2544–2549.

Walport, M.J. and Lynn, D.W. (2005) Research funding, partnership and strategy – a UK perspective. *Nature Reviews. Molecular Cell Biology*, **6**, 341–344.

Imaging

Aboagye, E.O. and Price, P.M. (2003) Use of positron emission tomography in anticancer drug development. *Investigational New Drugs*, **21**, 169–181.

Cai, W., Rao, J., Gambhir, S.S. and Chen, X. (2006) How molecular imaging is speeding up antiangiogenic drug development. *Molecular Cancer Therapeutics*, **5**, 2624–2633.

Galbraith, S.M. (2006) MR in oncology drug development. *NMR in Biomedicine*, **19**, 681–689.

Graham, K.C., Wirtzfeld, L.A., MacKenzie, L.T. *et al.* (2005) Three-dimensional high-frequency ultrasound imaging for longitudinal evaluation of liver metastases in preclinical models. *Cancer Research*, **65**, 5231–5237.

Griffin, L. and Kauppinen, R.A. (2007) Tumour metabolomics in animal models of human cancer. *Journal of Proteome Research*, **6**, 498–505.

Kabakci, N., Igci, E., Secil, M. *et al.* (2005) Echo contrast-enhanced power Doppler ultrasonography for assessment of angiogenesis in renal cell carcinoma. *Journal of Ultrasound in Medicine*, **24**, 747–753.

Kelloff, G.J., Hoffman, J.M., Johnson, B. *et al.* (2005) Progress and promise of FDG-PET imaging for cancer patient management and oncologic drug development. *Clinical Cancer Research*, **11** (8), 2785–2808.

Laking, G.R., West, C., Buckley, D.L. *et al.* (2006) Imaging vascular physiology to monitor cancer treatment. *Critical Reviews in Oncology/Hematology*, **58**, 95–113.

Martincich, L., Montemurro, F., De Rosa, G. *et al.* (2004) Monitoring response to primary chemotherapy in breast cancer using dynamic contrast-enhanced magnetic resonance imaging. *Breast Cancer Research and Treatment*, **83**, 67–76.

Seddon, B.M. and Workman, P. (2003) The role of functional and molecular imaging in cancer drug discovery and development. *British Journal of Radiology*, **76**, S128–S138.

Shockcor, J.P. and Holmes, E. (2002) Metabonomic applications in toxicity screening and disease diagnosis. *Current Topics in Medicinal Chemistry*, **2**, 35–51.

In vitro assays

Braunschweig, T., Chung, J. and Hewitt, S. (2005) Tissue microarrays: bridging the gap between research and the clinic. *Expert Review of Proteomics*, **2**, 325–336.

Carterson, A.J., Höner zu Bentrup, K., Ott, C.M. *et al.* (2005) A549 lung epithelial cells grown as three-dimensional aggregates: alternative tissue culture model for *Pseudomonas aeruginosa* pathogenesis. *Infection and Immunity*, **73** (2), 1129–1140.

Chen, J., Zhao, S., Nakada, K. *et al.* (2003) Dominant-negative hypoxia-inducible factor-1 reduces tumorigenicity of pancreatic cancer cells through the suppression of glucose metabolism. *American Journal of Pathology*, **162**, 1283–1291.

Coulton, G. (2004) Are histochemistry and cytochemistry 'Omics'? *Journal of Molecular Histology*, **35**, 603–613.

de Vries, A., Flores, E.R., Miranda, B. *et al.* (2002) Targeted point mutations of p53 lead to dominant-negative inhibition of wild-type p53 function. *Proceedings of the National Academy of Sciences of the United States of America*, **99**, 2948–2953.

Downward, J. (2004) RNA interference. *BMJ (Clinical Research Edition)*, **328**, 1245–1248.

Forster, K., Helbl, V., Lederer, T. *et al.* (1999) Tetracycline-inducible expression systems with reduced basal activity in mammalian cells. *Nucleic Acids Research*, **27**, 708–710.

Gossen, M. and Bujard, H. (1992) Tight control of gene expression in mammalian cells by tetracycline-responsive promoters. *Proceedings of the National Academy of Sciences of the United States of America*, **89**, 5547–5551.

Hasan, J., Shnyder, S.D., Bibby, M. *et al.* (2004) Quantitative angiogenesis assays in vivo – a review. *Angiogenesis*, **7**, 1–16.

Hewitt, S.M. (2006) The application of tissue microarrays in the validation of microarray results. *Methods in Enzymology*, **410**, 400–415.

Hofmann, A., Nolan, G.P. and Blau, H.M. (1996) Rapid retroviral delivery of tetracycline-inducible genes in a single autoregulatory cassette. *Proceedings of the National Academy of Sciences of the United States of America*, **93**, 5185–5190.

Jones, F.E. and Stern, D.F. (1999) Expression of dominant-negative ErbB2 in the mammary gland of transgenic mice reveals a role in lobuloalveolar development and lactation. *Oncogene*, **18**, 3481–3490.

Kawada, K., Yonei, T., Ueoka, H. *et al.* (2002) Comparison of chemosenstitivity tests: Clonogenic assay versus MTT assay. *Acta Medica*, **56**, 129–134.

Kim, J.B. (2005) Three-dimensional tissue culture models in cancer biology. *Seminars in Cancer Biology*, **15**, 365–377.

Laird, P.W. (2005) Cancer epigenetics. *Human Molecular Genetics*, **14**, R65–R66.

Shih, I.-M. and Wang, T.-L. (2005) Apply innovative technologies to explore cancer genome. *Current Opinion in Oncology*, **17**, 33–38.

L'Heureux, N., Pâquet, S., Labbé, R. *et al.* (1998) A completely biological tissue-engineered human blood vessel. *FASEB Journal*, **12**, 47–56.

Lu, P.Y., Xie, F. and Woodle, M.C. (2005) In Vivo application of RNA interference: from functional genomics to therapeutics. *Advances in Genetics*, **54**, 117–142.

Manning, A.T., Garvin, J.T., Shahbazi, R.I. *et al.* (2007) Molecular profiling techniques and bioinformatics in cancer research. *European Journal of Surgical Oncology*, **33**, 255–265.

Mobasheri, A., Airley, R., Foster, C.S. *et al.* (2004) Post-genomic applications of tissue microarrays: basic research, prognostic oncology, clinical genomics and drug discovery. *Histology and Histopathology*, **19**, 325–335.

Mosmann, T. (1983) Rapid colorimetric assay for cellular growth and survival: application to proliferation and cytotoxicity assays. *Journal of Immunological Methods*, **65**, 55–63.

Ngo, V.N., Davis, R.E., Lamy, L. *et al.* (2006) A loss-of-function RNA interference screen for molecular targets in cancer. *Nature*, **441**, 106–110.

No, D., Yao, T.P. and Evans, R.M. (1996) Ecdysone-inducible gene expression in mammalian cells and transgenic mice. *Proceedings of the National Academy of Sciences of the United States of America*, **93**, 3346–3351.

Pampaloni, F., Reynaud, E.G. and Stelzer, E.H. (2007) The third dimension bridges the gap between cell culture and live tissue. *Nature Reviews. Molecular Cell Biology*, **8**, 839–845.

Qian, X., LeVea, C.M., Freeman, J.K. *et al.* (1994) Heterodimerization of epidermal growth factor receptor and wild-type or kinase-deficient Neu: a mechanism of interreceptor kinase activation and transphosphorylation. *Proceedings of the National Academy of Sciences of the United States of America*, **91**, 1500–1504.

Sachse, C., Krausz, E., Krönke, A. *et al.* (2005) High-throughput RNA interference strategies for target discovery and validation by using synthetic short interfering RNAs: functional genomics investigations of biological pathways. *Methods in Enzymology*, **392**, 242–277.

Sausville, E.A. and Holbeck, S.L. (2004) Transcription profiling of gene expression in drug discovery and development: the NCI experience. *European Journal of Cancer*, **40**, 2544–2549.

Scudiero, D.A., Shoemaker, R.H., Paull, K.D. *et al.* (1988) Evaluation of a soluble tetrazolium/formazan assay for cell growth and drug sensitivity in culture using human and other tumor cell lines. *Cancer Research*, **48**, 4827–4833.

Shockett, P.E. and Schatz, D.G. (1996) Diverse strategies for tetracycline-regulated inducible gene expression. *Proceedings of the National Academy of Sciences of the United States of America*, **93**, 5173–5176.

Westbrook, T.F., Stegmeier, F. and Elledge, S.J. (2005) Dissecting cancer pathways and vulnerabilities with RNAi. *Cold Spring Harbor Symposia on Quantitative Biology*, **70**, 435–444.

Williams, N.S., Gaynor, R.B., Scoggin, S. *et al.* (2003) Identification and validation of genes involved in the pathogenesis of colorectal cancer using cDNA microarrays and RNA interference. *Clinical Cancer Research*, **9**, 931–946.

Wulfkuhle, J., Espina, V., Liotta, L. and Petricoin, E. (2004) Genomic and proteomic technologies for individualisation and improvement of cancer treatment. *European Journal of Cancer*, **40**, 2623–2632.

Yokoyama, T., Ohashi, K., Kuge, H. *et al.* (2006) In vivo engineering of metabolically active hepatic tissues in a neovascularized subcutaneous cavity. *American Journal of Transplantation*, **6**, 50–59.

Animal models

Bibby, S.M. and Bibby, M.C. (2005) 50 years of preclinical anticancer drug screening: empirical to target-driven approaches. *Clinical Cancer Research*, **11**, 971–981.

Brayton, C., Justice, M. and Montgomery, C.A. (2001) Evaluating mutant mice: anatomic pathology. *Veterinary Pathology*, **38**, 1–19.

Carver, B.S. and Pandolfi, P.P. (2006) Mouse modeling in oncologic preclinical and translational research. *Clinical Cancer Research*, **12**, 5305–5311.

Dobson, J.M., Samuel, S., Milstein, H. *et al.* (2002) Canine neoplasia in the UK: estimates of incidence rates from a population of insured dogs. *Journal of Small Animal Practice – English Edition*, **43**, 240–246.

Double, J., Barrass, N., Barnard, N.D. and Navaratnam, V. (2002) Toxicity testing in the development of anticancer drugs. *Lancet Oncology*, **3**, 438–442.

Ellies, L.G., Fishman, M., Hardison, J. *et al.* (2003) Mammary tumor latency is increased in mice lacking the inducible nitric oxide synthase. *International Journal of Cancer*, **106**, 1–7.

Finkle, D., Quan, Z.R., Asghari, V. *et al.* (2004) HER2-targeted therapy reduces incidence and progression of midlife mammary tumors in female murine mammary tumor virus huHER2-transgenic mice. *Clinical Cancer Research*, **10**, 2499–2511.

Fomchenko, E.I. and Holland, E.C. (2006) Mouse models of brain tumors and their applications in preclinical trials. *Clinical Cancer Research*, **12**, 2006.

Hansen, K. and Khanna, C. (2004) Spontaneous and genetically engineered animal models: use in preclinical cancer drug development. *European Journal of Cancer*, **40**, 858–880.

Hershey, A.E., Kurzman, I.D., Forrest, L.J. *et al.* (1999) Inhalation chemotherapy for macroscopic primary or metastatic lung tumors: proof of principle using dogs with spontaneously occurring tumors as a model. *Clinical Cancer Research*, **5**, 2653–2659.

Hollingshead, M.G., Alley, M.C., Camalier, R.F. *et al.* (1995) In vivo cultivation of tumor cells in hollow fibers. *Life Sciences*, **57**, 131–141.

Khanna, C., Lindblad-Toh, K., Vail, D. *et al.* (2006) The dog as a cancer model. *Nature Biotechnology*, **24**, 1065–1066.

Lawhead, J.B. and Baker, M. (2005) *Introduction to Veterinary Science*, Thomson Delmar Learning, Canada.

Lee, E.J., Jakacka, M., Duan, W.R. *et al.* (2001) Adenovirus-directed expression of dominant negative estrogen receptor induces apoptosis in breast cancer cells and regression of tumors in nude mice. *Molecular Medicine*, **7**, 773–782.

Mack, G.S. (2005) Cancer researchers usher in dog days of medicine. *Nature Medicine*, **11**, 1018.

Olive, K.P. and Tuveson, D.A. (2006) The use of targeted mouse models for preclinical testing of novel cancer therapeutics. *Clinical Cancer Research*, **12**, 5277–5287.

Papaioannou, V.E. and Behringer, RR. (2005) *Mouse Phenotypes: A Handbook of Mutation Analysis*, CSHL Press, Ohio, USA.

Phillips, R.M. and Bibby, M.C. (2001) Hollow fiber assay for tumor angiogenesis. Methods in molecular medicine, in *Angiogenesis Protocols*, Vol. **46** (ed. J.C. Murray), Humana Press Inc., Totowa, NJ, USA.

Phillips, R.M., Pearce, J., Loadman, P.M. *et al.* (1998) Angiogenesis in the hollow fiber tumor model influences drug delivery to tumor cells: implications for anticancer drug screening programs. *Cancer Research*, **58**, 5263–5266.

Rusk, A., Cozzi, E., Stebbins, M. *et al.* (2006) Cooperative activity of cytotoxic chemotherapy with antiangiogenic thrombospondin-I peptides, ABT-526 in pet dogs with relapsed lymphoma. *Clinical Cancer Research*, **12**, 7456–7464.

Sausville, E.A. and Burger, A.M. (2006) Contributions of human tumor xenografts to anticancer drug development. *Cancer Research*, **66**, 3351–3354.

Schiffer, S.P. (1997) Animal welfare and colony management in cancer research. *Breast Cancer Research and Treatment*, **46**, 313–331.

Sedivy, J.M. and Joyner, A.L. (1992) *Gene Targeting*, Oxford University Press, Oxford, UK.

Singh, M. and Johnson, L. (2006) Using genetically engineered mousemodels of cancer to aid drug development: an industry perspective. *Clinical Cancer Research*, **12**, 5312–5328.

Statistics of Scientific Procedures on Living Animals Great Britain 2004. December 2005 LONDON HMSO.

Vail, D.M. and Thamm, D.H. (2005) Cytotoxic chemotherapy: new players, new tactics. *Journal of the American Animal Hospital Association*, **41**, 209–214.

Wang, D., Pascual, J.M., Yang, H. *et al.* (2006) A mouse model for Glut-1 haploinsufficiency. *Human Molecular Genetics*, **15**, 1169–1179.

Withrow, S.J., Powers, B.E., Straw, R.C. and Wilkins, R.M. (1991) Comparative aspects of osteosarcoma dog versus man. *Clinical Orthopaedics and Related Research*, **270**, 159–168.

Clinical trials

Bland, J.M. and Altman, D.G. (1998) Survival probabilities (the Kaplan–Meier method). *BMJ (Clinical Research Edition)*, **317**, 1572.

Jagannath, S., Richardson, P.G., Barlogie, B. *et al.*; SUMMIT/CREST Investigators. (2006) Bortezomib in combination with dexamethasone for the treatment of patients with relapsed and/or refractory multiple myeloma with less than optimal response to bortezomib alone. *Haematologica*, **91**, 929–934.

Richardson, P.G., Sonneveld, P., Schuster, M.W. *et al.*; Assessment of Proteasome Inhibition for Extending Remissions (APEX) Investigators. (2005) Bortezomib or high-dose dexamethasone for relapsed multiple myeloma. *New England Journal of Medicine*, **352** (24), 2487–2498.

Romond, E.H., Perez, E.A., Bryant, J. *et al.* (2005) Trastuzumab plus adjuvant chemotherapy for operable HER2-positive breast cancer. *New England Journal of Medicine*, **353**, 1673–1684.

Hypoxia and bioreductive drugs

Airley, R., Loncaster, J., Davidson, S. *et al.* (2001) Glucose transporter Glut-1 expression correlates with tumor hypoxia and predicts metastasis-free survival in advanced carcinoma of the cervix. *Clinical Cancer Research*, **7**, 928–934.

Airley, R.E. and Mobasheri, A. (2007) Hypoxic regulation of glucose transport, anaerobic metabolism and angiogenesis in cancer: novel pathways and targets for anticancer therapeutics. *Chemotherapy*, **53**, 233–256.

Airley, R.E., Monaghan, J. and Stratford, I.J. (2000) Hypoxia and disease: opportunities for novel diagnostic and therapeutic prodrug strategies. *Pharmaceutical Journal*, **264**, 666–673.

Airley, R.E., Loncaster, J., Raleigh, J.A. *et al.* (2003) GLUT-1 and CAIX as intrinsic markers of hypoxia in carcinoma of the cervix: relationship to pimonidazole binding. *International Journal of Cancer*, **104**, 85–91.

Airley, R.E., Phillips, R.M., Evans, A.E. *et al.* (2005) Hypoxia-regulated glucose transporter Glut-1 may influence chemosensitivity to some alkylating agents: results of EORTC (First Translational Award) study of the relevance of tumour hypoxia to the outcome of chemotherapy in human tumour-derived xenografts. *International Journal of Oncology*, **26**, 1477–1484.

Albertella, M.R., Loadman, P.M., Jones, P.H. *et al.* (2008) Hypoxia-selective targeting by the bioreductive prodrug AQ4N in patients with solidtumors: results of a phase I study. *Clinical Cancer Research*, **14**, 1096–1104.

Ammons, W.S., Wang, J.W., Yang, Z. *et al.* (2007) A novel alkylating agent, glufosfamide, enhances the activity of gemcitabine in vitro and in vivo. *Neoplasia*, **9**, 625–633.

Babich, H. and Zuckerbraun, H.L. (2001) In vitro cytotoxicity of glyco-*S*-nitrosothiols. A novel class of nitric oxide donors. *Toxicology In Vitro*, **15**, 181–190.

Bleumer, I., Knuth, A., Oosterwijk, E. *et al.* (2004) A phase II trial of chimeric monoclonal antibody G250 for advanced renal cell carcinoma patients. *British Journal of Cancer*, **90**, 985–990.

Bleumer, I., Oosterwijk, E., Oosterwijk-Wakka, J.C. *et al.* (2006) A clinical trial with chimeric monoclonal antibody WX-G250 and low dose interleukin-2 pulsing scheme for advanced renal cell carcinoma. *Journal of Urology*, **175**, 57–62.

Briasoulis, E., Judson, I., Pavlidis, N. *et al.* (2000) Phase I trial of 6-hour infusion of glufosfamide, a new alkylating agent with potentially enhanced selectivity for tumors that overexpress transmembrane glucose transporters: a study of the European Organization for Research and Treatment of Cancer Early Clinical Studies Group. *Journal of Clinical Oncology*, **18**, 3535–3544.

Briasoulis, E., Pavlidis, N., Terret, C. *et al.* (2003) Glufosfamide administered using a 1-hour infusion given as first-line treatment for advanced pancreatic cancer. A phase II trial of the EORTC-new drug development group. *European Journal of Cancer*, **39**, 2334–2340.

Bui, M.H., Seligson, D., Han, K.R. *et al.* (2003) Carbonic anhydrase IX is an independent predictor of survival in advanced renal clear cell carcinoma: implications for prognosis and therapy. *Clinical Cancer Research*, **9**, 802–811.

Cantuaria, G., Magalhaes, A., Angioli, R. *et al.* (2000) Antitumor activity of a novel glyco-nitric oxide conjugate in ovarian carcinoma. *Cancer*, **88**, 381–388.

Carmeliet, P., Dor, Y., Herbert, J.M. *et al.* (1998) Role of HIF-1alpha in hypoxia-mediated apoptosis, cell proliferation and tumour angiogenesis. *Nature*, **394**, 485–490.

Chan, J.Y., Kong, S.K., Choy, Y.M. *et al.* (1999) Inhibition of glucose transporter gene expression by antisense nucleic acids in HL-60 leukaemia cells. *Life Sciences*, **65**, 63–70.

Chan, P., Milosevic, M., Fyles, A. *et al.* (2004) A phase III randomized study of misonidazole plus radiation vs. radiation alone for cervix cancer. *Radiotherapy and Oncology*, **70**, 295–299.

Chau, N.M., Rogers, P., Aherne, W. *et al.* (2005) Identification of novel small molecule inhibitors of hypoxia-inducible factor-1 that differentially block hypoxia-inducible factor-1 activity and hypoxia-inducible factor-1A induction in response to hypoxic stress and growth factors. *Cancer Research*, **65**, 4918–4928.

Chiorean, E.G., Dragovich, T., Hamm, J. *et al.* (2008) A Phase 1 dose-escalation trial of glufosfamide in combination with gemcitabine in solid tumors including pancreatic adeno-carcinoma. *Cancer Chemotherapy and Pharmacology*, **61**, 1019–1026.

Choi, H.J., Eun, J.S., Kim, B.G. *et al.* (2006) Vitexin, an HIF-1(inhibitor, has anti-metastatic potential in PC12 cells. *Molecules and Cells*, **22**, 291–299.

Dimmer, K.S., Friedrich, B., Lang, F. *et al.* (2000) The low-affinity monocarboxylate transporter MCT4 is adapted to the export of lactate in highly glycolytic cells. *Biochemical Journal*, **350**, 219–227.

Davis, I.D., Wiseman, G.A., Lee, F.T. *et al.* (2007) A phase I multiple dose, dose escalation study of cG250 monoclonal antibody in patients with advanced renal cell carcinoma. *Cancer Immunity*, **7**, 13.

Dittrich, C., Zandvliet, A.S., Gneist, M. *et al.* (2007) A phase I and pharmacokinetic study of indisulam in combination with carboplatin. *British Journal of Cancer*, **96**, 559–566.

Evans, A., Bates, V., Troy, H. *et al.* (2008) Glut-1 as a therapeutic target: increased chemore-sistance and HIF-1-independent link with cell turnover is revealed through COMPARE analysis and metabolomic studies. *Cancer Chemotherapy and Pharmacology*, **61**, 377–393.

Fang, J., Zhou, Q., Liu, L.Z. *et al.* (2007) Apigenin inhibits tumor angiogenesis through decreasing HIF-1α and VEGF expression. *Carcinogenesis*, **28**, 858–864.

Garcia, J.A. (2006) HIFing the brakes: therapeutic opportunities for treatment of human malignancies. *Science's STKE: Signal Transduction Knowledge Environment*, **2006**, pe25.

Giaccone, G., Smit, E.F., de Jonge, M. *et al.* (2004) Glufosfamide administered by 1-hour infusion as a second-line treatment for advanced non-small cell lung cancer; a phase II trial of the EORTC-New Drug Development Group. *European Journal of Cancer*, **40**, 667–672.

Guise, C.P., Wang, A.T., Theil, A. *et al.* (2007) Identification of human reductases that activate the dinitrobenzamide mustard prodrug PR-104A: a role for NADPH:cytochrome P450 oxidoreductase under hypoxia. *Biochemical Pharmacology*, **74**, 810–820.

Halestrap, A.P. and Price, N.T. (1999) The proton-linked monocarboxylate transporter (MCT) family: structure, function and regulation. *Biochemical Journal*, **343**, 281–299.

Höpfl, G., Wenger, R.H., Ziegler, U. *et al.* (2002) Rescue of hypoxia-inducible factor-1-deficient tumor growth by wild-type cells is independent of vascular endothelial growth factor. *Cancer Research*, **62**, 2962–2970.

Hou, Y., Wang, J., Andreana, P.R. *et al.* (1999) Targeting nitric oxide to cancer cells: cytotoxicity studies of glyco-*S*-nitrosothiols. *Bioorganic & Medicinal Chemistry Letters*, **9**, 2255–2258.

Huxham, L.A., Kyle, A.H., Baker, J.H. *et al.* (2008) Exploring vascular dysfunction caused by tirapazamine. *Microvascular Research*, **75**, 247–255.

Jaffar, M., Phillips, R.M., Williams, K.J. *et al.* (2003) 3-substituted-5-aziridinyl-1-methylindole-4,7-diones as NQO1-directed antitumour agents: mechanism of activation and cytotoxicity in vitro. *Biochemical Pharmacology*, **66**, 1199–1206.

Jain, V.K., Kalia, V.K., Sharma, R. *et al.* (1985) Effects of 2-deoxy-D-glucose on glycolysis, proliferation kinetics and radiation response of human cancer cells. *International Journal of Radiation Oncology, Biology, Physics*, **11**, 943–950.

Kim, H.L., Yeo, E.J., Chun, Y.S. and Park, J.W. (2006) A domain responsible for HIF-1 alpha degradation by YC-1, a novel anticancer agent. *International Journal of Oncology*, **29**, 255–260.

Koh, M.Y., Spivak-Kroizman, T., Venturini, S. *et al.* (2008) Molecular mechanisms for the activity of PX-478, an antitumor inhibitor of the hypoxia-inducible factor-1α. *Molecular Cancer Therapeutics*, **7**, 90–100.

Koukourakis, M.I., Giatromanolaki, A., Simopoulos, C. *et al.* (2005) Lactate dehydrogenase 5 (LDH5) relates to up-regulated hypoxia inducible factor pathway and metastasis in colorectal cancer. *Clinical & Experimental Metastasis*, **22**, 25–30.

Kurtoglu, M., Maher, J.C. and Lampidis, T.J. (2007) Differential toxic mechanisms of 2-deoxy-D-glucose versus 2-fluorodeoxy-D-glucose in hypoxic and normoxic tumor cells. *Antioxidants & Redox Signaling*, **9**, 1383–1390.

Lampidis, T.J., Kurtoglu, M., Maher, J.C. *et al.* (2006) Efficacy of 2-halogen substituted D-glucose analogs in blocking glycolysis and killing 'hypoxic tumor cells'. *Cancer Chemotherapy and Pharmacology*, **58**, 725–734.

Laudański, P., Dziecioł, J., Anchim, T. and Wołczyński, S. (2001) The influence of glyco-nitric oxide conjugate on proliferation of breast cancer cells in vitro. *Folia Histochemica et Cytobiologica*, **39** (Suppl. 2), 87–88.

Liu, Z., Smyth, F.E., Renner, C. *et al.* (2002) Anti-renal cell carcinoma chimeric antibody G250: cytokine enhancement of in vitro antibody-dependent cellular cytotoxicity. *Cancer Immunology, Immunotherapy*, **51**, 171–177.

Macpherson, G.R. and Figg, W.D. (2004) Small molecule-mediated anti-cancer therapy via hypoxia-inducible factor-1 blockade. *Cancer Biology & Therapy*, **3**, 503–504.

Maher, J.C., Wangpaichitr, M., Savaraj, N. *et al.* (2007) Hypoxia-inducible factor-1 confers resistance to the glycolytic inhibitor 2-deoxy-D-glucose. *Molecular Cancer Therapeutics*, **6**, 732–741.

Manning, A.T., Garvin, J.T., Shahbazi, R.I. *et al.* (2007) Molecular profiling techniques and bioinformatics in cancer research. *European Journal of Surgical Oncology*, **33**, 255–265.

Maschek, G., Savaraj, N., Priebe, W. *et al.* (2004) 2-deoxy-D-glucose increases the efficacy of adriamycin and paclitaxel in human osteosarcoma and non-small cell lung cancers in vivo. *Cancer Research*, **64**, 31–34.

McKeown, S.R., Cowen, R.L. and Williams, K.J. (2007) Bioreductive drugs: from concept to clinic. *Clinical Oncology*, **19**, 427–442.

Noguchi, Y., Saito, A., Miyagi, Y. *et al.* (2000) Supression of facilitative glucose transporter 1 mRNA can suppress tumour growth. *Cancer Letters*, **154**, 175–182.

Oh, S.H., Woo, J.K., Jin, Q. *et al.* (2008) Identification of novel antiangiogenic anticancer activities of deguelin targeting hypoxia-inducible factor-1 alpha. *International Journal of Cancer*, **122**, 5–14.

O'Rourke, M., Ward, C., Worthington, J. *et al.* (2008) Evaluation of the antiangiogenic potential of AQ4N. *Clinical Cancer Research*, **14**, 1502–1509.

Park, E.J., Kong, D., Fisher, R. *et al.* (2006) Targeting the PAS-A domain of HIF-1a for development of small molecule inhibitors of HIF-1. *Cell Cycle*, **5**, 1847–1853.

Patterson, A.V., Ferry, D.M., Edmunds, S.J. *et al.* (2007) Mechanism of action and preclinical antitumor activity of the novel hypoxia-activated DNA cross-linking agent PR-104. *Clinical Cancer Research*, **13**, 3922–3932.

Raghunand, N., Gatenby, R.A. and Gillies, R.J. (2003) Microenvironmental and cellular consequences of altered blood flow in tumours. *British Journal of Radiology*, **76**, S11–S12.

Rapisarda, A., Uranchimeg, B., Scudiero, D.A. *et al.* (2002) Identification of small molecule inhibitors of hypoxia-inducible factor 1 transcriptional activation pathway. *Cancer Research*, **62**, 4316–4324.

Rapisarda, A., Uranchimeg, B., Sordet, O. *et al.* (2004) Topoisomerase I-mediated inhibition of hypoxia-inducible factor 1: mechanism and therapeutic implications. *Cancer Research*, **64**, 1475–1482.

Rischin, D., Hicks, R.J., Fisher, R. *et al.* (2006) Prognostic significance of [18F]-misonidazole positron emission tomography-detected tumor hypoxia in patients with advanced head and neck cancer randomly assigned to chemoradiation with or without tirapazamine: a substudy of Trans-Tasman Radiation Oncology Group Study 98.02. *Journal of Clinical Oncology*, **24**, 2098–2104.

Rockwell, S., Sartorelli, A.C., Tomasz, M. and Kennedy, K.A. (1993) Cellular pharmacology of quinone bioreductive alkylating agents. *Cancer Metastasis Reviews*, **12**, 165–176.

Shepherd, F., Koschel, G., von Pawel, J. *et al.* (2000) Comparison of tirazone (Tirapazamine) and cisplatin vs. etoposide and cisplatin in advanced non-small cell lung cancer (NSCLC): final results of the international Phase III CATAPULT II Trial. *Lung Cancer*, **29** (Suppl. 1, Abstr 87), 28.

Siegel-Lakhai, W.S., Zandvliet, A.S., Huitema, A.D. *et al.* (2008) A dose-escalation study of indisulam in combination with capecitabine (Xeloda) in patients with solid tumours. *British Journal of Cancer*, **98**, 1320–1326.

Shin, D.H., Kim, J.H., Jung, Y.J. *et al.* (2007) Preclinical evaluation of YC-1, a HIF inhibitor, for the prevention of tumor spreading. *Cancer Letters*, **255**, 107–116.

Singh, D., Banerji, A.K., Dwarakanath, B.S. *et al.* (2005) Optimizing cancer radiotherapy with 2-deoxy-d-glucose dose escalation studies in patients with glioblastoma multiforme. *Strahlentherapie und Onkologie*, **181**, 507–514.

Song, C.W., Clement, J.J. and Levitt, S.H. (1976) Preferential cytotoxicity of 5-thio-D-glucose against hypoxic tumor cells. *Journal of the National Cancer Institute*, **57**, 603–605.

Song, C.W., Lee, C.K., Rhee, J.G. and Levitt, S.H. (1982) Comparison of the cytotoxicity of 5-thio-D-glucose and misonidazole on hypoxic cells in vitro. *International Journal of Radiation Oncology, Biology, Physics*, **8**, 749–752.

Subbarayan, P.R., Wang, P.G., Lampidis, T.J. *et al.* (2008) Differential expression of Glut 1 mRNA and protein levels correlates with increased sensitivity to the glyco-conjugated nitric oxide donor (2-glu-SNAP) in different tumor cell types. *Journal of Chemotherapy*, **20**, 106–111.

Sun, H.L., Liu, Y.N., Huang, Y.T. *et al.* (2007) YC-1 inhibits HIF-1 expression in prostate cancer cells: contribution of Akt/NF-kappaB signaling to HIF-1alpha accumulation during hypoxia. *Oncogene*, **26**, 3941–3951.

Supuran, C.T. (2008) Development of small molecule carbonic anhydrase IX inhibitors. *BJU International*, **101** (Suppl. 4), 39–40.

Svastová, E., Zilka, N., Zat'ovicová, M. *et al.* (2003) Carbonic anhydrase IX reduces E-cadherin-mediated adhesion of MDCK cells via interaction with beta-catenin. *Experimental Cell Research*, **290**, 332–345.

Swietach, P., Vaughan-Jones, R.D. and Harris, A.L. (2007) Regulation of tumor pH and the role of carbonic anhydrase 9. *Cancer Metastasis Reviews*, **26**, 299–310.

Talbot, D.C., von Pawel, J., Cattell, E. *et al.* (2007) A randomized phase II pharmacokinetic and pharmacodynamic study of indisulam as second-line therapy in patients with advanced non-small cell lung cancer. *Clinical Cancer Research*, **13**, 1816–1822.

Tan, C., de Noronha, R.G., Roecker, A.J. *et al.* (2005) Identification of a novel small-molecule inhibitor of the hypoxia-inducible factor 1 pathway. *Cancer Research*, **65**, 605–612.

Thiry, A., Dogné, J.M., Masereel, B. and Supuran, C.T. (2006) Targeting tumor-associated carbonic anhydrase IX in cancer therapy. *Trends in Pharmacological Sciences*, **27**, 566–573.

Ullah, M.S., Davies, A.J. and Halestrap, A.P. (2006) The plasma membrane lactate transporter MCT4, but not MCT1, is up-regulated by hypoxia through a HIF-1alpha-dependent mechanism. *Journal of Biological Chemistry*, **281**, 9030–9037.

van den Bent, M.J., Grisold, W., Frappaz, D. *et al.* (2003) European Organization for Research and Treatment of Cancer (EORTC) open label phase II study on glufosfamide administered as a 60-minute infusion every 3 weeks in recurrent glioblastoma multiforme. *Annals of Oncology*, **14**, 1732–1734.

Vaupel, P. (1990) Oxygenation of human tumors. *Strahlentherapie und Onkologie*, **166**, 377–386.

Vaupel, P., Kallinowski, F. and Okunieff, P. (1989) Blood flow, oxygen and nutrient supply, and metabolic microenvironment of human tumors: a review. *Cancer Research*, **49**, 6449–6465.

Vaupel, P., Kallinowski, F. and Okunieff, P. (1990) Blood flow, oxygen consumption and tissue oxygenation of human tumors. *Advances in Experimental Medicine and Biology*, **277**, 895–905.

von Pawel, J., von Roemeling, R., Gatzemeier, U. *et al.* (2000) Tirapazamine plus cisplatin versus cisplatin in advanced non–small-cell lung cancer: a report of the International CATAPULT I Study Group. *Journal of Clinical Oncology*, **18**, 1351–1359.

Vullo, D., Scozzafava, A., Pastorekova, S. *et al.* (2004) Carbonic anhydrase inhibitors: inhibition of the tumor-associated isozyme IX with fluorine-containing sulfonamides. The first sub-nanomolar CA IX inhibitor discovered. *Bioorganic & Medicinal Chemistry Letters*, **14**, 2351–2356.

Welch, S., Hirte, H.W., Carey, M.S. *et al.* (2007) UCN-01 in combination with topotecan in patients with advanced recurrent ovarian cancer: A study of the Princess Margaret Hospital Phase II consortium. *Gynecologic Oncology*, **106**, 305–310.

Welsh, S., Williams, R., Kirkpatrick, L. *et al.* (2004) Antitumor activity and pharmacodynamic properties of PX-478, an inhibitor of hypoxia-inducible factor-1α. *Molecular Cancer Therapeutics*, **3**, 233–244.

Williams, K.J., Telfer, B.A., Airley, R.E. *et al.* (2002) A protective role for HIF-1 in response to redox manipulation and glucose deprivation: implications for tumorigenesis. *Oncogene*, **21**, 282–290.

Williamson, S.K., Crowley, J.J., Lara, P.N., Jr. *et al.* (2005) Phase III trial of paclitaxel plus carboplatin with or without tirapazamine in advanced non–small-cell lung cancer: Southwest Oncology Group Trial S0003. *Journal of Clinical Oncology*, **23**, 9097–9104.

Yang, J., Zhang, L., Erbel, P.J. *et al.* (2005) Functions of the Per/ARNT/Sim domains of the hypoxia-inducible factor. *Journal of Biological Chemistry*, **280**, 36047–36054.

Yeo, E.J., Chun, Y.S., Cho, Y.S. *et al.* (2003) YC-1: a potential anticancer drug targeting hypoxia-inducible factor 1. *Journal of the National Cancer Institute*, **95**, 516–525.

Yeo, E.J., Chun, Y.S. and Park, J.W. (2004) New anticancer strategies targeting HIF-1. *Biochemical Pharmacology*, **68**, 1061–1069.

Ziello, J.E., Jovin, I.S. and Huang, Y. (2007) Hypoxia-inducible factor (HIF)-1 regulatory pathway and its potential for therapeutic intervention in malignancy and ischemia. *Yale Journal of Biology and Medicine*, **80**, 51–60.

Metastasis

Aguirre-Ghiso, J.A. (2007) Models, mechanisms and clinical evidence for cancer dormancy. *Nature Reviews Cancer*, **7**, 834–846.

Ayala, I., Baldassarre, M., Caldieri, G. and Buccione, R. (2006) Invadopodia: a guided tour. *European Journal of Cell Biology*, **85**, 159–164.

Bidard, F.C., Pierga, J.Y., Vincent-Salomon, A. and Poupon, M.F. (2008) A 'class action' against the microenvironment: do cancer cells, cooperate in metastasis? *Cancer Metastasis Reviews*, **7**, 5–10.

Bockhorn, M., Jain, R.K. and Munn, L.L. (2007) Active versus passive mechanisms in metastasis: do cancer cells crawl into vessels, or are they pushed? *Lancet Oncology*, **8**, 444–448.

Chambers, F., Groom, A.C. and MacDonald, I.C. (2002) Dissemination and growth of cancer cells in metastatic sites. *Nature Reviews Cancer*, **2**, 563–572.

Christofori1, G. (2006) New signals from the invasive front. *Nature*, **441**, 444–450.

DeNardo, D.G., Johansson, M. and Coussens, L.M. (2008) Immune cells as mediators of solid tumor metastasis. *Cancer Metastasis Reviews*, **27**, 11–18.

Duffy, M.J., McGowan, P.M. and Gallagher, W.M. (2008) Cancer invasion and metastasis: changing views. *Journal of Pathology*, **214**, 283–293.

Fokas, E., Engenhart-Cabillic, R., Daniilidis, K. *et al.* (2007) Metastasis: the seed and soil theory gains identity. *Cancer Metastasis Reviews*, **26**, 705–715.

Gimona, M. and Buccione, R. (2006) Adhesions that mediate invasion. *International Journal of Biochemistry & Cell Biology*, **38**, 1875–1892.

Grossmann, J. (2002) Molecular mechanisms of 'detachment-induced apoptosis – Anoikis'. *Apoptosis*, **7**, 247–260.

Hasan, N.M., Adams, G.E., Joiner, M.C. *et al.* (1998) Hypoxia facilitates tumour cell detachment by reducing expression of surface adhesion molecules and adhesion to extracellular matrices without loss of cell viability. *British Journal of Cancer*, **77**, 1799–1805.

Kalluri, R. and Zeisberg, M. (2006) Fibroblasts in cancer. *Nature Reviews. Cancer*, **6**, 392–401.

Kaplan, R.N., Rafii, S. and Lyden, D. (2006) Preparing the 'soil': the premetastatic niche. *Cancer Research*, **66**, 11089–11093.

Kirfel, G., Rigort, A., Borm, B. and Herzog, V. (2004) Cell migration: mechanisms of rear detachment and the formation of migration tracks. *European Journal of Cell Biology*, **83**, 717–724.

Kopfstein, L. and Christofori, G. (2006) Metastasis: cell-autonomous mechanisms versus contributions by the tumor microenvironment. *Cellular and Molecular Life Sciences*, **63**, 449–468.

Linder, S. (2007) The matrix corroded: podosomes and invadopodia in extracellular matrix degradation. *Trends in Cell Biology*, **17**, 107–117.

Liotta, L.A. and Kohn, E.C. (2001) The microenvironment of the tumour–host interface. *Nature*, **411**, 375–379.

Liotta, L.A., Rao, C.N. and Wewer, U.M. (1986) Biochemical interactions of tumor cells with the basement membrane. *Annual Review of Biochemistry*, **55**, 1037–1057.

Lyons, A.J. and Jones, J. (2007) Cell adhesion molecules, the extracellular matrix and oral squamous carcinoma. *International Journal of Oral and Maxillofacial Surgery*, **36**, 671–679.

Mehlen, P. and Puisieux, A. (2006) Metastasis: a question of life or death. *Nature Reviews Cancer*, **6**, 449–458.

Miles, F.L., Pruitt, F.L., van Golen, K.L. and Cooper, C.R. (2008) Stepping out of the flow: capillary extravasation in cancer metastasis. *Clinical & Experimental Metastasis*, **25**, 305–324.

Naumov, G.N., Akslen, L.A. and Folkman, J. (2006) Role of angiogenesis in human tumor dormancy: animal models of the angiogenic switch. *Cell Cycle*, **5**, 1779–1787.

Orimo, A. and Weinberg, R.A. (2006) Stromal fibroblasts in cancer: a novel tumor-promoting cell type. *Cell Cycle*, **5**, 1597–1601.

Papadopoulos, M.C., Saadoun, S. and Verkman, A.S. (2008) Aquaporins and cell migration. *Pflugers Archiv: European Journal of Physiology*, **456**, 693–700.

Pepper, M.S., Tille, J.C., Nisato, R. and Skobe, M. (2003) Lymphangiogenesis and tumor metastasis. *Cell and Tissue Research*, **314**, 167–177.

Rennebeck, G., Martelli, M. and Kyprianou, N. (2005) Anoikis and survival connections in the tumor microenvironment: is there a role in prostate cancer metastasis? *Cancer Research*, **65**, 11230–11235.

Stetler-Stevenson, W.G., Aznavoorian, S. and Liotta, L.A. (1993) Tumor cell interactions with the extracellular matrix during invasion and metastasis. *Annual Review of Cell Biology*, **9**, 541–573.

Steeg, P.S. (2005) Cancer biology: emissaries set up new sites. *Nature*, **438**, 750–751.

Tchou-Wong, K.M., Fok, S.Y., Rubin, J.S. *et al.* (2006) Rapid chemokinetic movement and the invasive potential of lung cancer cells; a functional molecular study. *BMC Cancer*, **6**, 151.

Valentijn, A.J., Zouq, N. and Gilmore, A.P. (2004) Anoikis. *Biochemical Society Transactions*, **32**, 421–425.

Verkman, A.S., Hara-Chikuma, M. and Papadopoulos, M.C. (2008) Aquaporins – new players in cancer biology. *Journal of Molecular Medicine*, **86**, 523–529.

Voura, E.B., Sandig, M. and Siu, C.H. (1998) Cell–cell interactions during transendothelial migration of tumor cells. *Microscopy Research and Technique*, **43**, 265–275.

Weiss, L. and Ward, P.M. (1983) Cell detachment and metastasis. *Cancer Metastasis Reviews*, **2**, 111–127.

Wong, S.Y. and Hynes, R.O. (2006) Lymphatic or hematogenous dissemination: how does a, metastatic tumor cell decide? *Cell Cycle*, **5**, 812–817.

Wyckoff, J.B., Wang, Y., Lin, E.Y. *et al.* (2007) Direct visualization of macrophage-assisted tumor cell intravasation in mammary tumours. *Cancer Research*, **67**, 2649–2656.

Xian, X., Håkansson, J., Ståhlberg, A. *et al.* (2006) Pericytes limit tumor cell metastasis. *Journal of Clinical Investigation*, **116**, 642–651.

Yamaguchi, H., Wyckoff, J. and Condeelis, J. (2005) Cell migration in tumours. *Current Opinion in Cell Biology*, **17**, 559–564.

Yamaguchi, H., Pixley, F. and Condeelis, J. (2006) Invadopodia and podosomes in tumor invasion. *European Journal of Cell Biology*, **85**, 213–218.

Zeisberg, E.M., Potenta, S., Xie, L. *et al.* (2007) Discovery of endothelial to mesenchymal transition as a source for carcinoma-associated fibroblasts. *Cancer Research*, **67**, 10123–10128.

Angiogenesis

Eccles, S.A. (2004) Parallels in invasion and angiogenesis provide pivotal points for therapeutic intervention. *International Journal of Developmental Biology*, **48**, 583–598.

Folkman, J. (1971) Tumor angiogenesis: therapeutic implications. *New England Journal of Medicine*, **285**, 1182–1186.

Folkman, J. (1974) Tumor Angiogenesis Factor. *Cancer Research*, **34**, 2109–2113.

Folkman, J., Merler, E., Abernathy, C. and Williams, G. (1971) Isolation of a tumor factor responsible for angiogenesis. *Journal of Experimental Medicine*, **133**, 275–288.

Goodall, C.M., Sanders, A.G. and Shubik, P. (1965) Studies of vascular patterns in living tumors with a transparent chamber inserted in hamster cheek pouch. *Journal of the National Cancer Institute*, **35**, 497–521.

Holleb, A.I. and Folkman, J. (1972) Tumor angiogenesis. *CA: A Cancer Journal for Clinicians*, **22**, 226–229.

Kisucka, J., Butterfield, C.E., Duda, D.G. *et al.* (2006) Platelets and platelet adhesion support angiogenesis while preventing excessive hemorrhage. *Proceedings of the National Academy of Sciences of the United States of America*, **103**, 855–860.

Roskoski, R. (2007) Vascular endothelial growth factor (VEGF) signaling in tumor progression. *Critical Reviews in Oncology/Hematology*, **62**, 179–213.

Sadar, M.D., Akopian, V.A. and Beraldi, E. (2002) Characterization of a new in vivo hollow fiber model for the study of progression of prostate cancer to androgen independence. *Molecular Cancer Therapy*, **1**, 629–637.

Staton, C.A., Stribbling, S.M., Tazzyman, S. *et al.* (2004) Current methods for assaying angiogenesis in vitro and in vivo. *International Journal of Experimental Pathology*, **85**, 233–248.

Anti-angiogenic agents

Aragon-Ching, J.B., Li, H., Gardner, E.R. and Figg, W.D. (2007) Thalidomide Analogues as Anticancer Drugs. *Recent Patents on Anti-Cancer Drug Discovery*, **2**, 167–174.

Bartlett, J.B., Dredge, K. and Dalgleish, A.G. (2004) The evolution of thalidomide and its IMiD derivatives as anticancer agents. *Nature Reviews Cancer*, **4**, 314–322.

Cohen, M.H., Gootenberg, J., Keegan, P. and Pazdur, R. (2007) FDA drug approval summary: bevacizumab (Avastin) plus Carboplatin and Paclitaxel as first-line treatment of advanced/metastatic recurrent nonsquamous non-small cell lung cancer. *Oncologist*, **12**, 713–718.

Deplanque, G. and Harris, A.L. (2000) Anti-angiogenic agents: clinical trial design and therapies in development. *European Journal of Cancer*, **36**, 1713–1724.

Eichhorn, M.E., Kleespies, A., Angele, M.K. *et al.* (2007) Angiogenesis in cancer: molecular mechanisms, clinical impact. *Langenbeck's Archives of Surgery/Deutsche Gesellschaft fur Chirurgie*, **392**, 371–379.

Friess, H., Langrehr, J.M., Oettle, H. *et al.* (2006) A randomized multi-center phase II trial of the angiogenesis inhibitor Cilengitide (EMD 121974) and gemcitabine compared with gemcitabine alone in advanced unresectable pancreatic cancer. *BMC Cancer*, **6**, 285.

Gutheil, J.C., Campbell, T.N., Pierce, P.R. *et al.* (2000) Targeted Antiangiogenic Therapy for Cancer Using Vitaxin: A Humanized Monoclonal Antibody to the Integrin anb3. *Clinical Cancer Research*, **6**, 3056–3061.

Hinnen, P. and Eskens, F.A. (2007) Vascular disrupting agents in clinical development. *British Journal of Cancer*, **96**, 1159–1165.

Khosravi Shahi, P. and Fernández Pineda, I. (2008) Tumoral Angiogenesis: Review of the Literature. *Cancer Investigation*, **26**, 104–108.

Lien, S. and Lowman, H.B. (2008) Therapeutic anti-VEGF antibodies, in *Handbook of Experimental Pharmacology*, (181), Springer, Berlin, pp. 131–150.

Lippert, J.W. 3rd (2007) Vascular disrupting agents. *Bioorganic and Medicinal Chemistry*, **15**, 605–615.

MacDonald, T.J., Stewart, C.F., Kocak, M. *et al.* (2008) Phase I clinical trial of cilengitide in children with refractory brain tumors: Pediatric Brain Tumor Consortium Study PBTC-012. *Journal of Clinical Oncology*, **26**, 919–924.

Melchert, M. and List, A. (2007) The thalidomide saga. *The International Journal of Biochemistry & Cell Biology*, **39**, 1489–1499.

Moy, B., Kirkpatrick, P., Kar, S. and Goss, P. (2007) Lapatinib. *Nature Reviews Drug Discovery*, **6**, 431–432.

Nabors, L.B., Mikkelsen, T., Rosenfeld, S.S. *et al.* (2007) Phase I and correlative biology study of cilengitide in patients with recurrent malignant glioma. *Journal of Clinical Oncology*, **25**, 1651–1657.

Nemeth, J.A., Nakada, M.T., Trikha, M. *et al.* (2007) Alpha-v integrins as therapeutic targets in oncology. *Cancer Investigation*, **25**, 632–646.

Overall, C.M. and Kleifeld, O. (2006) Validating matrix metalloproteinases as drug targets and anti-targets for cancer therapy. *Nature Reviews Cancer*, **6**, 227–239.

Podar, K., Tonon, G., Sattler, M. *et al.* (2006) The small-molecule VEGF receptor inhibitor pazopanib (GW786034B) targets both tumor and endothelial cells in multiple myeloma. *Proceedings of the National Academy of Sciences of the United States of America*, **103**, 19478–19483.

Rao, K.V. (2007) Lenalidomide in the treatment of multiple myeloma. *American Journal of Health-System Pharmacy*, **64**, 1799–1807.

Sandler, A. (2007) Bevacizumab in non-small cell lung cancer. *Clinical Cancer Research*, **13**, s4613–s4616.

Shih, T. and Lindley, C. (2006) Bevacizumab: an angiogenesis inhibitor for the treatment of solid malignancies. *Clinical Therapeutics*, **28**, 1779–1802.

Sridhar, S.S. and Shepherd, F.A. (2003) Targeting angiogenesis: a review of angiogenesis inhibitors in the treatment of lung cancer. *Lung Cancer*, **42** (Suppl. 1), S81–S91.

Tabruyn, S.P. and Griffioen, A.W. (2007) Molecular pathways of angiogenesis inhibition. *Biochemical and Biophysical Research Communications*, **355**, 1–5.

Tozer, G.M., Kanthou, C. and Baguley, B.C. (2005) Disrupting tumour blood vessels. *Nature Reviews Cancer*, **5**, 423–435.

Wilhelm, S., Carter, C., Lynch, M. *et al.* (2006) Discovery and development of sorafenib: a multikinase inhibitor for treating cancer. *Nature Reviews Drug Discovery*, **5**, 835–844.

Wu, M., Rivkin, A. and Pham, T. (2008) Panitumumab: human monoclonal antibody against epidermal growth factor receptors for the treatment of metastatic colorectal cancer. *Clinical Therapeutics*, **30**, 14–30.

Yano, S., Matsumori, Y., Ikuta, K. *et al.* (2006) Current status and perspective of angiogenesis and antivascular therapeutic strategy: non-small cell lung cancer. *International Journal of Clinical Oncology/Japan Society of Clinical Oncology*, **11**, 73–81.

Inhibitors of receptor tyrosine and signal transduction protein kinases

Adjei, A.A. (2006) Farnesyltransferase inhibitors. *Update on Cancer Therapeutics*, 1, 17–23.

Alinari, L., Lapalombella, R., Andritsos, L. *et al.* (2007) Alemtuzumab (Campath-1H) in the treatment of chronic lymphocytic leukemia. *Oncogene*, 26, 3644–3653.

Altomare, D.A. and Testa, J.R. (2005) Perturbations of the AKT signaling pathway in human cancer. *Oncogene*, 24, 7455–7464.

Argiris, A., Cohen, E., Karrison, T. *et al.* (2006) A phase II trial of perifosine, an oral alkylphospholipid, in recurrent or metastatic head and neck cancer. *Cancer Biology & Therapy*, 5, 766–770.

Arora, A. and Scholar, E.M. (2005) Role of tyrosine kinase inhibitors in cancer therapy. *Journal of Pharmacology and Experimental Therapeutics*, 315, 971–979.

Bailey, H.H., Alberti, D.B., Thomas, J.P. *et al.* (2007) Phase I trial of weekly paclitaxel and BMS-214662 in patients with advanced solid tumors. *Clinical Cancer Research*, 13, 3623–3629.

Baselga, J. (2006) Targeting tyrosine kinases in cancer: the second wave. *Science*, 312, 1175–1178.

Buchanan, S.G. (2003) Protein structure: discovering selective protein kinase inhibitors. *Targets*, 2, 101–108.

Buolamwini, J.K. (1999) Novel anticancer drug discovery. *Current Opinion in Chemical Biology*, 3, 500–509.

Burris, H.A. 3rd. (2004) Dual kinase inhibition in the treatment of breast cancer: initial experience with the EGFR/ErbB-2 inhibitor lapatinib. *Oncologist*, 9 (Suppl. 3), 10–15.

Cabebe, E. and Wakelee, H. (2007) Role of anti-angiogenesis agents in treating NSCLC: focus on bevacizumab and VEGFR tyrosine kinase inhibitors. *Current Treatment Options in Oncology*, 8, 15–27.

Cabebe, E. and Wakelee, H. (2006) Sunitinib: a newly approved small-molecule inhibitor of angiogenesis. *Drugs of Today*, 42, 387–398.

Cartenì, G., Fiorentino, R., Vecchione, L. *et al.* (2007) Panitumumab a novel drug in cancer treatment. *Annals of Oncology*, 18 (Suppl. 6), vi16–vi21.

Cartron, G., Blasco, H., Paintaud, G. *et al.* (2007) Pharmacokinetics of rituximab and its clinical use: thought for the best use? *Critical Reviews in Oncology/Hematology*, 62, 43–52.

Chang, J.C. (2007) HER2 inhibition: from discovery to clinical practice. *Clinical Cancer Research*, 13, 1–3.

Chang, Y.M., Kung, H.J. and Evans, C.P. (2007) Nonreceptor Tyrosine Kinases in Prostate Cancer. *Neoplasia*, 9, 90–100.

Chen, Y.L., Law, P.Y. and Loh, H.H. (2004) Inhibition of Akt/protein kinase B signaling by naltrindole in small cell lung cancer cells. *Cancer Research*, 64, 8723–8730.

Cheng, J.Q., Lindsley, C.W., Cheng, G.Z. *et al.* (2005) The Akt/PKB pathway: molecular target for cancer drug discovery. *Oncogene*, 24, 7482–7492.

Chow, L.Q., Eckhardt, S.G., O'Bryant, C.L. *et al.* (2007) A phase I safety, pharmacological, and biological study of the farnesyl protein transferase inhibitor, lonafarnib (SCH 663366), in combination with cisplatin and gemcitabine in patients with advanced solid tumors. *Cancer Chemotherapy and Pharmacology*, 62 (4), 631–646.

Coiffier, B. (2007) Rituximab therapy in malignant lymphoma. *Oncogene*, 26, 3603–3613.

Cox, A.D. and Der, C.J. (2002) Ras family signaling: therapeutic targeting. *Cancer Biology & Therapy*, **1**, 599–606.

Dagher, R., Cohen, M., Williams, G. *et al.* (2002) Approval summary: imatinib mesylate in the treatment of metastatic and/or unresectable malignant gastrointestinal stromal tumors. *Clinical Cancer Research*, **8**, 3034–3038.

Dalgarno, D., Stehle, T., Narula, S. *et al.* (2006) Structural basis of Src tyrosine kinase inhibition with a new class of potent and selective trisubstituted purine-based compounds. *Chemical Biology and Drug Design*, **67**, 46–57.

Duursma, A.M. and Agami, R. (2003) Ras interference as cancer therapy. *Seminars in Cancer Biology*, **13**, 267–273.

Elrod, H.A., Lin, Y.D., Yue, P. *et al.* (2007) The alkylphospholipid perifosine induces apoptosis of human lung cancer cells requiring inhibition of Akt and activation of the extrinsic apoptotic pathway. *Molecular Cancer Therapeutics*, **6**, 2029–2038.

Feldman, R.I., Wu, J.M., Polokoff, M.A. *et al.* (2005) Novel small molecule inhibitors of 3-phosphoinositide-dependent kinase-1. *Journal of Biological Chemistry*, **280**, 19867–19874.

Festuccia, C., Gravina, G.L., Muzi, P. *et al.* (2008) Akt down-modulation induces apoptosis of human prostate cancer cells and synergizes with EGFR tyrosine kinase inhibitors. *Prostate*, **68**, 965–974.

Floryk, D. and Thompson, T.C. (2008) Perifosine induces differentiation and cell death in prostate cancer cells. *Cancer Letters*, **266**, 216–226.

Fouladi, M., Nicholson, H.S., Zhou, T. *et al.* (2007) A phase II study of the farnesyl transferase inhibitor, tipifarnib, in children with recurrent or progressive high-grade glioma, medulloblastoma/primitive neuroectodermal tumor, or brainstem glioma: a Children's Oncology Group study. *Cancer*, **110**, 2535–2541.

Friday, B.B. and Adjei, A.A. (2008) Advances in targeting the Ras/Raf/MEK/Erk mitogen-activated protein kinase cascade with MEK inhibitors for cancer therapy. *Clinical Cancer Research*, **14**, 342–346.

García-Echeverría, C., Traxler, P. and Evans, D.B. (2000) ATP site-directed competitive and irreversible inhibitors of protein kinases. *Medicinal Research Reviews*, **20**, 28–57.

Geahlen, R.L., Handley, M.D. and Harrison, M.L. (2004) Molecular interdiction of Src-family kinase signaling in hematopoietic cells. *Oncogene*, **23**, 8024–8032.

Gibbs, J.B., Graham, S.L., Hartman, G.D. *et al.* (1997) Farnesyltransferase inhibitors versus Ras inhibitors. *Current Opinion in Chemical Biology*, **1**, 197–203.

Grimaldi, A.M., Guida, T., D'Attino, R. *et al.* (2007) Sunitinib: bridging present and future cancer treatment. *Annals of Oncology*, **18** (Suppl. 6), vi31–vi34.

Gschwind, A., Fischer, O.M. and Ullrich, A. (2004) The discovery of receptor tyrosine kinases: targets for cancer therapy. *Nature Reviews. Cancer*, **4**, 361–370.

Gunningham, S.P., Currie, M.J., Han, C. *et al.* (2001) VEGF-B expression in human primary breast cancers is associated with lymph node metastasis but not angiogenesis. *Journal of Pathology*, **193**, 325–332.

Haluska, P., Dy, G.K. and Adjei, A.A. (2002) Farnesyl transferase inhibitors as anticancer agents. *European Journal of Cancer*, **38**, 1685–1700.

Hanrahan, E.O. and Heymach, J.V. (2007) Vascular endothelial growth factor receptor tyrosine kinase inhibitors vandetanib (ZD6474) and AZD2171 in lung cancer. *Clinical Cancer Research*, **13**, s4617–s4622.

Ho, Q.T. and Kuo, C.J. (2007) Vascular endothelial growth factor: Biology and therapeutic applications. *International Journal of Biochemistry & Cell Biology*, **39** (7–8), 1349–1357.

Hsieh, A.C. and Moasser, M.M. (2007) Targeting HER proteins in cancer therapy and the role of the non-target HER3. *British Journal of Cancer*, **97**, 453–457.

Hubbard, S.R. and Till, J.H. (2000) Protein tyrosine kinase structure and function. *Annual Review of Biochemistry*, **69**, 373–398.

Johnston, S.R.D. (2001) Farnesyl transferase inhibitors: a novel targeted therapy for cancer. *Lancet Oncology*, **2**, 18–26.

Kantarjian, H., Jabbour, E., Grimley, J. and Kirkpatrick, P. (2006) Dasatinib. *Nature Reviews Drug Discovery*, **5**, 717–718.

Kloog, Y. and Cox, A.D. (2000) RAS inhibitors: potential for cancer therapeutics. *Molecular Medicine Today*, **6**, 398–402.

Kopetz, S., Shah, A.N. and Gallick, G.E. (2007) Src continues aging: current and future clinical directions. *Clinical Cancer Research*, **13**, 7232–7236.

Kumar, A., Petri, E.T., Halmos, B. and Boggon, T.J. (2008) Structure and clinical relevance of the epidermal growth factor receptor in human cancer. *Journal of Clinical Oncology*, **26**, 1742–1751.

Leonard, J.P. and Goldenberg, D.M. (2007) Preclinical and clinical evaluation of epratuzumab (anti-CD22 IgG) in B-cell malignancies. *Oncogene*, **26**, 3704–3713.

Levitzki, A. (1999) Protein tyrosine kinase inhibitors as novel therapeutic agents. *Pharmacology & Therapeutics*, **82**, 231–239.

Mazieres, J., Pradines, A. and Favre, G. (2004) Perspectives on farnesyl transferase inhibitors in cancer therapy. *Cancer Letters*, **206**, 159–167.

Neet, K. and Hunter, T. (1996) Vertebrate non-receptor protein-tyrosine kinase families. *Genes to Cells*, **1**, 147–169.

Noble, M.E., Endicott, J.A. and Johnson, L.N. (2004) Protein kinase inhibitors: insights into drug design from structure. *Science*, **303**, 1800–1805.

Park, J.W., Kirpotin, D.B., Hong, K. *et al.* (2001) Tumor targeting using anti-her2 immunoliposomes. *Journal of Controlled Release*, **74**, 95–113.

Paul, M.K. and Mukhopadhyay, A.K. (2004) Tyrosine kinase – role and significance in Cancer. *International Journal of Medical Sciences*, **1**, 101–115.

Posadas, E.M., Gulley, J., Arlen, P.M. *et al.* (2005) A phase II study of perifosine in androgen independent prostate cancer. *Cancer Biology & Therapy*, **4**, 1133–1137.

Qian, X., LeVea, C.M., Freeman, J.K. *et al.* (1994) Heterodimerization of epidermal growth factor receptor and wild-type or kinase-deficient Neu: a mechanism of interreceptor kinase activation and transphosphorylation. *Proceedings of the National Academy of Sciences of the United States of America*, **91**, 1500–1504.

Reid, T.S. and Beese, L.S. (2004) Crystal structures of the anticancer clinical candidates R115777 (Tipifarnib) and BMS-214662 complexed with protein farnesyltransferase suggest a mechanism of FTI selectivity. *Biochemistry*, **43**, 6877–6884.

Salven, P., Lymboussaki, A., Heikkilä, P. *et al.* (1998) Vascular endothelial growth factors VEGF-B and VEGF-C are expressed in human tumours. *American Journal of Pathology*, **153**, 103–108.

Scapin, G. (2002) Structural biology in drug design: selective protein kinase inhibitors. *Drug Discovery Today*, **7**, 601–611.

Schittenhelm, M.M., Shiraga, S., Schroeder, A. *et al.* (2006) Dasatinib (BMS-354825), a dual SRC/ABL kinase inhibitor, inhibits the kinase activity of wild-type, juxtamembrane, and activation loop mutant KIT isoforms associated with human malignancies. *Cancer Research*, **66**, 473–481.

Schlessinger, J. (2000) Cell signaling by receptor tyrosine kinases. *Cell*, **103**, 211–225.

Sebti, S.M. and Hamilton, A.D. (2000) Farnesyltransferase and geranylgeranyltransferase I inhibitors and cancer therapy: lessons from mechanism and bench-to-bedside translational studies. *Oncogene*, **19**, 6584–6593.

Sequist, L.V. (2007) Second-generation epidermal growth factor receptor tyrosine kinase inhibitors in non-small cell lung cancer. *Oncologist*, **12**, 325–330.

Summy, J.M. and Gallick, G.E. (2003) Src family kinases in tumor progression and metastasis. *Cancer Metastasis Reviews*, **22**, 337–358.

Takimoto, C.H. and Awada, A. (2008) Safety and anti-tumor activity of sorafenib (Nexavar®) in combination with other anti-cancer agents: a review of clinical trials. *Cancer Chemotherapy and Pharmacology*, **61** (4), 535–548.

Tatton, L., Morley, G.M., Chopra, R. and Khwaja, A. (2003) The Src-selective kinase inhibitor PP1 also inhibits Kit and Bcr-Abl tyrosine kinases. *The Journal of Biological Chemistry*, **278**, 4847–4853.

Theodore, C., Geoffrois, L., Vermorken, J.B. *et al.* (2005) Multicentre EORTC study 16997: Feasibility and phase II trial of farnesyl transferase inhibitor & gemcitabine combinationin salvage treatment of advanced urothelial tract cancers. *European Journal of Cancer*, **41**, 1150–1157.

Tokarski, J.S., Newitt, J.A., Chang, C.Y. *et al.* (2006) The structure of Dasatinib (BMS-354825) bound to activated ABL kinase domain elucidates its inhibitory activity against imatinib-resistant ABL mutants. *Cancer Research*, **66**, 5790–5797.

Vera, J.C., Reyes, A.M., Velásquez, F.V. *et al.* (2001) Direct inhibition of the hexose transporter GLUT1 by tyrosine kinase inhibitors. *Biochemistry*, **40**, 777–790.

Weisberg, E., Manley, P., Mestan, J. *et al.* (2006) AMN107 (nilotinib): a novel and selective inhibitor of BCR-ABL. *British Journal of Cancer*, **94** (12), 1765–1769.

Wong, S.F. (2005) Cetuximab: an epidermal growth factor receptor monoclonal antibody for the treatment of colorectal cancer. *Clinical Therapeutics*, **27**, 684–694.

Xu, J.M., Paradiso, A. and McLeod, H.L. (2004) Evaluation of epidermal growth factor receptor tyrosine kinase inhibitors combined with chemotherapy: Is there a need for a more rational design? *European Journal of Cancer*, **40**, 1807–1809.

Yarden, Y. and Ullrich, A. (1988) Growth factor receptor tyrosine kinases. *Annual Review of Biochemistry*, **57**, 443–478.

Zwick, E., Bange, J. and Ullrich, A. (2001) Receptor tyrosine kinase signalling as a target for cancer intervention strategies. *Endocrine-Related Cancer*, **8**, 161–173.

Epigenetic targets

Atmaca, A., Al-Batran, S.E., Maurer, A. *et al.* (2007) Valproic acid (VPA) in patients with refractory advanced cancer: a dose escalating phase I clinical trial. *British Journal of Cancer*, **97**, 177–182.

Blum, W., Klisovic, R.B., Hackanson, B. *et al.* (2007) Phase I study of decitabine alone or in combination with valproic acid in acute myeloid leukemia. *Journal of Clinical Oncology*, **25**, 3884–3891.

Ciossek, T., Julius, H., Wieland, H. *et al.* (2008) A homogeneous cellular histone deacetylase assay suitable for compound profiling and robotic screening. *Analytical Biochemistry*, **372**, 72–81.

de Ruijter, A.J., van Gennip, A.H., Caron, H.N. *et al.* (2003) Histone deacetylases (HDACs): characterization of the classical HDAC family. *The Biochemical Journal*, **370**, 737–749.

Dokmanovic, M. and Marks, P.A. (2005) Prospects: Histone Deacetylase Inhibitors. *Journal of Cellular Biochemistry*, **96**, 293–304.

Fenaux, P. (2005) Inhibitors of DNA methylation: beyond myelodysplastic syndromes. *Nature Clinical Practice Oncology*, **2** (Suppl. 1), S36–S44.

Fouladi, M., Furman, W.L., Chin, T. *et al.* (2006) Phase I study of depsipeptide in pediatric patients with refractory solid tumors: a Children's Oncology Group Report. *Journal of Clinical Oncology*, **24**, 3678–3685.

Gallinari, P., Di Marco, S., Jones, P. *et al.* (2007) HDACs, histone deacetylation and gene transcription: from molecular biology to cancer therapeutics. *Cell Research*, **17**, 195–211.

Goffin, J. and Eisenhauer, E. (2002) DNA methyltransferase inhibitors—state of the art. *Annals of Oncology*, **13**, 1699–1716.

Hess-Stumpp, H., Bracker, T.U., Henderson, D. and Politz, O. (2007) MS-275, a potent orally available inhibitor of histone deacetylases – the development of an anticancer agent. *International Journal of Biochemistry & Cell Biology*, **39**, 1388–1405.

Hildmann, C., Riester, D. and Schwienhorst, A. (2007) Histone deacetylases – an important class of cellular regulators with a variety of functions. *Applied Microbiology and Biotechnology*, **75**, 487–497.

Ishihama, K., Yamakawa, M., Semba, S. *et al.* (2007) Expression of HDAC1 and CBP/p300 in human colorectal carcinomas. *Journal of Clinical Pathology*, **60**, 1205–1210.

Issa, J.P. (2007) DNA methylation as a therapeutic target in cancer. *Clinical Cancer Research*, **13**, 2007.

Khan, N., Jeffers, M., Kumar, S. *et al.* (2008) Determination of the class and isoform selectivity of small-molecule histone deacetylase inhibitors. *Biochemical Journal*, **409**, 581–589.

Kostrouchová, M., Kostrouch, Z. and Kostrouchová, M. (2007) Valproic acid, a molecular lead to multiple regulatory pathways. *Folia Biologica*, **53**, 37–49.

Luo, R.X. and Dean, D.C. (1999) Chromatin Remodeling and Transcriptional Regulation. *Journal of the National Cancer Institute*, **91**, 1288–1294.

Mack, G.S. (2006) Mack epigenetic cancer therapy makes headway. *Journal of the National Cancer Institute*, **98**, 1443–1444.

Mann, B.S., Johnson, J.R., He, K. *et al.* (2007) Vorinostat for treatment of cutaneous manifestations of advanced primary cutaneous T-cell lymphoma. *Clinical Cancer Research*, **13**, 2318–2322.

Marks, P.A., Richon, V.M. and Rifkind, R.A. (2000) Histone deacetylase inhibitors: inducers of differentiation or apoptosis of transformed cells. *Journal of the National Cancer Institute*, **92**, 1210–1216.

Münster, P., Marchion, D., Bicaku, E. *et al.* (2007) Phase I trial of histone deacetylase inhibition by valproic acid followed by the topoisomerase II inhibitor epirubicin in advanced solid tumors: a clinical and translational study. *Journal of Clinical Oncology*, **25**, 1979–1985.

Ramalingam, S.S., Parise, R.A., Ramanathan, R.K. *et al.* (2007) Phase I and pharmacokinetic study of vorinostat, a histone deacetylase inhibitor, in combination with carboplatin and paclitaxel for advanced solid malignancies. *Clinical Cancer Research*, **13**, 3605–3610.

Takai, N., Desmond, J.C., Kumagai, T. *et al.* (2004) Histone deacetylase inhibitors have a profound antigrowth activity in endometrial cancer cells. *Clinical Cancer Research*, **10**, 1141–1149.

Velculescu, V.E., Zhang, L., Vogelstein, B. and Kinzler, K.W. (1995) Serial analysis of gene expression. *Science*, **270**, 484–487.

Wijermans, P.W., Rüter, B., Baer, M.R. *et al.* (2008) Efficacy of decitabine in the treatment of patients with chronic myelomonocytic leukemia (CMML). *Leukemia Research*, **32**, 587–591.

Wilson, A.J., Byun, D.S., Popova, N. *et al.* (2006) Histone deacetylase 3 (HDAC3) and other class I HDACs regulate colon cell maturation and p21 expression and are deregulated in human colon cancer. *Journal of Biological Chemistry*, **281**, 13548–13558.

Xu, W.S., Parmigiani, R.B. and Marks, P.A. (2007) Histone deacetylase inhibitors: molecular mechanisms of action. *Oncogene*, **26**, 5541–5552.

Molecular chaperones and the proteasome

Bagatell, R. and Whitesell, L. (2004) Altered Hsp90 function in cancer: A unique therapeutic opportunity. *Molecular Cancer Therapeutics*, **3**, 1021–1030.

Brown, M.A., Zhu, L., Schmidt, C. and Tucker, P.W. (2007) Tucker. Hsp90 – from signal transduction to cell transformation. *Biochemical and Biophysical Research Communications*, **363**, 241–246.

Goetz, M.P., Toft, D.O., Ames, M.M. and Erlichman, C. (2003) The Hsp90 chaperone complex as a novel target for cancer therapy. *Annals of Oncology*, **14**, 1169–1176.

Heath, E.I., Gaskins, M., Pitot, H.C. *et al.* (2005) Phase II trial of 17-allylamino-17-demethoxy-geldanamycin (17-AAG) in patients with hormone-refractory metastatic prostate cancer. *Clinical Prostate Cancer*, **4**, 138–141.

Kreusch, A., Han, S., Brinker, A. *et al.* (2005) Crystal structures of human HSP90a-complexed with dihydroxyphenylpyrazoles. *Bioorganic & Medicinal Chemistry Letters*, **15**, 1475–1478.

Plescia, J., Salz, W., Xia, F. *et al.* (2005) Rational design of shepherdin, a novel anticancer agent. *Cancer Cell*, **7**, 457–468.

Powers, M.V. and Workman, P. (2006) Targeting of multiple signalling pathways by heat shock protein 90 molecular chaperone inhibitors. *Endocrine-Related Cancer*, **13** (Suppl. 1), S125–S135.

Rechsteiner, M. and Hill, C.P. (2005) Mobilizing the proteolytic machine: cell biological roles of proteasome activators and inhibitors. *Trends in Cell Biology*, **15**, 27–33.

Richardson, P.G., Hideshima, T., Mitsiades, C. and Anderson, K. (2004) Proteasome inhibition in hematologic malignancies. *Annals of Medicine*, **36**, 304–314.

Richardson, P.G., Mitsiades, C., Hideshima, T. and Anderson, K.C. (2005) Proteasome inhibition in the treatment of cancer. *Cell Cycle*, **4**, 290–296.

Roos-Mattjus, P. and Sistonen, L. (2004) The ubiquitin–proteasome pathway. *Annals of Medicine*, **36**, 285–295.

Sharp, S. and Workman, P. (2006) Inhibitors of the HSP90 Molecular Chaperone: Current Status. *Advances in Cancer Research*, **95**, 323–348.

Stebbins, C.E., Russo, A.A., Schneider, C. *et al.* (1997) Crystal structure of an Hsp90-geldana-mycin complex: targeting of a protein chaperone by an antitumor agent. *Cell*, **89**, 239–250.

mTOR

Chan, S. (2004) Targeting the mammalian target of rapamycin (mTOR): a new approach to treating cancer. *British Journal of Cancer*, **91**, 1420–1424.

Edinger, A.L., Linardic, C.M., Chiang, G.G. *et al.* (2003) Differential effects of rapamycin on mammalian target of rapamycin signaling functions in mammalian cells. *Cancer Research*, **63**, 8451–8460.

Feng, Z., Zhang, H., Levine, A.J. and Jin, S. (2005) The coordinate regulation of the p53 and mTOR pathways in cells. *Proceedings of the National Academy of Sciences of the United States of America*, **102**, 8204–8209.

Gore, M.E. (2007) Temsirolimus in the treatment of advanced renal cell carcinoma. *Annals of Oncology*, **18** (Suppl 9), ix87–ix88

Hay, N. and Sonenberg, N. (2004) Upstream and downstream of mTOR. *Genes and Development*, **18**, 1926–1945.

Huang, J., Zhu, H., Haggarty, S.J. *et al.* (2004) Finding new components of the target of rapamycin (TOR) signaling network through chemical genetics and proteome chips. *Proceedings of the National Academy of Sciences of the United States of America*, **101**, 16594–16599.

Hudes, G., Carducci, M., Tomczak, P. *et al.*; Global ARCC Trial. (2007) Temsirolimus, interferon alfa, or both for advanced renal-cell carcinoma. *New England Journal of Medicine*, **356**, 2271–2281.

Hudson, C.C., Liu, M., Chiang, G.G. *et al.* (2002) Regulation of hypoxia-inducible factor 1alpha expression and function by the mammalian target of rapamycin. *Molecular and Cellular Biology*, **22**, 7004–7014.

Land, S.C. and Tee, A.R. (2007) Hypoxia-inducible factor 1alpha is regulated by the mammalian target of rapamycin (mTOR) via an mTOR signaling motif. *The Journal of Biological Chemistry*, **282**, 20534–20543.

Le Tourneau, C., Faivre, S., Serova, M. and Raymond, E. (2008) mTORC1 inhibitors: is temsirolimus in renal cancer telling us how they really work? *British Journal of Cancer*, **99**, 1197–1203.

Motzer, R.J., Hudes, G.R., Curti, B.D. *et al.* (2007) Phase I/II trial of temsirolimus combined with interferon alfa for advanced renal cell carcinoma. *Journal of Clinical Oncology*, **25**, 3958–3964.

Noh, W.C., Mondesire, W.H., Peng, J. *et al.* (2004) Determinants of rapamycin sensitivity in breast cancer cells. *Clinical Cancer Research*, **10**, 1013–1023.

Proud, C.G. (2002) Regulation of mammalian translation factors by nutrients. *European Journal of Biochemistry*, **269**, 5338–5349.

Ravikumar, B., Stewart, A., Kita, H. *et al.* (2003) Raised intracellular glucose concentrations reduce aggregation and cell death caused by mutant huntingtin exon 1 by decreasing mTOR phosphorylation and inducing autophagy. *Human Molecular Genetics*, **12**, 985–994.

Rowinsky, E.K. (2004) Targeting the molecular target of rapamycin (mTOR). *Current Opinion in Oncology*, **16**, 564–575.

Telomerase inhibitors

Biroccio, A. and Leonetti, C. (2004) Telomerase as a new target for the treatment of hormone-refractory prostate cancer. *Endocrine-Related Cancer*, **11**, 407–421.

Corey, D.R. (2002) Telomerase inhibition, oligonucleotides, and clinical trials. *Oncogene*, **21**, 631–637.

Dahse, R., Fiedler, W. and Ernst, G. (1997) Telomeres and telomerase: biological and clinical importance. *Clinical Chemistry*, **43**, 708–714.

Damm, K., Hemmann, U., Garin-Chesa, P. *et al.* (2001) A highly selective telomerase inhibitor limiting human cancer cell proliferation. *EMBO Journal*, **20**, 6958–6968.

Hahn, W.C. (2003) Role of telomeres and telomerase in the pathogenesis of human cancer. *Journal of Clinical Oncology*, **21**, 2034–2043.

Hiyama, E. and Hiyama, K. (2002) Clinical utility of telomerase in cancer. *Oncogene*, **21**, 643–649.

Ince, T.A. and Crum, C.P. (2004) Telomerase: promise and challenge. *Human Pathology*, **35**, 393–395.

Keith, W.N., Bilsland, A., Evans, T.R. and Glasspool, R.M. (2002) Telomerase-directed molecular therapeutics. *Expert Reviews in Molecular Medicine*, **4**, 1–25.

Kelland, L.R. (2001) Telomerase: biology and phase I trials. *Lancet Oncology*, **2**, 95–102.

Meyerson, M. (2000) Role of telomerase in normal and cancer cells. *Journal of Clinical Oncology*, **18**, 2626–2634.

Nicol Keith, W., Jeffry Evans, T.R. and Glasspool, R.M. (2001) Telomerase and cancer: time to move from a promising target to a clinical reality. *Journal of Pathology*, **195**, 404–414.

Plentz, R.R., Wiemann, S.U., Flemming, P. *et al.* (2003) Telomere shortening of epithelial cells characterises the adenoma-carcinoma transition of human colorectal cancer. *Gut*, **52**, 1304–1307.

Ulaner, G.A. (2004) Telomere maintenance in clinical medicine. *The American Journal of Medicine*, **117**, 262–269.

Pharmaceutical problems in cancer chemotherapy

Allwood, N., Stanley, A. and Wright, P. (eds) (2002) *Cytotoxics Handbook*, 4th edn, Radcliffe Publishing, Slough, UK.

American Society of Clinical Oncology, Kris, M.G., Hesketh, P.J., Somerfield, M.R. *et al.* (2006) American Society of Clinical Oncology guidelines for antiemetics in oncology: update 2006. *J. Clin. Oncol.*, **24**, 2932–2947.

Atadja, P., Watanabe, T., Xu, H. and Cohen, D. (1998) PSC-833, a frontier in modulation of P-glycoprotein mediated multidrug resistance. *Cancer Metastasis Reviews*, **17**, 163–168.

Bowman, K.J., Newell, D.R., Calvert, A.H. and Curtin, N.J. (2001) Differential effects of the poly (ADP-ribose) polymerase (PARP) inhibitor NU1025 on topoisomerase I and II inhibitor cytotoxicity in L1210 cells in vitro. *British Journal of Cancer*, **84**, 106–112.

Calabrese, C.R., Almassy, R., Barton, S. *et al.* (2004) Anticancer chemosensitization and radiosensitization by the novel poly(ADP-ribose) polymerase-1 inhibitor AG14361. *Journal of the National Cancer Institute*, **96**, 56–67.

Delaney, C.A., Wang, L.Z., Kyle, S. *et al.* (2000) Potentiation of temozolomide and topotecan growth inhibition and cytotoxicity by novel poly(adenosine diphosphoribose) polymerase inhibitors in a panel of human tumor cell lines. *Clinical Cancer Research*, **6**, 2860–2867.

Griffin, R.J., Srinivasan, S., Bowman, K. *et al.* (1998) Resistance-modifying agents. 5. Synthesis and biological properties of quinazolinone inhibitors of the DNA repair enzyme poly(ADP-ribose) polymerase (PARP) *Journal of Medicinal Chemistry*, **41**, 5247–5256.

Haince, J.F., Rouleau, M., Hendzel, M.J. *et al.* (2005) Targeting poly(ADP-ribosyl)ation: a promising approach in cancer therapy. *Trends in Molecular Medicine*, **11**, 456–463.

Helleday, T., Lo, J., van Gent, D.C. and Engelward, B.P. (2007) DNA double-strand break repair: from mechanistic understanding to cancer treatment. *DNA Repair*, **6**, 923–935.

Kelland, L.R. and Tonkin, K.S. (1989) The effect of 3-aminobenzamide in the radiation response of three human cervix carcinoma xenografts. *Radiotherapy and Oncology*, **15**, 363–369.

Leonard, G.D., Fojo, T. and Bates, S.E. (2003) The role of ABC transporters in clinical practice. *Oncologist*, **8**, 411–424.

Madhusudan, S. and Hickson, I.D. (2005) DNA repair inhibition: a selective tumour targeting strategy. *Trends in Molecular Medicine*, **11**, 503–511.

Miwa, M. and Masutani, M. (2007) PolyADP-ribosylation and cancer. *Cancer Science*, **98**, 1528–1535.

Modok, S., Mellor, H.R. and Callaghan, R. (2006) Modulation of multidrug resistance efflux pump activity to overcome chemoresistance in cancer. *Current Opinion in Pharmacology*, **6**, 350–354.

Mullin, S., Mani, N. and Grossman, T.H. (2004) Inhibition of antibiotic efflux in bacteria by the novel multidrug resistance inhibitors biricodar (VX-710) and timcodar (VX-853). *Antimicrobial Agents and Chemotherapy*, **48**, 4171–4176.

National Comprehensive Cancer Network guidelines. http://www.nccn.org/professionals/physician_gls/PDF/antiemesis.pdf.

Rabik, C.A., Njoku, M.C. and Dolan, M.E. (2006) Inactivation of O6-alkylguanine DNA alkyltransferase as a means to enhance chemotherapy. *Cancer Treatment Reviews*, **32**, 261–276.

Saeki, T., Nomizu, T., Toi, M. *et al.* (2007) Dofequidar fumarate (MS-209) in combination with cyclophosphamide, doxorubicin, and fluorouracil for patients with advanced or recurrent breast cancer. *Journal of Clinical Oncology*, **25**, 411–417.

Virág, L. and Szabó, C. (2002) The therapeutic potential of poly(ADP-ribose) polymerase inhibitors. *Pharmacological Reviews*, **54**, 375–429.

Inhibitors of the MDM2–p53 interaction

Chène, P. (2004) Inhibition of the p53–MDM2 interaction: targeting a protein-protein interface. *Molecular Cancer Research*, **2**, 20–28.

Fischer, P.M. and Lane, D.P. (2004) Small-molecule inhibitors of the p53 suppressor HDM2: have protein–protein interactions come of age as drug targets? *Trends in Pharmacological Sciences*, **25**, 343–346.

Hardcastle, I.R., Ahmed, S.U., Atkins, H. *et al.* (2005) Isoindolinone-based inhibitors of the MDM2–p53 protein–protein interaction. *Bioorganic & Medicinal Chemistry Letters*, **15**, 1515–1520.

Pagliaro, L., Felding, J., Audouze, K. *et al.* (2004) Emerging classes of protein-protein interaction inhibitors and new tools for their development. *Current Opinion in Chemical Biology*, **8**, 442–449.

Vassilev, L.T. (2004) Small-molecule antagonists of p53–MDM2 binding: research tools and potential therapeutics. *Cell Cycle*, **3**, 419–421.

Index